LITTLE,
BROWN

PRIME-TIME HEALTH

HEALTH

A Scientifically Proven Plan
for Feeling Young and Living Longer

William Sears, MD
with Martha Sears, RN

Foreword by Dean Ornish, MD

LITTLE, BROWN AND COMPANY
LARGE PRINT EDITION

Little, Brown and Company
Hachette Book Group
237 Park Avenue, New York, NY 10017
www.hachettebookgroup.com

FIRST LARGE PRINT EDITION: JANUARY 2010

Little, Brown and Company is a division of Hachette Book Group, Inc. The Little,
Brown name and logo are trademarks of Hachette Book Group, Inc.

This book is intended to supplement, not replace, the advice of a trained health
professional. If you know or suspect that you have a health problem, you should
consult a health professional. The author and publisher specifically disclaim any
liability, loss, or risk, personal or otherwise, which is incurred as a consequence,
directly or indirectly, of the use and application of any of the contents of this book.

Illustrations by Debbie Maze

ISBN 978-0-316-07401-8
LCCN 2009938671

10 9 8 7 6 5 4 3 2 1

RRD-IN

Book design by Fearn Cutler deVicq

Printed in the United States of America

To our children and grandchildren:

James
Robert
Peter
Hayden
Erin
Matthew
Stephen
Lauren
Lea
Jonathan
Andrew
Alex
Joshua
Ashton
Morgan
Thomas

Following the Prime-Time Health plan in this book will help us be there for you.

CONTENTS

CONTENTS

CONTENTS

FOREWORD

When my son Lucas was born, nine years ago, I was determined to be the best father I could be. So, I must have read just about every child-care book ever written, or at least it felt that way. I was getting a little discouraged with the conflicting advice, some of which seemed misguided or even downright cruel ("Leave your baby in another room, and let him cry himself to sleep").

Fortunately, I came across the books of Bill and Martha Sears. They were like a breath of fresh air — authoritatively written and scientifically based but tempered by the real-world wisdom the authors gained raising eight kids. Bill and Martha speak from experience, both personal and clinical, and their books became my field guides.

Their recommendations mirrored my intuitive and scientific understanding of the importance of attachment parenting, good nutrition (especially omega-3 fatty acids), the countless benefits of breast-feeding, and so on. I knew that when children are loved, held, cuddled, touched, and bonded with, they become more confident, healthy, and independent, not spoiled. So it felt affirming when I read, "Spoiling is what happens when you leave something (or some person) alone on the shelf — it spoils."

I thought, *Too bad the Searses haven't written a book to show grown-ups how to stay healthy and enjoy life*. Now, in *Prime-Time Health*, they have.

In this book they apply their decades of clinical experience to show how diet and lifestyle changes can turn around your illness issues — and much faster than had once been thought possible — so you can enjoy living longer and healthier.

Dr. Sears also shares his personal story about how being diagnosed with colon cancer was a wake-up call, a catalyst for transforming his own life for the better. His experience mirrors that of many patients who have told me, "Being diagnosed with a life-threatening illness was the best thing that ever happened to me." Why? Because it was a powerful motivator for making changes in their lifestyle that made life so much more joyful, healthful, and meaningful.

For more than thirty years, my colleagues and I at the nonprofit Preventive Medicine Research Institute have conducted a series of research studies showing that changes in diet and lifestyle can make a powerful difference in our health and well-being, how quickly these changes may occur, and how dynamic these mechanisms can be.

Because these mechanisms are so dynamic, people who make comprehensive lifestyle changes usually find, as Dr. Sears eloquently describes, that they feel so much better, so quickly, that they reframe the reason for making lifestyle changes from fear of dying to joy of living. We've learned that joy, pleasure, and freedom are what make lifestyle changes sustainable and worth doing.

Many people tend to think of a breakthrough in medicine as a new drug, laser, or high-tech surgical procedure. They have a hard time believing that the simple choices that we make in our daily lives — what we eat, how we respond to stress, whether or not we smoke cigarettes, how much exercise we get, and the quality of our relationships and social support — can be as powerful as drugs and surgery, but they often are. And often, the results are even better.

We used high-tech, state-of-the-art measures

to prove the power of simple, low-tech, and low-cost interventions. We showed that comprehensive lifestyle changes can stop or even reverse the progression of coronary artery disease, prostate cancer (and, by extension, breast cancer), diabetes, hypertension, obesity, hypercholesterolemia, and other chronic conditions.

Often, I hear people say, "Oh, I've got bad genes. There's not much I can do." It turns out that even our genes are more dynamic than had once been realized. In our research, we found that changing your lifestyle changes your genes as well — "turning on" hundreds of genes that help prevent diseases, and "turning off" genes that promote heart disease, prostate cancer, breast cancer, and other illnesses. We published this study in the *Proceedings of the National Academy of Sciences*. We also found that changing your lifestyle increases telomerase and thus the length of telomeres, the ends of our chromosomes that control how long we live. Even drugs have not been shown to do this. Dr. Sears describes these findings in chapter 2, and they are giving many people new hope and new choices.

The theme of *Prime-Time Health* has been a

guiding principle of all of my work: your body often has a remarkable capacity to begin healing itself if you stop doing what's causing the problem. To a large degree, these underlying causes are the lifestyle choices we make each day — for better and for worse.

In my experience, people who really understand something can make it simple without being simplistic. In *Prime-Time Health*, Bill and Martha Sears do just that. They describe clearly and simply not only how to live longer but also how to live better and enjoy life more fully every day. Awareness is the first step in healing, and this book is a powerful way of increasing awareness. Read it, and it will transform your life for the better.

— Dean Ornish, MD
Founder and President, Preventive Medicine Research Institute; Clinical Professor of Medicine, University of California, San Francisco; author of *The Spectrum, Dr. Dean Ornish's Program for Reversing Heart Disease,* and *Eat More, Weigh Less.*

INTRODUCTION

Prime time can be the best part of your life. What does *prime time* mean to you? My wife, Martha, defines prime time as "the second half of life." I consider it a time of less pressure, when the kids are out of the house — if not yet out of your pocket. You've raised your family, built your career, developed your social networks, and, most important, accumulated a whole lot of memories. It's an opportunity to enjoy those memories and to make more. It's a time when the "want to dos" can start to replace the "must dos."

We should look forward to prime time. Yet most of us dread getting older as we hit middle age because we think it will mean a prolonged period of disease and disability. I hope this book will relieve any fears you have about aging and help you prepare for one of the most pleasurable stages of life. I put together the Prime-Time Health plan after my own midlife health crisis. Based on my experiences and sound medical science, it contains all the health and wellness advice I give my own children as they reach middle age.

In the early decades of adulthood, you work to fulfill your family obligations and do what you have to do professionally, socially, and economically, which leaves you with few resources for yourself. In prime time, you finally have some of those resources. Will you have the health to enjoy them? It depends on how well you prepare.

Consider the story of our close friends Jim and Susan. They each worked hard and diligently put money into their retirement plans. Susan loved to travel to exotic and exciting places; Jim loved weekends on their boat. The problem was that Jim and Susan led their lives differently. They both saved money, but only Susan saved her body. She worked long hours at her job as a nurse, but she also worked out regularly, watched what she ate, and maintained her health. Jim was a TV addict. He sat a lot, drank a lot, smoked, and thought exercise was a waste of time. He loved his Texas-size grilled steaks, and "burn a big one" was how he ate. But it turns out he was grilling his body too — on the inside. At fifty Jim got diabetes; at fifty-five he had a coronary bypass; at sixty-two knee replacement surgery. He has to take pills for his highs: high blood pressure, high blood cholesterol, and high blood sugar; and also for his lows: depression. For Jim, prime time is sick time, not the best time in his life. Jim and Susan's hopes for their future are dwindling. Susan spends much of her time caring for Jim, and about the only travel his health permits is to and from the hospital or a doctor's office, or an occasional golf game when his legs can take it.

Like Jim, many folks spend much of their prime time coping with the three Ds: disease, disability, and doctors. This book is written for the Jims of this world and for prime timers who want to avoid these Ds.

I could have been a Jim, but when faced with a medical crisis twelve years ago, I turned a corner and discovered the benefits of prime-time health.

Longevity means a long and healthful life. I love that word! I don't like *antiaging*, the term used in most healthy-aging books. Think about it: if you don't age, you die. That reminds me of a card my son Matthew gave me on my sixty-fifth birthday. It read, "Getting older isn't so bad when you consider the alternative." Early in my research to develop my Prime-Time Health plan, I figured out that longevity comes down to four factors, which I remember with the acronym LEAN:

- Lifestyle: how we *live*
- Exercise: how we *move*
- Attitude: how we *think*
- Nutrition: how we *eat*

Let me give you a brief overview of what you can expect from this book. First, you will learn why and how I put this health plan together. Then you will learn the simplest explanation of aging you've ever heard and the secrets of people who age well. Next, I will take you on a journey through your body so you can help yourself age more healthfully. Last, you will get a crash course on prime-time well-being: how to eat, sleep, manage stress, and enjoy better sex.

Realizing that even when you practice the Prime-Time Health plan you will eventually get some illnesses, I'll also teach you about the pills-and-skills model of health care. In partnership with your doctor, you will be able to take charge of your health. And as part of your health-care program, you will learn a doable and enjoyable fitness and weight-management regimen.

While this book is for all audiences, I wrote it mainly for three groups of readers:

1. The forty- to fiftysomething prime timers who are in the *prevent* mind-set. They wisely want to keep their bodies in good working order before they start to wear out. They want to prepare so they can be there for their children and grandchildren.

2. Prime timers who are in the *repair* mode. This group didn't take the best care of their bodies, some parts of which are starting to wear out. *Prime-Time Health* can give you a second chance. Fortunately, the body is resilient.

3. Young parents who want to give a gift to their own parents. The loving message: "Mom and Dad, we want you to be around for your grandchildren's weddings. Please read this book — and follow it!"

Reading alarming headlines about Medicare soon going bankrupt and people using all of their savings to pay medical bills motivated me even more. I concluded that the answer to our country's health-care crisis is *self-care.*

SHOW ME THE SCIENCE!

As I was putting together my own Prime-Time Health plan, I realized that there have been volumes written about aging, and hundreds of youth-promising supplements touted. Yet few claims are based on solid science. Studies that "prove" that one diet works are later refuted by other studies showing that it doesn't. Who's a prime timer to trust? I've made sure that everything in *Prime-Time Health* is backed up by common sense and credible science. I am a science-based physician, and my patients and my readers trust me to have thoroughly researched what I write about and teach. So, here's my promise to you: this health plan is based on what I learned during twelve years of study of scientific research.

Visualize how you would like to spend your prime time. Imagine being able to enjoy the delights of the world, the pleasure of walking along a beach, a pain-free day, and the mental clarity to remember and enjoy the experiences and resources you've accumulated. Or, do you want your prime-time years to be brief and your calendar littered with doctors' appointments? Do you want your life's savings to go to co-pays on drugs that fill your medicine cabinet? The choice is yours.

This book is both a life plan and a health plan, and with it you can add years to your life and life to your years.

Here's to your prime-time health!

HOW TO READ THIS BOOK

To get the most dramatic benefits from *Prime-Time Health*, we suggest that you follow these steps:

1. Take a health break. Go to a relaxing place for a week or a weekend. Read the book cover to cover, highlighting topics you find especially relevant. Reading the entire book first will show you how your organs and tissues work together, like well-tuned instruments in an orchestra. When they are in harmony, beautiful music — health — results. You will see how the health of one organ affects that of another and appreciate the common themes that make each operate at its prime. You may think, *I don't have a knee problem, so I'll skip that chapter.* Don't! You need to know how to *prevent* a knee problem, because painful knees could eventually lead to a hurting heart.

2. Pick the parts. Go back and choose the concerns that are most pressing for your own health. Practice the whole Prime-Time Health plan or just part of it. It's okay to pick and choose. The best part of the plan for you is the one you will consistently do.

3. Put together your plan. Turn to chapter 24 to customize your own personal Prime-Time Health plan.

Because the field of prime-time health is changing so quickly, we will provide frequent updates at AskDrSears.com/Prime-TimeHealth. Featured at our website are:

- a list of recommended nutritional supplements
- video clips that elaborate on many of the important points in this book, including fitness tips, breathing techniques, nasal flushing, and personal messages from Dr. Bill
- reports on new scientific breakthroughs in prime-time health
- recommended books, websites, and other resources

And now, on to prime time.

PART I

Are You Ready for Prime Time?

In this section I will share with you how I researched, formulated, and live the Prime-Time Health plan and how I enjoy better health in nearly every organ of my body because of it. I will show you how you can do it too. You will learn what steps to take to make health your hobby. You will also learn about the usual changes that occur as you age during prime time and, even more important, how you can positively influence these changes. Let's begin by putting together your personal prime-time plan for health.

CHAPTER 1

Invest in Your Personal Prime-Time Health Plan

The scene opens on a cruise ship in the Pacific Ocean. I was a guest speaker and had been scheduled to talk about healthy aging. When it was my turn to speak, I opened with a question: "Now that you're in the prime of your life, how many of you have a retirement plan, such as an individual retirement account, or IRA?" Nearly every hand went up. Next I asked, "How many of you have set up an Individual Retirement Account for *Health,* an I-R-A-*H*?" No hands went up, yet the look on people's faces revealed what they were thinking: *I'm not sure what a health retirement plan is, but I should have one!* After the seminar, many folks thanked me for opening their eyes. They had saved money for retirement, but they had not saved their bodies to better enjoy it.

PLANNING FOR PRIME TIME:
THE FABULOUS FOUR

1. Save enough *money.*
2. Save enough *time.*
3. Nurture your *relationships.*
4. Maintain your *health.*

Consider health the vital ingredient in your prime-time plan. Not everyone can save as much money as they'd like or have as much free time as they want. But you *can* work to save your health. I wrote this book to help you prepare your very own Individual Retirement Account for Health.

Certainly, I had an IRA (as a father of eight, and needing to pay for all those braces and help three of our children get through medical school, I wish I could have saved more). After forty years as a hard-working physician, I looked forward to my prime time. This book, which took me more than a decade to finish, was written on the job as I was formulating my own IRAH, a plan that I wish I had started earlier.

MY STORY

Even though I am a doctor, my health habits used to leave a lot to be desired. I grew up as an overweight overeater. I still cringe at the memory of my mother taking me into a department store to buy huskies, those big-waisted pants that chubby kids wore. My nickname was Templeton, after the overeating rat in the book *Charlotte's Web*. My first date with Martha, my coauthor and wife of forty-three years, was at an all-you-can-eat buffet — I figured that if the date was a dud, I'd at least be able to eat.

For most of our married life, Martha tried to change my eating habits. I remember asking her on one of our weekly "date nights" (when we put the kids to bed early and enjoyed a romantic dinner for two) what we were having for dinner. "Stroganoff," she said. Ah, my favorite. When I sat down to eat what looked and smelled like beef stroganoff, I took a bite and complained, "Martha, this tastes like dog food!" (She'd substituted tofu for beef.)

Cancer caused me to care. I should have listened to Martha and eaten the tofu, because in

April 1997, at the age of fifty-seven, I underwent surgery, chemotherapy, and radiation therapy for colon cancer. During my recovery, I realized that I had been neglecting a vital aspect of planning for prime time — my health. Cancer caused me to care. Before that, I'd been a "wuss" (*wait until you get sick — stupid!*).

I vowed that I would not squander my health. I had too much to live for. As a physician, I knew that the human body is resilient and can bounce back and repair itself in many ways — with the right care. So I began my journey back to health. I wanted to be an asset, not a liability, to my wife and children. I wanted to be active, pain free, and disease free, and to not only be at my grandchildren's weddings but to dance at them. I wanted to be a healthy prime timer. Here's how I got started.

MAKE HEALTH YOUR HOBBY

In preparation for developing my health plan, I decided to study success stories — testimonies of people who survived major illnesses like cancer and became healthier. They all had one thing in common: *they had made a project out of their problem.* They studied their illness and researched ways they could help heal themselves. I realized that after I got one cancer, I was at a higher risk of getting another cancer, especially since my body had been polluted by chemotherapy and burned by radiation therapy, and even more so because my father died of colon cancer at age seventy-five.

Next, I consulted the experts. I studied the secrets of centenarians, people who live to be a hundred or more. What did these folks do to live longer and healthier? In addition to healthy eating and habits, centenarians had one thing in common: *they made health their hobby.*

So I was determined to make health my hobby too. We all need a hobby, and the older we get, the more important hobbies become. What more wonderful pastime could a person choose than to become a health nut? Why not focus more energy on the one thing that matters most?

Health span is more important than lifespan. What impressed me most about the centenarians was not only their quantity of life but also their *quality* of life. Researchers who study the health habits of cultures with the highest longevity focus less on lifespan and more on health span (the number of disability-free years we live in reasonably good health). We read that human beings are living longer now than ever. In most developed countries people over eighty-five are the fastest-growing segment of the population. Yet, that statistic is misleading. The fact is that we are living longer but not better.

Enjoy more time at the top. The standard American model of aging is health until age fifty,

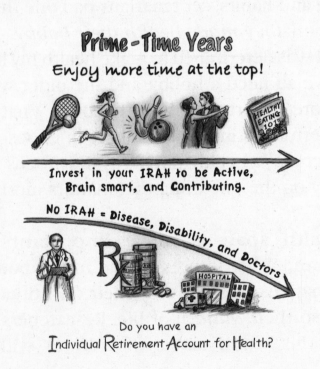

Prime-Time Years

Enjoy more time at the top!

Invest in your IRAH to be Active, Brain smart, and Contributing.

NO IRAH = Disease, Disability, and Doctors

Do you have an Individual Retirement Account for Health?

wearing down from fifty to sixty-five, and gradually falling apart after that. According to this model, many of us miss prime time entirely. But we don't have to follow this pattern. Consider prime time your opportunity to spend more time at the top in good health. How long we spend at the top depends, in large part, on how we plan for it. We can focus on the ABCs, seeking to remain *a*ctive, *b*rain smart, and *c*ontributing. Or, we can do nothing and look forward to the three Ds: *d*isease, *d*isability, and *d*octors. Which will you choose?

DISTURBING PRIME-TIME STATS

These health statistics are hard pills to swallow:

- More than 50 percent of all insured adults in the United States take prescription medicines regularly for chronic health problems.
- On average, Americans buy more medicine per person than do the people of any other country.
- Three out of four people over age sixty-five take medication for chronic illness.
- Twenty-five percent of people over age sixty-five take *five* or more medicines regularly.

THE BENEFITS OF MY PRIME-TIME PLAN FOR HEALTH

Within three months of beginning my health plan, I noticed big changes from head to toe. And at this writing, I continue to enjoy medication-free, disability-free prime-time living.

Clearer thinking. My brain got better faster than my body. I experienced a lot of mental perks from the program: my thought processes were clearer, and my memory improved. I noticed fewer mood swings, and I managed my feelings more easily. I was more consistently upbeat and handled stress better. My brain seemed more focused. All of this makes scientific sense. The brain is affected by eating and lifestyle changes — for better or for worse — more than any other organ in the body, so it stands to reason that it would show improvement first.

Clearer vision. My eyesight improved. I used to wear glasses to read the scoreboard at baseball games. One night a few months into this program, I forgot my glasses. Surprisingly, I could read the scoreboard clearly without them.

This makes sense because the eyes are really an extension of the brain. What is good for the brain is also good for the eyes.

More sensitive nose. Pardon the comparison, but in wild animals the nose is the organ of survival, hunting, and danger alert. The same is true of humans. Hazardous vapors are supposed to warn us to get away from the source before they harm our health. Most prime timers have lost this nasal alarm system, but you can get it back. My sense of smell became *more discerning*. Smelly substances in the air bothered me more. I went out of my way while driving to avoid following buses and trucks that spewed out irritating exhaust fumes. I could sniff out a smoker before entering a room. These irritants did not bother me before, but they should have. My garbage-avoidance system was working better.

More sensitive hearing. Prolonged exposure to loud, high-pitched noise is the main cause of ARHL (age-related hearing loss). Noises such as train horns and grandkids' screeching, which before cancer — BC — I rarely noticed, now began to really bother me. One day I had to

A PATIENT'S STORY

A few years ago I got scared thinking about the aches and pains, the multitude of medications, and the illnesses that my mother experienced (not to mention her dementia and Parkinson's), realizing that all that might be in store for me. I also watched friends who were unwilling to change their diet and lifestyle suffering from diabetes and heart disease.

As I searched for ways to keep this from happening to me, I began reading lots of self-help books, taking minerals and supplements, and doing moderate exercise. Nothing worked, not even the strong urgings from my doctor, who eventually resorted to a last-ditch solution—giving me more drugs. Then Dr. Bill told me that he didn't take any medications and gave me an opportunity to read his work.

Most of my life I have had to fight weight gain, and for the past thirty-five years I have used the on-again, off-again low-carb dieting approach. The older I got, the more difficult it was to lose weight and to maintain weight loss. After each period of weight loss, I ended up with a higher baseline weight, and along with it came diabetes and high blood pressure. Each year, I depended more and more on drugs. Then I began reading Dr. Bill's manuscript and was so inspired by his personal story that I began using his techniques and wound up completely changing my eating and my lifestyle.

Dr. Bill's stories, wit, insight, and simple yet easy-to-remember rules for healthy living made this a fun, informative, and motivating read. The more ideas I tried, the more confident I became. Now I will try almost any new food, and I've discovered a whole world of very tasty foods that I would not have considered eating even a year ago.

With a goal of extending my life and living more comfortably and healthily, I figured I had to lose sixty pounds. As I write this, I have reached three-quarters of my goal and am slightly ahead of my plan. More important, my blood sugar readings have dropped dramatically, as has my blood pressure and cholesterol—all while enjoying more and better food!

As my waist shrank from forty-four inches to thirty-eight inches, I gave all my pants to my son-in-law, along with an early copy of *Prime-Time Health*. There is no doubt in my mind that I will reach my goal and be able to maintain a healthy lifestyle and enjoy eating at the same time. I can honestly say that the Prime-Time Health plan has resulted in the best change in my life, one for which I will be forever grateful. At age sixty-nine, I am happy to hear my personal physician say that I look a lot younger, and when people ask me how I'm feeling I can honestly say that I feel terrific.

— Bill Bridegroom, healthier prime timer

tell my four-year-old granddaughter, "That hurts Grandpa's ears." This protective perk prompted me to deliberately avoid loud noise whenever possible to keep my hearing healthy.

Healthier teeth and gums, and improved sense of taste. For many years I had suffered from severe gum problems (gingivitis). After I spent about a year on my new health plan, my dentist noticed the difference and remarked, "Your gums look great! What are you doing differently?" Even my tongue became healthier, or at least the taste buds on it did. Artificially sweetened foods became increasingly distasteful; I craved the taste of real food.

Better breathing. As my body was getting into better biochemical balance, so was my breathing. I noticed I was automatically breathing more slowly and deeply, and more from the belly than from the chest. While at rest most people take about ten to fourteen breaths per minute, I average six breaths per minute. (On page 210 you will learn how this pattern of breathing is good for both mind and body.)

Leaner body. My waist size went from thirty-seven inches to thirty-four inches, which, as you will learn in chapter 3, is more significant than scale weight. When a friend inquired, "You look so healthy! What diet are you on?" I replied, "The real-food diet!" "What's that?" asked my puzzled friend. I cleared up the confusion: "You know, the foods that grow in fields, swim in the sea, run on the land, and spend very little time in factories; and most of them don't even have a food label."

Good gut feelings. Perhaps the greatest changes were in my gut. I experienced firsthand the effects of a nutritional concept called *metabolic programming,* which you will learn about on page 575. After a few months of healthy eating, my gut became increasingly selective. When I would indulge in junk food, it would scream, "You should not have eaten that." I'm convinced that millions of nerves in the gut and intestinal lining that register food as good for you or bad for you had been turned on again. Years of unhealthy eating had squelched these helpful signals. It's as if they were saying, "He's not going to listen to us anyway. We'll stop telling him what's good and bad to eat." Now my gut and brain began working together, telling me, "If you eat food that's good for you, you'll feel good!"

Tastes and cravings changed. I went through a stage of *taste reshaping*. Initially, I made a list of the prime foods that were best for my body, such as spicy turmeric and chili peppers, and started eating them, whether or not I liked the taste. After a few months, I actually craved these previously disliked foods. For example, after craving curry and turmeric, I found studies showing these spices help suppress colon cancer and inflammation. One day I was browsing the produce department at Trader Joe's and noticed that pomegranates were in season. That inner voice prompted me to buy a case. Smart gut voice! As you will learn in chapter 5, the body has a built-in survival mechanism that says, "Feed me what's good, and you'll develop a taste for it."

Meal patterns changed. Not only did my newly turned-on gut voice tell me *what* to eat, it prompted me *how* to eat. This gut voice started giving me three messages:
- Eat more *often.*

- Eat *less.*
- Chew *longer.*

I practiced and preached *Dr. Bill's Rule of Twos:* Eat *twice* as often, eat *half* as much, and chew *twice* as long. When you eat more often, in smaller minimeals — a pattern called *grazing* — you won't feel hungry or uncomfortably full.

Eat less, and enjoy food more. Once I started craving quality foods, I noticed I was satisfied with less. After a lifetime of acting like Templeton the rat, a chronic overeater, I was amazed by this change. Why was my belly brain telling me to eat less? *Calorie restriction.* There is a huge amount of research attesting to the fact that people who eat less live longer and healthier. I didn't want to be known as a calorie restrictor, yet it made sense: eating less means less food to metabolize, less "oxidation" (or wear and tear on the body), and healthier aging. It's a simple concept. I theorized — and found scientific support in studies on calorie restriction — that the body becomes more *efficient* with less food. It is sort of like trading in your gas-guzzling SUV for a hybrid or getting a tune-up. You burn less fuel, produce less exhaust, and your engine lasts longer.

Finer dining. Within six months of changing my eating habits, I had become a *picky eater* — in a good way. I was particularly selective about the quality of food I put in my gut. Fruits and vegetables had to be fresh or frozen, not canned (I'll never eat canned soup again!). I stayed away from processed foods, which were far too sweet or salty for my more sensitive taste buds. Sauces had to be lighter and less greasy. Seafood had to be wild, not farmed. Salad greens had to be green, not pale. Bread had to be whole grain, not white. My body was demanding quality food. This would be the beginning, not the end, of fine dining.

In my precancer years, I never cared for spicy foods. Why all of a sudden was I craving chili peppers and dishes with curry, turmeric, and garlic? My body seemed to know these spicy foods are full of phytos, natural anticancer, antiaging, and anti-inflammatory substances. I even enjoyed eating tofu — a food I once made fun of.

One day our eight-year-old, Lauren, said, "Daddy, I liked it better before you got cancer. We got more junk food." A year later Lauren helped me plant a garden of greens, herbs, and, of course, red-hot chili peppers. All of these good foods found their way into our meals, and even Lauren enjoyed them. Our kids and grandkids watch our health habits. Lauren learned that her daddy had made some poor health choices and got sick, but now he was making healthier choices and getting well.

Some inner switch turned on. I also became reacquainted with a sixth sense, the *wisdom of the body,* a concept I heard way back in medical school but dismissed as some fanciful notion a philosopher made up. We are all born with this wise voice, but decades of not listening to it cause our awareness of it to fade. When you do start listening, the voice gets stronger and you become more tuned in to it. It will help you make this plan a way of life for you and your family, because your body will crave what it needs. After I started following my health plan, I'd walk toward a salad bar, and an internal switch would turn on and nudge, "Ah, health food — gotta eat it." My body started prompting me to take up lots of other health-boosting habits. For example, if I saw lemon or lime wedges, I would automatically squeeze some fresh juice in my water or on my salad. After this lemon-juice switch turned on, I went to the books to find out why it was good for me. (See answer, page 369.) I discovered there is a psychological term for these "gotta have it" and "gotta do it" urges: *positive addiction.*

What is this wisdom of the body exactly? And what's its source? I don't know, but I'm certain it is the biochemical basis for the phrase "it's in the blood." I believe that when the body is in biochemical balance and hormonal harmony (concepts you will learn about later), an internal *switch* gets turned on or some biochemical magic circulates throughout the body telling it what to do and what not to do. That's what this Prime-Time Health plan will do for you.

Healthier skin. For years in our medical practice, I've noticed that people with healthier diets have more beautiful skin. Now I was experiencing this for myself. My skin was less flaky and dry, especially during the low-humidity winter months. I attributed this change to my seafood indulgence. Even my fingernails started to get stronger and grow more rapidly. Many of our friends said, "You look so much younger!"

Heightened healing. Because I tend to move fast and often get a bit klutzy, I ding myself a lot. Close friends have dubbed me "Doctor Band-Aid." With aging, blood supply to the skin diminishes, leaving it less able to repair itself. After a couple of years on my program, I noticed speedier and more complete healing of cuts. Besides healing faster on the outside, I was healthier on the inside. My immune system worked better than ever. Colds went away faster. Over twelve years, except for scheduled checkups, colonoscopies every few years, and dental care, I haven't had to seek additional medical care.

Taller body, longer feet. Around eight years into the program, I noticed that I was developing calluses at the ends of my big toes. Initially, I ignored them. Then the calluses got bigger. Then I noticed my toes were touching the ends of my shoes. My shoes were too small! But I've worn the same brand and size of running shoes for years. Could my feet have grown at age sixty-five? Sure enough, measurements showed that my shoe size had increased from size 11½ to size 12. And, while prime timers are supposed to shrink as they age, my height has actually increased a half inch, mostly due to improved posture and muscle strength. It seems I walked my way to a stronger skeletal system.

More energy. Three months into my program, I was becoming a healthier person. My resting heart rate and breathing rate were lower. My body was acting like an engine that was now well tuned and more energy efficient. With this new vitality, Martha and I actually beat younger couples in a swing dance contest. Martha calls me "the Energizer Bunny." I just keep going and going.

Feeling in control. With all these positives, I gradually gained a sense of control over my health. Now I believed I could greatly influence my destiny — aging healthfully or painfully. I no longer feared growing old. No longer did I fret about those S words: *sore, stiff, sick,* and *senile.* Once I knew that I could help my body make its own longevity medicines, I looked forward to retirement as a time to do more, not less. I was being given a choice about what sort of prime timer I would become. In fact, helping your body make its own internal medicines is the central theme of the Prime-Time Health plan.

Doctors were amazed. At age sixty-five when I was updating my life insurance policy, I had to go through a series of tests, including an electrocardiogram, blood pressure, and a lipid blood panel. A few days later I got a call from one of the doctors at the insurance company who began the conversation by

SHARE THE HEALTH PLAN WITH YOUR KIDS

While writing this book, I envisioned happily presenting the completed publication to each one of our children before they turned forty, with a little doctorly and fatherly advice: "Please read it and do it. Our grandchildren deserve it."

Once you get your health plan going, brag about it, and share your story with your grandchildren: "Grandma made some unwise choices. My joints hurt, and my big middle slows me down. But now I know better, and I'm eating better and exercising more." Or, when they visit and notice a fridge full of health food and a home gym you call your "playroom," you could proudly say, "That's what smart grandmas do!"

THE PRIME-TIME PLAN AT A GLANCE

Here's a preview of the vital parts of the Prime-Time Health plan. Check those that most concern you. While you may be tempted to read ahead, I recommend that you *read the entire book first,* since so many chapters are interdependent. Later, reread the topics you've checked.

- ❏ Make health your hobby, page 6.
- ❏ Have a healthy heart, page 49.
- ❏ Stay smart, page 99.
- ❏ Be good to your gut, *how* to eat, page 140.
- ❏ Avoid "bad words" on food labels, page 158.
- ❏ Follow the Rule of Twos: eat *twice* as often, eat *half* as much, and chew *twice* as long, page 150.
- ❏ Get plenty of antioxidants by eating the three Ss: seafood, salads, and smoothies.
- ❏ Keep the pollutants—from the air you breathe, the food you eat, and the thoughts you think—out of your body.

saying, "The computer flagged your policy because your total cholesterol was high. The reason your total cholesterol was so high was that your *good* cholesterol was eighty. We seldom see sixty-five-

- ❑ Improve your Eye-Q, page 175.
- ❑ Tune up your hearing, page 187.
- ❑ Enjoy better breathing, page 199.
- ❑ Be good to your gums, page 215.
- ❑ Build better bones, page 222.
- ❑ Give joy to your joints, page 245.
- ❑ Have smoother skin, page 290.
- ❑ Enjoy superfoods: *what* to eat, page 305.
- ❑ Sleep soundly, page 372.
- ❑ Reduce stress, page 397.
- ❑ Enjoy better sex, page 426.
- ❑ Practice the pills-and-skills model of health care and self-care, page 449.
- ❑ Lower your highs: high blood pressure, high blood sugar, high blood cholesterol, page 486.
- ❑ Cut your chances of getting cancer, page 533.
- ❑ Stay lean, page 567.
- ❑ Move! Stay fit, page 614.
- ❑ Enjoy a fall-safe home, page 659.

year-old men with such a healthy cholesterol profile. Would you mind telling me what your secret is?" Imagine, a life insurance company inquiring about the secret to healthy aging and longevity.

ARE YOU AT RISK FOR A SHORTER PRIME TIME?

If any of these items describe you, you need the Prime-Time Health plan:

- Do you have a prime-time *potbelly?*
- Do you do *less than two hours* of moderate exercise weekly?
- Do you eat more *animal-based foods* than seafood and plant-based foods?
- Do you eat *fast, large* meals?
- Do you spend much of your time *indoors?*
- Do you spend much of your time *sitting?*

JUST DO IT!

You'll be aware of two phases in the Prime-Time Health plan. In the first few months, you will need to persevere with all the steps. This is the got-to-do-it stage. Then you will notice how good your body feels and how well it works, and an inner switch will be flipped on. Now, you are in the want-to-do-it stage and will *crave* this lifestyle. Once you reach this point, you'll never look back.

CHAPTER 2

Understand How Your Body Changes during Prime Time

One day I was playing golf with a friend who collects cars. He also loves a few drinks at lunch and dinner, smokes, and says he never gets enough sleep. He was boasting about how a few of his vintage cars run as well as they did when they were made. Ah, the perfect opening for some prime-time preaching.

"So, what's your secret? Why are your cars in such good shape?" I asked.

"I take good care of them," Mark responded.

"What do you do?"

"I put the best fuel and oil in them. I get regular tune-ups. I don't let the wear and tear get out of hand. It's really quite easy. You just know what a car needs, and you take care of it."

"Okay, Mark, why don't you take care of your

body the same way? Otherwise, soon your kids are going to inherit your cars."

Mark realized how foolish it was to take better care of his cars than himself.

When you read articles on aging, you will notice the term *age-related* keeps cropping up: age-related cognitive decline, age-related hearing loss, age-related macular degeneration. The list of age-related challenges is long. These conditions are portrayed as a normal part of the aging process. But that is not necessarily so.

Now we'll take you deep inside your body, even inside your cells, to show you why prime-time aging occurs. After you learn what can go wrong, the rest of the book will help you make it right.

THE SIMPLEST EXPLANATION OF AGING YOU'VE EVER HEARD

Call it my sticky-stuff/garbage-disposal theory of aging. Aging has two main causes: too much sticky stuff (garbage) accumulates in the body, and the body's garbage-disposal system weakens so it can't get rid of the sticky stuff. *Health*, therefore, is simply keeping the sticky stuff out of your body and strengthening your garbage-disposal system. The longer we live, the more garbage gets into our bodies through the food we eat, the air we breathe, and the stress we store. And, as we age, our body's garbage-disposal system (immune system) weakens. The garbage that accumulates in our bodies causes the sticky stuff (oxidation, inflammation, and glycation) to build up in our blood and to pile up in our tissues. People who maintain their garbage-disposal systems and put less garbage into their bodies age better than those who do not.

The blood tests your doctor may order for you during a checkup — cholesterol, homocysteine, C-reactive protein, and so on — measure the levels of sticky stuff collecting in your blood.

Garbage accumulates in two vital places: inside the cells, damaging the mitochondria, the cells' microscopic power plants; and outside the cells on the surfaces of the tissues. While over time the body cleverly adapts its garbage-disposal systems to changing diets and lifestyles, it can't keep pace with the garbage. Garbage just keeps piling up. And this leads to unhealthy aging. A classic example of garbage accumulation, called amyloid deposits, is seen in Alzheimer's disease.

The Prime-Time Health plan focuses on keeping the sticky stuff out of your body and maintaining your garbage-disposal system.

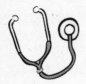

DR. SEARS SAYS...
My prescription for healthy aging: Keep the sticky stuff out of your body, and strengthen your garbage-disposal system.

FIVE REASONS WHY WE AGE

Prime-time health means a *balance* between wear and tear and repair. The focus of our plan is to slow down normal wear and tear and to strengthen the body's repair mechanisms. With unhealthy aging, wear and tear overwhelms repair.

Simply speaking, three main mechanisms cause us to age, and two other factors play a role as well. Let's start with the big three:

Oxidation: rust
Inflammation: wear and tear
Glycation: stiff and sticky stuff accumulates
    in the bloodstream

These "-tions"—which, as their names suggest, we should *shun*—are agers that account for the illnesses that make prime time *sick* time for so many: they contribute to cardiovascular disease, hardening of the arteries, and "-itis" illnesses such as arthritis, bronchitis, dermatitis, colitis, and one I dub cognitivitis (Alzheimer's). These "-tions" also cause cancer, perhaps the scariest of all prime-time illnesses. They damage the genetic control mechanism of cells, causing them to mutate and multiply out of control. In addition, as we get older, genes that influence aging get quirky, and some of our hormones get out of balance.

Here's an overview of what happens to most of us during prime time:

1. We Rust

Our bodies are oxygen-burning machines. Every minute, countless biochemical reactions throughout the body generate exhaust called *oxidants*, or free radicals. Trillions of times a day, these free radicals hit your cells and tissues like miniature hammers, whittling away at them. They're responsible for hardened arteries, stiff joints, blurry vision, and wrinkled skin. So the key to aging well is to lessen the number of hits. Throughout this book, you will learn how to avoid hard hitters, the habits and foods that pound away at your body like sledgehammers.

Normally, our bodies handle free radicals by producing antiexhaust chemicals called *antioxidants*. But when the body builds up more oxidants than antioxidants, the garbage backs up and increases the wear and tear on the tissues. As we age, our bodies tend to produce fewer antioxidants. So as we get older we need to eat more foods that contain them.

Picture a fresh, crisp apple. Inside that apple are oxidants and antioxidants. Over time, as the oxidants outnumber the antioxidants, the apple gets softer, browner, and more wrinkled. The apple ages.

Now cut an apple in half and place it on the counter. Pour lemon juice (an antioxidant) on one half. In a few hours, the lemon-juice-protected half still looks good. In contrast, the unprotected half looks brown, definitely older. It oxidized, or rusted. Our bodies are in a constant state of rust versus antirust. The Prime-Time Health plan is an *antirust* maintenance program, sort of like lemon juice on an apple.

2. Our Immune System Weakens

During prime time, our body's maintenance crew, the immune system, usually starts to get out of balance, making our tissues more prone to wear and tear, or inflammation — a medical buzzword you will hear a lot about during your prime-time years. Inflammation is the main cause of unhealthy aging. Dubbed *inflammaging* in this context, it makes prime timers more susceptible to "-itis" illnesses, such as arthritis and colitis. In autoimmune diseases such as these, the immune system attacks its own tissues. Here's how the self-destruction happens: Unhealthy lifestyle and dietary habits cause the cells to change their genetic code. In addition, that stiff and sticky stuff (inflammatory changes) from years of unhealthy living and eating accumulates in tissues and changes their structure. The immune system reacts to these unfamiliar cells and tissues by saying, in effect, "This sticky stuff doesn't belong here! It must be a foreign substance, like a germ." The mixed-up immune system then attacks the sticky stuff lining the blood vessels, joints, and other tissues; imagine millions of miniature Pac-Men eating away at your body — not a pretty picture. But there is good news: you can teach your body to produce just the right kind and amount of anti-inflammatories when you need them.

When the body is healthy, its inflammatory reactions — wear and tear and repair — are in perfect balance. Just as a well-maintained road stays smooth because the wear and tear is fixed as it occurs, so does a body in balance stay healthier longer. But when the wear and tear overcomes the internal repair crew's ability to maintain a certain tissue or organ, aging occurs. (In chapter 18, you will learn how to keep your body from accumulating inflammatory chemicals we call "iBods" and how to balance your immune system.)

3. We Produce AGEs

When you eat like a typical teenager, excess sugar molecules in your blood attach to proteins, changing their structure and making them stiff and sticky. These "aging proteins" are called advanced glycation end products, or AGEs. This sludge in the tissues of your body prevents healthy growth and the repair of new tissues. Two obvious examples of AGEs' effects are wrinkles, which appear when excess sugar attaches to the collagen in your skin, and the stiffening of arteries, which occurs when AGEs stick to artery linings. As we get older, our cells become less sensitive to insulin, which leaves a higher level of glucose in the bloodstream. So, unless you take the proper steps as you enter prime time, you could soon be considered prediabetic.

I'm not going to bash the word *sugar,* because there are good sugars and bad sugars. In fact, it's nutritionally correct to say that the body runs well on a diet that's 50 percent sugars, but that's when the sugars are good slow-release sugars, the ones that nature makes. Nature makes the right fuel for the body; factories don't.

These three basic mechanisms of aging — oxidation, inflammation, and glycation — underlie nearly all of the controllable processes of aging. And they are at the root of two other theories of aging that we'll cover next.

THE STICKY-STUFF CYCLE OF AGING

One "-tion" leads to another. *Glycation* alters proteins, which the body in turn perceives as foreign, which triggers *inflammation,* which triggers *oxidation*—more sticky stuff.

---

4. Our Genes Get Quirky

Our cells are constantly reproducing and repairing themselves. But some of the trillions of reproductions that occur throughout the day go wrong, and the DNA gets damaged. Normally, the body repairs damaged DNA, but as we age the cellular repair system becomes less efficient; this is called *genetic aging.* Our Prime-Time Health plan is aimed at strengthening the cellular repair system, as well as avoiding cellular pollutants that damage DNA. We are able to "help you fit into your genes" because of an exciting new field of research called *nutrigenomics,* which studies how food communicates to genes, telling them to stay young, and how junk foods turn on the "grow old fast" genes.

For a better understanding of how your genes age, here's a theory that makes sense: At the end of each chromosome dangles a *telomere,* somewhat like the end of a shoelace. Telomeres are the biologic clock in the cell's genetic code for aging. The longer the telomeres stay intact, the less quickly the cells age. Genetically speaking, aging is thought to be caused by all the garbage that gets into the body and gradually snips away at these telomeres. As your telomeres get *shorter,* your life gets shorter.

Dr. Dean Ornish, founder and president of the Preventive Medicine Research Institute in Sausalito, California, and author of the healthy-aging book *The Spectrum,* conducted a study that showed that the length of the repair enzyme telomerase increased by an average of nearly 30 percent after just three months in patients who improved their lifestyle, exercise, attitude, and nutrition. This makes sense since healthy food and healthy lifestyles support the chromosomes and tell them to stay younger longer.

Living long and well is influenced more by how you live than by the genes you were born with. Geriatric specialists estimate that the so-called longevity gene (the genes you may have inherited from your parents and grandparents) only influence how long you live by less than 33 percent (compared to other influences).

5. Hormones Become Helpless

The endocrine theory of aging teaches that hormones, our body's control systems, slow down as we get older. Insulin, the master hormone, is especially important. As we age, the microscopic doors (receptor sites) on cell membranes get stiff, or resistant to letting insulin escort sugar into the cells. In chapter 3, you will learn why stable insulin levels are a key to your health, and why hormonal balance is the essence of the Prime-Time Health plan.

SECRETS OF CENTENARIANS

What are the health secrets of the experts, people who live — and live healthily — to at least one hundred years old? These are all longevity-boosting habits that most centenarians have in common:

They move. Vigorous centenarians spend much of their day doing physical exercise, whether in their gardens or on a golf course. Their joints don't have a chance to get stiff or their bones and muscles frail.

> *Motion is your best joint lotion.*
> —WALDO McBURNEY, FORMER MARATHON
> RUNNER, AGE 101

They love. They have deep intimate relationships.

They're lean. As they aged, they neither gained fat nor lost muscle. Because of their healthy living and eating habits, centenarians have higher blood levels of adiponectin, a hormone that regulates metabolism and acts like a natural anti-inflammatory. Centenarians are not skinny; they are *lean,* which means they have just the right amount of body fat for their body type. They maintain their weight by maintaining muscle.

They eat less. Centenarians tend to eat 10 to 20 percent fewer daily calories than people on the standard American diet.

They graze. They eat smaller meals more often and take more time to eat.

They eat pure. They eat real foods (mostly fruits, vegetables, and fish) and shun processed, packaged foods and chemical additives.

> *We dig our graves with our teeth.*
> — WALDO MCBURNEY

They laugh. They enjoy themselves. Humor is therapeutic.

They pray. Spiritual beliefs and practices occupy much of their time and thoughts. They enjoy a sense of spiritual belonging.

They're flexible. "The most adaptable live the longest," said Henry Rempel, my friend who lived to be one hundred years old.

They serve. Volunteering and ministering to others' needs is high on their "to do" list. They thrive on the helper's high.

They're musical. Music mellows the mind. For an uplifting DVD that I guarantee will leave you laughing and admiring active seniors, see the documentary *Young at Heart*.

They swim. Water is a wonderful refuge, calming the mind and soothing the body.

They think. Mental exercise, such as Sudoku and crossword puzzles, keeps their minds active.

They go slow. Okinawans, people who live the longest and healthiest, accuse Americans of having a "hurry sickness."

They're fun. They are fun-loving but not foolish in their activities.

They sleep. Quality sleep is very important.

They're up! They are positive thinkers, not worrywarts. They figure, "If I can't change it, I'm not going to worry about it."

They work. "I need a project" is a common refrain. They have a reason to wake up in the morning.

They're sexy. Longevity research has found that couples who engage in the most sexual activity tend to live the longest.

They plan. When I asked centenarian Henry Rempel for his advice to prime timers, he said, "Most young people aren't preparing well for their next ten years."

Most centenarians enjoy a long life of abilities and a short end-of-life period of disabilities. Men, take note: Female centenarians outnumber males by a ratio of nine to one. In the United

States only one male in twenty thousand attains the age of one hundred. Why does longevity seem to favor women? Researchers theorize that women tend to eat better, socialize more, and engage less in risky behaviors. The oldest documented supercentenarian was a French woman, Jeanne Calment, who died in 1997 at the blessed age of 122.

Which column do you want to be in? Do you want to take control of your health during prime time? Tired of hearing all those S words: *slower, stickier, stiffer, smaller, softer,* and *shorter*? Sorry, they're ultimately unavoidable. Yet, we can slow down the aging process.

PRIME-TIME CHANGES: WHAT'S LIKELY TO HAPPEN AND WHAT OUR PLAN CAN DO

From head to toe, here are the typical changes that can occur with age. In the following chapters you will learn, step by step, how to slow down these changes.

Typical Prime Timers	Prime Timers on the Prime-Time Health Plan
Heart muscle becomes *stiffer*. Blood vessels get *sticky* stuff inside and narrow.	Arteries widen; vessel walls stay *smooth* and *soft*. Heart stays *strong*.
Brain *tissue shrinks*. Speed of nerve transmission *slows*.	Nerve transmission stays *fast*. Thinking stays *sharp*.
Gut digestion *slows*, causing constipation, reflux (heartburn), and indigestion.	Digestion *hastens*, increasing nutrient absorption, stomach emptying, and waste passage.
Eyes accumulate *sticky stuff*. Vessels clot. Vision gets cloudy.	Vision is maintained and may even improve.
Hearing lessens. Tiny vibrating bones get *stiff*. Ear ringing (tinnitus) increases.	Hearing stays *strong*; tinnitus decreases.

(continued) Typical Prime Timers	Prime Timers on the Prime-Time Health Plan
Lungs get *stiff*. Airways *narrow*. Oxygen intake lessens as does energy.	More oxygen is inhaled with each breath. Energy *increases*.
Teeth and gums weaken.	Gums are healthy; less gingivitis. Teeth are strong.
Bones *weaken,* causing osteoporosis and fractures. Stature *shortens*.	Bones *strengthen,* reducing fractures. You retain your height and stay *mobile*.
Joints stiffen, making movement painful.	Joints stay mobile, and movement is comfortable.
Skin gets *rough* and *wrinkly*.	Skin stays *smoother*.
Muscle gets *weaker;* replaced by increased body *fat*.	Muscle stays *strong;* body stays *lean*.
Kidneys *weaken*. Bladder weakens. More nighttime trips to bathroom.	Kidneys stay *strong;* fewer bathroom breaks.

(continued) **Typical Prime Timers**	**Prime Timers on the** **Prime-Time Health Plan**
Sex drive fizzles. Erectile dysfunction (ED) is common in men.	Less ED; sexual activity maintained.
Immunity weakens; more infections, more "-itis" illnesses, more *pills*.	Fewer infections and pills; more *self-care skills*.
Mood disorders cause more Ds: depression, bipolar disorder.	Moods more stable; fewer Ds.
Hormones become *unbalanced;* more diabetes, more highs: high blood sugar, high blood pressure, and high cholesterol.	Stable insulin levels, fewer highs: normal blood sugar, blood pressure, and blood cholesterol.

PART II

Keeping Your Body at Its Prime

In part II, you will learn how to think better, feel better, move better, and enjoy better health. We will help you develop a health plan *before* these vital organs and tissues start to wear out:

- heart
- brain
- gut
- eyes
- ears

- lungs
- gums
- bones
- joints
- skin

After my health crisis, I figured if I could improve the health of each one of these organs and tissues, then I would enjoy my prime-time years even more. I was right.

We'll begin by looking at the heart, brain, and gut, the three most influential body parts in healthy prime-time living. Most heart disease begins in the gut, and most brain illnesses begin in the blood vessels, so these "big three" go together and determine overall health. We'll start by showing you the single most important health change you can make in preparing for prime time: protecting your blood vessels against endothelial dysfunction.

CHAPTER 3

Have a Healthy Prime-Time Heart

Y ou're only as young and healthy as your blood vessels" is the granddaddy of medical truisms. This makes sense since each organ in the body relies on the blood vessels supplying it. That's why we're starting our health plan with an explanation of how to keep your vessels healthy. Prime-time heart health means keeping your blood vessels at their prime.

HOW YOUR CARDIOVASCULAR SYSTEM AGES

The term *cardiovascular* means the whole blood-delivery system: the pump (cardio or heart) and the vessels (vascular). The more you know about how blood vessel health contributes to longevity, the more motivated you will be to take care of your blood vessels. Here's what you should know about those miles of blood-transporting highways that keep your body, shall we say, in its prime.

Healthy Prime Time	Unhealthy Prime Time
Vessels stay *wide* open.	Vessels *narrow*.
Vessel lining stays *smooth*.	Vessel lining gets *rough*.
Vessel walls stay *flexible*.	Vessel walls become *stiff*.
Heart muscle stays *strong*.	Heart muscle *weakens*.
Blood *flows better*.	Blood becomes *sticky*, clots too fast.

During middle age four changes typically occur that slow the blood flow through the arteries and increase the strain on the heart:

1. **Arteries narrow.** Gradually, sticky stuff builds up, narrowing the arteries and impeding blood flow.

2. **Arteries harden.** The vessel walls and the lining of the vessels become more rigid and less elastic. The heart has to pump harder to force blood through these stiff arteries, which leads to high blood pressure.

3. **Arteries become rough.** The lining of the blood vessels, the *endothelium,* becomes sticky (like Velcro, instead of smooth, like Teflon). This leads to buildup of sticky stuff, or plaque, and contributes to further hardening of the arteries.

4. **Blood thickens.** Blood cells become less flexible and stickier, so they clump together and have more difficulty squeezing through the tiny blood vessels. In cardiologist-speak, as we age the blood of most people "clots too fast." Blood is supposed to clot only when it leaks out of a vessel, as in a cut finger, not inside the vessel.

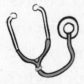

DR. SEARS SAYS...
Women, take note: The risk of death from heart disease is higher in women than in men.

FOUR HEART PARTS
EVERY PRIME TIMER MUST KNOW

Heart health depends on the health of four areas of your cardiovascular system:
- the endothelium, or lining, of your blood vessels
- the walls of your blood vessels
- the blood
- the heart

1. Go Easy on Your Endothelium

Prime-time quiz: What's the largest endocrine organ in your body?
A. pancreas
B. thyroid
C. adrenal glands
D. endothelium

Answer: D, endothelium. In fact, if you were to open up all the blood vessels in the human body and lay them out flat, they would occupy a surface area larger than several tennis courts. I believe that the most exciting medical discovery in the past decade is that the lining of the blood vessels — the endothelium — is your body's largest internal medicine pharmacy. Searching for your fountain of youth? It's inside your blood vessels. A person with healthy endothelium could rightly be called "young on the inside." Your one-cell-layer-thick endothelium is a true silver lining.

As recently as ten years ago, even some doctors considered blood vessels nothing more than an elaborate system of hoses. Most people believed that the heart pumped blood into one end of a big hose, that the blood came out the ends of little hoses to nourish all the tissues, and that nothing else happened to the blood on its journey. Not true!

The billions of cells that line your arteries don't just sit there; they do something. The lining of healthy blood vessels is like a smooth highway over which the traffic of the blood passes. This lining contains metabolically active cells that function like microscopic medicine bottles, releasing hormones and other substances to help maintain the blood vessels' health. The hormones released by the endothelium act like chemical messengers, telling the arteries and other organs and tissues to behave in a healthful way.

Your endothelial pharmacy dispenses dozens of medicines that regulate:

- blood flow and blood pressure
- blood clotting
- cholesterol
- inflammation
- growth and repair of blood vessels

The endothelium has a built-in self-maintenance system that keeps the surface smooth. This vascular highway automatically expands during rush-hour traffic, such as when you exercise, to let more blood flow more smoothly.

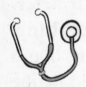

DR. SEARS SAYS...
Your endothelium is your personal blood-chemistry monitor. Care for it!

My lunch with Dr. Lou. While practicing what I preach—making health my hobby—I befriended top experts in healthy aging. One of the most educational three hours of my life was a lunch with Dr. Lou Ignarro, who shared the Nobel Prize in Physiology or Medicine in 1998 for his discovery of how healthy endothelium releases nitric oxide (NO) in just the right amount to regulate blood flow to tissues. (I admit I began to address Dr. Lou as Dr. NO.) Nitric oxide is the body's natural vasodilator; it widens arteries and increases blood flow to meet the body's increased need for energy, such as during exercise. It's interesting that his discovery led to the formulation of the drug Viagra, which works by releasing NO to increase blood flow to the penis. (More about how NO perks up the penis in chapter 16.) If the body can muster extra NO when the penis needs it, it can certainly do so for other organs, such as the brain, heart, intestines, and muscles.

Intuitively, I have always suspected that the body can make the medicines it needs, but I didn't know how or where. After hearing about Dr. Ignarro's research, I said: "Lou, nitric oxide is the body's natural internal medicine for cardiovascular health." He thanked me for simplifying his discovery, and he put my quote on the back cover of his book, *NO More Heart Disease*. I believe, and Dr. Ignarro agreed, that the release of NO by the endothelium may be the body's own healthy-aging medicine.

IS YOUR PRIME-TIME PHARMACY CLOSED OR OPEN?

Notice the prime timer who sits too much and eats too much of the wrong foods *(top):* Blood cells stick together and form clots, and sticky stuff accumulates over the medicine bottles of the endothelium so they can't open. This prime timer's pharmacy is *closed*, and the artery is narrower. As a result, both health span and lifespan will be shortened.

Notice what's going on in the prime timer who moves more and eats more fruits and vegetables and seafood rich in (anti–sticky stuff) antioxidants *(bottom):* The blood flows freely, and there is no sticky stuff accumulating on top of the medicine bottles in the endothelium. This allows the endothelium to dispense the right medicines at the right time and in the right dosage. This pharmacy stays *open* long hours, resulting in longer and healthier life.

So, how can you tap into your own personal pharmacy? Two habits influence whether those microscopic medicine bottles open and dispense the right medicine in the right dose at the right time:

- *How you eat.* You have to keep the sticky stuff out of your bloodstream so it doesn't

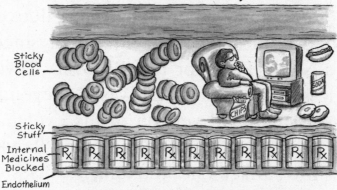

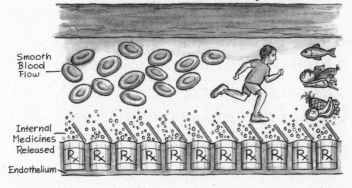

form a plaque over the surface of the "lids" and prevent them from opening.

- *How you move.* This is the discovery that won Dr. Ignarro the Nobel Prize.

At my lunch with Dr. Ignarro, I drew a simple picture on a napkin (that was the basis for the one on page 57) and said, "So we eat right to keep the 'sticky stuff' from accumulating on the lids of medicine bottles, but how does exercise open the lids?" I imagined that since he won a Nobel Prize for the discovery, I was in for a lesson in physics that was far beyond me. Here's a simplified version of his explanation of the value of exercise: When blood flows fast across the surface endothelium, it causes what is known as a shear force (frictional force). The cells (medicine bottles) lining the endothelium sense this extra blood flow and squirt out extra NO, which dilates the arteries, optimizes blood pressure, and delivers more blood flow and nutrients to the organs downstream.

Dr. NO, who begins his day in the gym at 6 a.m., went on to say, "Once you become a regular exerciser, you will literally begin to 'train' your endothelial cells to make more nitric oxide, even when you're not working out. Exercise is the only known process that causes a consistent and continuous production of nitric oxide by the endothelial cells, long after you have done your last sit-up or taken your last step on the treadmill for the day."

This NO concept (see illustration on page 57, one of the most important in this whole book) sums up the Prime-Time Health plan in a nutshell. I had always heard the platitudes "Eat right" and "Exercise more for good health," but no one had ever explained to me what exercise actually does. What I learned from Dr. Lou has forever motivated me to move — and I trust it will do the same for you.

Your endothelium regulates blood pressure. The health of your heart depends on normal blood pressure. If your blood pressure is too low, you won't get enough blood to nourish your tissues; if it's too high, the blood vessels wear out too soon and leak or pop, causing a stroke. Taking care of your endothelial lining is like planting a superefficient blood pressure monitor in your circulatory system. Microscopic blood-pressure-monitor cells in the endothelium release substances called vasodilators, which open up (dilate) the arteries to let more blood flow through.

One of these natural blood pressure-monitoring substances is *NO* (known in cardiology research circles as endothelial-derived relaxing factor, or EDRF). Do you remember seeing a grandparent popping nitroglycerin pills to relieve the chest pains of angina? A healthy endothelium does the same thing naturally. Regulating NO is like self-medicating your blood pressure, without unpleasant side effects.

Your endothelium regulates blood clotting. Besides monitoring blood pressure, those internal medicines released by your endothelium also monitor blood clotting. Blood needs to be unsticky enough to flow freely, yet able to become sticky to readily clot when you get a cut. If you're explaining blood vessel health to your children or grandchildren, tell them that healthy blood flow should be like a Slip 'n Slide. The smoother the surface, the faster you slide and the better your blood flows.

Your endothelium is self-healing. Your blood vessel pharmacy secretes a grow-and-repair substance called vascular endothelial growth factor (VEGF). Just as traffic causes wear and tear on the surface of a road, so can the constant beating of the blood against the sensitive endothelial lining cause tiny tears in the vessel walls. When this happens, the "road crew," which is standing by 24/7 to make repairs, rushes into action in what's called an *inflammatory response*. If a pothole develops, the road crew quickly fills it. To keep traffic flowing smoothly, the pothole must be filled precisely — no rough edges and no overfilling.

Throughout this book, you will learn about inflammation. Many of the diseases of aging are due to the body's inflammatory system, or repair crew, going wrong. Excess inflammation is an *overrepair* and is one of the top causes of premature aging. When healthy, the endothelium makes sure potholes are filled correctly. If there are rough edges or an uneven surface, platelets (the blood cells responsible for blood clotting when you cut a finger) get stuck and gradually build up a clot. The tiny balls of fat molecules (called low-density lipoprotein, or LDL, cholesterol) from that marbled sirloin steak you just ate could also get stuck on the rough edges of the pothole. The fat plus the sticky platelets form a bump in the road. This is known as *plaque*, the number one cause of fatal "traffic accidents" in the bloodstream. Plaque can build up gradually over years and slow or stop the blood flow to the organs, or break off and cause a traffic jam (clot), resulting in a heart attack or stroke.

A healthy endothelial maintenance crew sees this bump developing and rushes to remove the plaque and clean up the pothole. Sometimes an overzealous immune system removes the plaque so quickly that it breaks off, travels downstream, and gets lodged in a smaller blood vessel, where it blocks blood flow to an area. (If this happens in the brain, it causes a stroke.) In contrast, a healthy road crew knows how to quickly repair potholes in the endothelium so that the traffic keeps moving and there are no bumps to break off.

Of course, the endothelial lining of the blood vessels, like the surface of roads, eventually wears out and needs to be resurfaced. The endothelial lining also has a group of cells that secrete resurfacing substances called *growth factors,* which replace worn-out lining cells with fresh ones.

So you see, it's vitally important for arterial health and longevity to feed and care for the "road crew" in your endothelium. As you will learn later, two conditions (high blood sugar and high body fat, especially excess abdominal fat) stimulate the endothelium to release factors called plasminogen activator inhibitor 1, or PAI-1 — we'll call it "sticky stuff" — and other substances that promote blood clotting and the buildup of plaque in the arteries. These bad highs (high blood sugar and high belly fat) themselves function as endocrine organs and work like a bunch of highway bandits who injure the maintenance crew and keep it from doing its job. What's the lining of your arteries like? Sticky like Velcro or smooth like Teflon?

PRIME-TIME ED

What's the number one prime-time dysfunction? It's ED! A clue: Women also get it, and it's not erectile dysfunction, as the television ads would have you believe. It's *endothelial* dysfunction. The drugs to treat it are found in your body's own pharmacy. And the good news is, you don't have to ask your doctor if this drug is right for you. It's right for *every* body.

2. Keep the Walls of Your Blood Vessels Healthy

Not only is it vital to have the lining of your arteries stay smooth like Teflon, it's life-saving to keep the muscular walls of your vessels from getting stiff.

Keep the blood vessel walls flexible. The dreaded disease that prime timers worry about is arteriosclerosis, or hardening of the arteries. Arteries become stiff and harden because of two main causes: inflammation and stress. We've already discussed inflammation in the endothelium, the lining of the arteries. The same thing happens in the walls of the arteries: sticky stuff in the blood piles up, then plaque forms and works its way into the arterial walls, making the arteries stiff. The more hardening, the higher the blood pressure and the harder the heart has to work. The higher pressure against the already roughened endothelium damages the arteries even more, making them even stiffer, which requires the heart to work still harder. Eventually the pump gives out — heart failure.

3. Keep Your Blood Less Sticky

The third key to heart health is to keep the blood thin and moving. The thicker the blood, the slower it flows. In fact, arterial aging is often referred to as *thick blood syndrome.* Red blood cells are like thin, flexible, microscopic wafers and are able to change shape and squeeze through the capillaries, the tiniest blood vessels, to deliver oxygen to the tissues. As we age, our blood cells can become more rigid and sticky, so they have difficulty squeezing through tiny blood vessels. Later you will learn how poor nutrition can cause these blood cells to become stiff, which keeps them from changing shape and squeezing through vessels. Poor nutrition can also damage the flexible membranes of these blood cells. Instead of tumbling through the blood vessels like socks in a clothes dryer, they stack up like Pringles potato chips and stick together.

Unstick the sticky cells. Platelets contribute to making the blood thick like sludge rather than thin like water. Normally, these sticky cells flow freely throughout the bloodstream and don't come together unless called on to seal a leak or to form a clot, for instance, to plug a cut. A healthy endothelium squirts out anticlotting substances to keep platelets from sticking together, but a damaged endothelium does not prevent the cells from sticking together, so platelets pile up and contribute to sluggish blood flow.

Sludge forms clots and blocks arteries, leading to heart attack and stroke. Fat particles further contribute to sludge and blood clotting.

This mechanism, dubbed *steakhouse syndrome* (see page 76), can cause people to suffer a stroke or heart attack following a high-fat meal. Doctors prescribe low doses of anticoagulants, such as a baby aspirin a day, to many prime timers to help keep the blood from getting too sticky. You will soon learn how to help your body make its own "aspirin" to keep your blood moving.

4. Keep Your Heart Strong

Like any other muscle, your heart follows the "use it or lose it" principle of health. Athletes have strong arm and leg muscles, and they also have strong heart muscles and wide-open arteries. Movers have stronger heart muscles; sitters have weaker heart muscles.

Stiffness of the arteries overloads the heart and slows blood flow, leading to fatigue, one of the main reasons many older folks can't walk or run as fast or as long as younger people whose arteries are more flexible. This has to do with a property of the heart called *stroke volume output,* which simply means the amount of blood a heart is able to pump with each contraction. When you move fast, demand is put on the heart to pump more blood, and the vessels dilate, or open up, thereby making the heart's work easier. The stiffer the arteries, the lower the stroke volume output. Cardiovascular fitness depends on the heart's ability to increase stroke volume output to meet demand. If the stroke volume output decreases as we age, the heart can't increase blood flow to meet increased demand, so we tire more easily during exercise.

SEVEN WAYS TO KEEP YOUR CARDIOVASCULAR SYSTEM HEALTHY

While on a fishing trip in Alaska, I was standing on a riverbank and made two observations that had a profound impact on my understanding of cardiovascular health. In this pristine environment, the water was clean and clear. But even more striking was the appearance of the stones on the riverbank: they were clean and smooth. This was a stark contrast to the polluted waters of the muddy Mississippi where I grew up. That water is like sludge, and there the rocks are grungy with sediment. I want my circulatory system to be like the rivers in Alaska: clean and flowing, with smooth artery walls. If we dump a bunch of junk into the bloodstream, sludge forms, and the arterial walls get rough. Basically, putting junk in our mouths is like dumping pollutants in a river. We may not feel the effects of arterial pollution right away, but over time it builds up until the artery gets clogged.

If you walked into my office and said, "Doctor, tell me in ten seconds or less what I can do to help my heart," I'd quickly answer:

- Eat a right-fat diet.
- Eat more plants.
- Eat more potassium and less sodium.
- Graze.
- Stay lean.
- Relax.
- Move.

1. Eat a Right-Fat Diet

Science says: Eat a *right*-fat diet, not necessarily a *low*-fat diet. The biggest scientific breakthrough in the prevention of cardiovascular disease is that the *type* of fat in your diet is more significant in maintaining a healthy heart than the *amount* of fat in your diet.

Next time you're on vacation and see an advertisement to swim with dolphins, do it. The skin of dolphins has a smooth, slippery feel. It's exactly what you want the inside of your blood vessels to be like so the blood can easily slide through. Like putting high-quality lubricants on moving parts of your car engine to improve its performance, the better the oils you eat, the smoother your blood flows; it's as simple as that. You will now learn about "young" oils that are heart-healthy and "old" oils that contribute to aging.

My fish story. In June 2006, I had the opportunity to spend a week on a fishing trip in Norway with Dr. Jorn Dyerberg, who is deservedly known

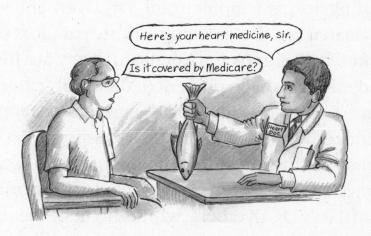

as the "father of omega-3s." As past president of the International Society for the Study of Fatty Acids and Lipids (ISSFAL), Dr. Dyerberg has published more studies on the health benefits of seafood than any other researcher. After hearing about his thirty-plus years of research on omega-3s, I came home jazzed not only to have our family eat more fish but also to share this research with my readers.

In the early 1970s, the correlation between a high-fat diet and a high incidence of heart disease became an increasingly popular theory. The fat-is-bad-for-you fad persisted until the late 1990s, when doctors started realizing that the fats in seafood are actually *good* for the heart.

When the fat-is-bad-for-you campaign was starting to gain momentum, Dr. Dyerberg was fascinated by the seeming health paradox presented by Eskimos in Greenland. They ate high-fat diets (around 60 percent of their daily calories come from fat — double the percentage recommended by the American Heart Association) yet had one of the lowest incidences of heart disease (as well as arthritis and diabetes) in the world.

In 1968 Dr. Dyerberg wrote the first scientific

paper on omega-3s, "The Eskimo Experience." He noticed that coronary artery disease was the cause of death in 40 percent of Americans, 34 percent of Danes, but only 5 percent of Eskimos. In subsequent papers and studies, he found that high omega-3 diets (rich in fish such as salmon) even raised high-density lipoprotein (HDL), the "healthy" cholesterol. He took 130 samples of blood from the Eskimos and compared it with blood from the Danish and found differences in their blood lipid profiles.

Nutrients	Eskimos	Danes
Omega-3s	High	Low
Omega-6s	Low	High
Omega-6:omega-3	0.4:1	3.3:1
Cholesterol in diet (mg/1,000 calories)	245	139

Eskimos ate many more omega-3s than omega-6s (the opposite of the standard American diet). In the typical Western diet, the ratio of omega-6s to omega-3s can be as high as 20:1. Real foods tend to be high in omega-3s. Processed foods tend to be high in omega-6s. Numerous studies have shown that lowering the ratio of omega-6s to omega-3s to between 1:1 and 3:1 translates into valuable health benefits.

Hmm! Eating a lower cholesterol diet than the Eskimos but having a higher rate of heart disease? Something's different in Denmark! That something is too many omega-6s and too few omega-3s. Over thirty years ago, Dr. Dyerberg raised a question that still divides cardiologists today: could the ratio of omega-6s to omega-3s in the diet be even more of a risk factor for heart disease than cholesterol?

Intrigued by findings that the Eskimos ate more fat yet had a healthier fatty-acid profile and enjoyed a lower incidence of heart disease, Dr. Dyerberg wanted to know why. He noticed that Eskimos experienced a lot of nuisance nosebleeds, perhaps a side effect of the high omega-3 diet. That observation became a clue. He then went on to find that the Eskimos' blood clotted (thrombosis) more slowly than the Danes' blood. The omega-3s were antithrombotic, the omega-6s prothrombotic. He concluded that more omega-3s produce less thrombosis and that less thrombosis in the coronary arteries lowers the incidence of heart disease, stroke, and other cardiovascular diseases. By the end of my fishing trip, Dr. Dyerberg's stories prompted me to further investigate why seafood is such a top superfood.

PRIME-TIME PERK: GO FISHING FOR YOUR HEART

Statistics show that people who eat fatty fish, such as wild salmon, at least twice a week can cut their risk of heart attack nearly in *half*. (For more information on the health benefits of seafood and how much to eat, see page 308.)

Go fish! Seafood is our top prime-time food. Fish fats are the healthiest fats. Since the oil in fish is like antifreeze in a car engine, cold-water fish, such as salmon and tuna, have the healthiest

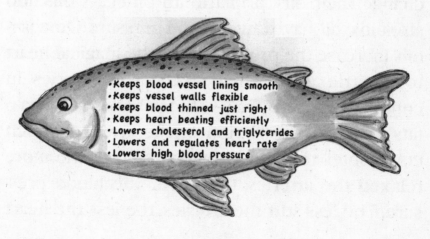

- Keeps blood vessel lining smooth
- Keeps vessel walls flexible
- Keeps blood thinned just right
- Keeps heart beating efficiently
- Lowers cholesterol and triglycerides
- Lowers and regulates heart rate
- Lowers high blood pressure

fats: omega-3s. Now I tell my patients, "To keep the lining of your arteries slippery like a fish, eat fish." The omega-3 oils in seafood act as heart-healthy medicines.

Omega-3s can lower your blood pressure. The systolic reading (the top number of your blood pressure) relates to the pounding of your arteries with every heartbeat. The higher the number, the higher the pounding pressure. The diastolic number, the bottom number, is the artery pressure at rest. People with high blood pressure have both high systolic and diastolic numbers. As a result, their arteries are subjected to constant high-pressure pounding with every heartbeat and don't get sufficient rest between heartbeats. Studies have shown that people who change their oils, primarily to omega-3 oils and also olive oil, have lower blood pressure. Omega-3 oils increase the production of the magical heart tonic nitric oxide, which relaxes your arteries. In contrast, unhealthy oils — those high in omega-6 fats — cause constriction of the arteries, which contributes to higher blood pressure. The more relaxed the arteries, the lower the blood pressure. The less stiff the arteries, the less the heart has to work to pump blood through them. Nitric oxide is the "open-up" molecule. It makes blood vessels dilate for improved blood flow; it opens bronchial airways for better breathing; and, as you will learn in chapter 16, it even increases blood flow to the sex organs during arousal.

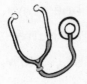

DR. SEARS SAYS…
Eat salad and salmon to your heart's content.

Omega-3s rest the heart. Omega-3s not only lower your resting heart rate, they also blunt the heart-stimulating effects of increased stress hormones. Imagine how much less wear and tear there would be on your heart and blood vessels if you could just lower your heart rate a few beats per minute. This could translate into a million fewer heartbeats a year. Saving a few heartbeats per minute could add more heartbeats to your life.

Omega-3s act like anti-inflammatories and anticoagulants. Omega-3s act the same way that some prescription drugs do but without

SALMON VS. SIRLOIN

When ordering surf and turf, consider asking the waiter to hold the turf and double the surf. My interest in the prevalence of severe heart attacks following high-fat meals began when a close friend suffered a massive heart attack and nearly died after dinner at a famous steakhouse. (Cardiologists call this correlation the *steakhouse syndrome*. Happily, there is no such correlation for seafood.) After you eat a high-fat meal, especially one heavy in saturated fats, such as a marbled steak with a butter-based sauce, your arteries go berserk, as if to say, "How could you do this to us?" The blood goes into a hypersticky state (sludging), and the vessels constrict (narrow), both of which restrict blood flow to vital organs. The triglycerides (fats) in the blood shoot way up, and blood pressure also tends to rise. Also, fibrinogen levels increase. (Fibrinogen is important for normal blood clotting.) All those particles in the bloodstream adhere to the fibrinogen, causing millions of tiny thrombotic molecules—more sticky stuff—to travel throughout the bloodstream and gradually clump together to form blood clots. This can lead to coronary thrombosis (heart attack) or stroke.

Also, high blood fats after a high-fat meal (medically known as *postprandial lipemia,* or PPL) cause the endothelium to release substances that constrict the arteries and cause the blood to get sticky and to become prone to clot.

A big high-fat meal causes big fat damage to the blood vessels. The high circulating fats irritate the lining of the blood vessels, causing them to harden and clog. Omega-3 oils blunt this effect.

After a meal of salmon, less PPL occurs. The omega-3s work by increasing lipoprotein lipase (LPL) activity. LPL is the enzyme that helps clear triglycerides from the bloodstream, thereby reducing the PPL response. Heart-healthy omega-3 oils thin the blood and dilate the arteries, just the opposite of the sirloin meal. In fact, an interesting study showed that taking four grams of omega-3 fish-oil supplements after a high-fat meal reduced the level of PPL. Favor fish. Instead of surf and turf, hold the turf and double the surf. A similar PPL blunting effect has been noticed with olive oil. So, instead of a coronary bypass, simply bypass the meat on the menu and go directly to the seafood and salad section.

Eat More

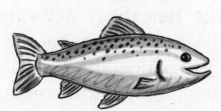

Eat Less

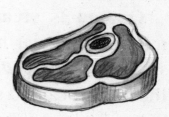

the unpleasant side effects. They prompt the endothelial lining to squirt substances into the bloodstream that decrease wear and tear (anti-inflammatories) and keep the blood thin and moving (anticoagulants). Omega-3 oils lessen clotting and damage to the arterial walls, keeping the surface smooth and the blood flowing.

Omega-3s can lower cholesterol and triglycerides. Eat fat to lower fat? Yes! A diet high in omega-3 fats (from seafood) and monounsaturated fats (such as olive oil) and low in saturated fats has been shown to lower cholesterol levels. Not only do these healthy oils lower the bad cholesterol (LDL), but they can even raise HDL, the good, or protective, cholesterol. While you may hear a lot about cholesterol, the most artery-clogging fats are known as triglycerides, and omega-3 fish oils lower their levels too.

Omega-3s steady the heartbeat. Arrhythmias, or irregular heartbeats, can contribute to *sudden cardiac death,* a sudden stopping of the heart. Seafood steadies the electrical system of the heart, decreasing the likelihood of a misfire. It's a mystery why this happens, yet studies

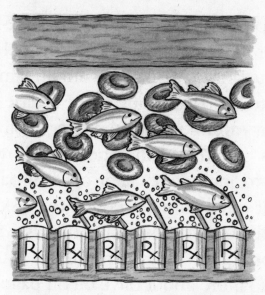

Notice how omega-3s (here represented by fish) ride along on blood cells, keeping them from sticking together and helping the blood flow. Omega-3s release nitric oxide, which prevents the sticky stuff from the meal you just ate from collecting on the walls of your arteries.

show that omega-3s can lower the risk of fatal arrhythmias.

Go olive oil. People who have a lot of olive oil in their diet have less heart disease than people who use a lot of processed vegetable oils, such as corn, cottonseed, sunflower, and safflower. This seems to be because olive oil is rich in monounsaturated fatty acids (MUFAs), which lower LDL cholesterol and exert blood-pressure-lowering and other heart-healthy effects by helping NO work better. Also, MUFAs are anti-inflammatories and help to keep the lining of the arteries smooth. That's why cardiologists often refer to olive oil and fish oil as "liquid aspirin." The FDA allows manufacturers to include a claim on food labels that states that olive oil may reduce the risk of heart disease. Be sure you use olive oil *instead of,* not in addition to, the heart-harmful oils listed in the box. (Read more about olive oil on page 355.)

PRIME-TIME OIL CHANGES FOR HEART MAINTENANCE

"Young" Oils: Heart-Healthy Oils	"Old" Oils: Heart-Harmful Oils
Fish oils	"Partially hydrogenated" oils
Flax oil	Corn oil
Olive oil	Cottonseed oil
Nut oils	Palm kernel oil
	Sunflower oil
	Safflower oil
	Soybean oil

Go nuts. Nuts are also high in heart-healthy monounsaturated fats, which lower LDL cholesterol. Even though they are high in fat, they're unlikely to be translated into a lot of body fat since they have a *high satiety factor,* meaning they fill you up quickly (a palmful of nuts is a perfect portion), so you're less likely to overeat them. (For more about the health benefits of nuts and why we list raw nuts as a superfood, see page 321.)

2. Eat More Plant-Based Foods

Food from plants keeps your arteries soft and smooth; food from animals makes them stiff and sticky. One fact that all doctors and nutritionists agree on is that *plant eaters outlive animal eaters.* Your risk of just about every illness you don't want to get is lower when you eat more salads and less sirloin. Eating more plant-based foods and less meat is especially helpful in lowering high blood pressure, high blood cholesterol, and high blood sugar. Of course, many of us don't want to give up bacon, ribs, pork chops, and beef, so here are my suggestions for helping your heart better tolerate the effects of meat:

Eat plant-based foods along with meat. When we eat a high-fat, junk-food meal, we not only bloat our intestines with indigestion, we also bloat our bloodstream with artery-clogging fats. Remember postprandial lipemia? (You learned about PPL on page 76.) That's sticky stuff in the blood. Delaying PPL is an important part of heart-healthy eating, and it is becoming the subject of much research. Studies show that if we eat a high-fat meal, our blood fats peak between *four and six hours* later and don't start to go down until almost eight hours later.

What's even more heart-threatening is what science says about endothelial dysfunction following a high-fat meal. After a high-fat meal, vascular reactivity (cardiology-speak for the ability of the blood vessels to open up and widen to allow more blood flow) decreases in vital organs, such as the coronary arteries — there's that steakhouse syndrome again. Blood pressure goes up as well. All the studies come to one simple conclusion: Gorging on a high-fat meal is hard on the heart. However, eating plant-based foods before and during a meal with meat keeps some of that stiff and sticky stuff from hardening your arteries and wearing out your heart. Researchers

BETTER SEX? SKIP THE SIRLOIN TONIGHT

Some sexy science: Because of PPL, erectile dysfunction is more common after a high-fat meal. "Not tonight, dear, I've had too much steak."

While you may have heard that the best way to a man's heart is through his stomach, his penis may be more persuasive. For many men, prime time is not when the penis is at its prime. Erectile dysfunction—the inability to get or maintain an erection—is a common nuisance in men over forty and is much more likely to occur if a man has cardiovascular disease. After all, for erections to occur, blood vessels need to be healthy. So, the same seven prime-time habits that maintain a healthy heart can also maintain a healthy erection.

---

have shown that PPL is *lessened* by eating more plant-based foods along with meat.

Eat fruits first. Fruits, especially berries, are full of phytos — antirust nutrients that lower PPL. A bowl of fruit before or while you enjoy bacon and eggs is just what the heart doctor ordered. A study in the February 2008 issue of *American Journal of Clinical Nutrition* showed why blueberries merit being called the "heart berry." Middle-aged men and women with cardiovascular risk factors who ate berries twice a day showed lower blood pressure, higher HDL, and less-sticky platelets, perhaps due to the naturally occurring antioxidants in berries.

Savor salad before the steak. Salads are full of phytos. Studies show that eating foods high in vitamins C, E, and folic acid can mellow out PPL so you don't get such a high spike in artery-clogging blood fats. Because blood pressure can shoot up after a high-fat meal, eat a multivegetable spinach salad as a first course. The fiber in salads slows the absorption of fat, a good reason to put more color on your plate. Enjoying a generous salad also may prompt you to eat less steak. (See "Go Green," page 320.) What you dress your salad with can help lower the level of the sticky stuff in your blood from the steak too. Studies show that olive oil lowers PPL. Of course, if you do choose to eat steak, remove excess fat.

Chase with chocolate. Enjoy a nibble of *dark* chocolate for dessert. This treat is also full of heart-healthy polyphenols (see page 423).

3. Consume More Potassium and Less Sodium

A 2008 study from Harvard Medical School showed that people who ate twice as much potassium as sodium could cut their risk of cardiovascular disease in half. Wow! Yet, the standard American diet is just the opposite: too high in sodium and too low in potassium. A high potassium/low sodium diet works by lowering high blood pressure, a prime cause of the heart wearing out. For an explanation

---

IS A LITTLE WINE GOOD FOR THE HEART?

Wine, in moderation, can be healthy for the heart in these ways:

- The grape skins used to make red wine contain flavonoids and polyphenols, powerful antioxidants that keep blood platelets from getting too sticky and can dilate arteries.
- Alcohol may slightly raise HDL, the good cholesterol.

If you want a nonalcoholic drink, enjoy a glass of pomegranate juice or grape juice, both of which are high in antioxidants. (See "Safe-Alcohol-Drinking Tips," page 671.)

---

of this heart-healthy strategy and a list of high-potassium foods to eat and high-sodium foods to avoid, see chapter 19.

4. Graze

Grazers have healthier hearts than gorgers. The older we get, the more frequently we should eat, and the smaller our meals should be.

Grazers have:

- lower blood cholesterol
- less PPL (high blood levels of artery-clogging fats after eating)
- less after-meal vasoconstriction (less artery narrowing)
- more stable blood sugar and blood insulin levels
- lower levels of stress hormones
- leaner bodies

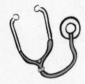

DR. SEARS SAYS...
To become a *lean*ager, don't eat like a teenager.

Big meals can cause big biochemical problems, especially for prime timers. The physiologic principle behind grazing can be summed up in

HEART-HEALTHY EATING TIP

Dr. Bill's rule of twos: Eat *twice* as often, eat *half* as much, and chew *twice* as long.

these three words: *stable insulin levels*. Grazing throughout the day on frequent minimeals rather than binging on three big meals keeps the body and the brain in biochemical balance, or hormonal harmony.

Grazing lowers the risk of after-meal heart attacks because the heart doesn't have to pump harder and faster like it does after we gorge on a big meal. Also, there's no sudden spike in after-meal blood fats, which cause arteries to go into spasm, slowing the blood flow. So, shoot for six small meals rather than three squares. And take more time to dine. If you do indulge in a high-fat meal, be sure to eat salad and vegetables and eat more slowly; doing so allows more time for those salad phytos to get to work and lower PPL.

5. Stay Lean

Leanness promotes longevity. The fatter you are, the more you overload your heart. You may think that extra fat around the middle is just globs of extra tissue sitting there doing nothing but slowing you down. But those extra fat cells are chemical factories pumping out proinflammatory substances. All these inflammatory fighters increase the wear and tear on the lining of the blood vessels, giving you Velcro rather than Teflon arterial linings. Shedding extra fat sheds years of potential disability.

6. Relax

Don't stress out your heart. The cardiovascular system and the nervous system are intimately connected. A large network of nerves encircles your arteries, helping them to relax and open up when more blood is needed in certain areas of the body. The brain and the heart are energy-delivering teammates. If the brain is upset, so is the heart. Optimists and people who are generally more relaxed and handle stress better have a lower incidence of cardiovascular disease. Stress is tough on your ticker. Chronic stress causes the brain to pour out stress hormones that stimulate the nerves around the vessels to constrict, resulting in high blood pressure and eventually causing the heart to wear out. When the stock market crashed in 2008, so did the cardiovascular health of many. My friend David died of a heart attack after spending hours each day watching — and worrying about — the declining value of his stocks.

7. Move

Why are diet and exercise the dynamic duo for preventing cardiovascular disease? Simply put, a healthy diet keeps the sticky stuff off the lining of the arteries so it doesn't build up and keep the internal medicine bottles from opening; exercise opens these medicine bottles (see illustration on page 57). Here are some great reasons why movement is your best heart medicine:

Movement helps blood vessels muster up their own internal medicine. Movement (such as walking, dancing, or swimming) gets the blood flowing faster over the lids of the medicine bottles in your arteries and releases your internal medicines. The NO mechanism you learned about earlier in the chapter is one of the most powerful total-body benefits of exercise. Think of exercise as a promoter of the pharmaceutical response of your arteries; it's like walking into your pharmacy and picking up a bunch of free cardiovascular medicines that help your heart but have absolutely no harmful side effects. Even if the endothelium is damaged, exercise helps access whatever internal medicine it has and gradually restores much of the endothelium to better health. Exercise and diet are the best preventive medicines for endothelial dysfunction.

Movement prevents clogging of vessels. Three main components contribute to the clogging and hardening of arteries: the buildup of fatty deposits (cholesterol, triglycerides, and other blood fats), the waste products left behind when the immune system tries to attack these fatty buildups (inflammation), and the excessive stickiness of the blood cells forming clots. The increased blood flow prompted by exercise opens the endothelial pharmacy, which in turn releases three internal medicines that reduce fatty buildup, control an overzealous inflammatory response, and lessen the stickiness of blood cells.

Movement reopens clogged vessels. Besides building new vessels, movement reopens old vessels that are partially clogged with fatty deposits, a process called *vascular remodeling*. Prolonged exercise can widen blood vessels, increase their elasticity, and, when combined with an overall heart-health program, can partially dissolve plaque buildup, sort of like a plumber cleaning out a pipe. Remember our highway analogy? Well, unlike road surfaces, blood vessels enjoy a physiologic quirk in which increased traffic actually makes them smoother, wider, and less congested. Even if the endothelium is damaged, exercise helps restore it and improves its function. This is one reason why people who suffer a heart attack and then make movement their medicine live longer and healthier.

Movement makes your internal medicine stronger. Not only does movement train muscles, it also trains blood vessels. Habitual movement keeps blood vessels relaxed longer. This *exercise-induced reactivity* of blood vessels means that once blood vessels get used to lots of exercise and lots of fast blood flow, they become more reactive and open up wider in response to exercise. Cardiovascular researchers call this *upregulation,* which simply means that when the vessel wall gets used to the increased blood

TOXIC WAIST

Suppose you went for a checkup but your doctor had time to take only *one measurement* to most accurately assess your overall health. The doctor would measure your waist size. This could be your most important vital sign. Recent research shows that waist size is one of the most controllable risk factors of heart attack. One of the quirks of prime time is that we tend to accumulate more *abdominal adipocytes* (fat-storage cells) around the middle. Before age forty, testosterone in men and estrogen in women distribute body fat more evenly and keep it from collecting around the middle. Between the ages of forty and fifty, these hormones usually decline, causing buildup of belly fat. During menopause, women have higher circulating levels of insulin and therefore tend to store extra body fat. Here's a scary statistic: men whose waists measure more than forty inches are twelve times more likely to develop diabetes.

Excess abdominal fat is just the tip of the iceberg. The more fat that shows around the waistline, the more likely it is that excess fat is being stored inside the abdomen. *Visceral fat,* or "middle fat," behaves like a different animal chemically. It is a metabolically hyperactive fat, which means it releases health-harming chemicals into the bloodstream that cause premature aging and increase your risk of:

Increased highs. An increase in abdominal fat can cause an increase in blood levels of cholesterol, blood sugar, and triglycerides, and can elevate blood pressure. This excess fat tissue releases chemicals that foul up the way the liver processes cholesterol and insulin. It also releases chemicals that can make cells more resistant to the effects of insulin, leading to type 2 diabetes. The shape of your waist often mirrors the quality of your health.

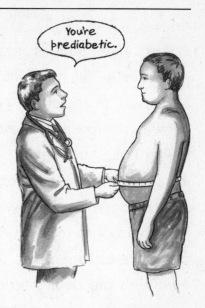

You're prediabetic.

Increased lows. Excess abdominal fat can interfere with neurochemicals, resulting in depression.

Weak heart. These metabolically active fat cells can release chemicals that cause blood clots to form in the capillaries, reducing the amount of blood that can flow to vital organs, such as the brain and coronary arteries. They can also block the release of NO, the body's natural vasodilator that relaxes the pressure inside the arteries. Lower NO levels in the bloodstream lead to high blood pressure. A 2005 study in the medical journal *Lancet* concluded that the higher the waist-to-hip ratio, the greater the risk of heart attack. New research has also shown that cardiovascular disease begins in childhood. Ultrasound studies on the arteries of obese children revealed early stages of endothelial dysfunction from the accumulation of sticky stuff on the artery walls.

(continued)

Less male. Studies reveal that men who carry around excess belly fat tend to have lower testosterone levels. Lower testosterone can trigger other agers, such as decreased muscle, cholesterol reversals (lower HDL and higher LDL), and higher triglycerides. Excess belly fat also increases female hormones like estrogen: an enzyme called aromatase that lives in the excess fat cells converts male hormones to female hormones. That's right—more fat, more estrogen, *less* testosterone. That explains why men with big bellies tend to have bigger breasts. Men, here's a motivator: a recent poll by *Men's Health* magazine revealed that the number one body change that women would like to see in their men is a flatter belly.

---

flow from lots of movement, it relaxes more easily with less movement. An increase in vascular reactivity is one way people with coronary artery disease who exercise regularly show improvement.

Movement lowers blood cholesterol. Movement is the only cholesterol-lowering medication that has no side effects. As you will learn in chapter 19, healthy cholesterol (HDL) acts as a sort of ferryboat garbage collector, shuttling

Cancer. These toxic fat cells can manufacture chemicals that increase the risk of getting all cancers, especially breast and colorectal cancers (see page 533).

Increased risk of "-itis." Toxic waist cells spew cytokines, proinflammatory chemicals, into the bloodstream, resulting in premature aging.

Strive for nice numbers. Women, keep your waist measurement under thirty-five inches; men, under forty inches.

Middle fat is a good news/bad news scenario. The good news is that while it's easiest to put on fat around the middle by eating too much or moving too little during prime time, middle fat is also the *first to go* when you follow the Prime-Time Health plan.

---

excess blood cholesterol back to the liver before it has a chance to be deposited in the arteries or damage the endothelium. LDL cholesterol, the so-called bad (or less healthy) cholesterol, is the sticky stuff that works its way into and through the lining of the arteries, and is a main contributor to arteriosclerosis, or hardening of the arteries. (I dislike the term *bad cholesterol.* Our bodies need some LDL. It's the *excess* that makes LDL cholesterol bad.) This buildup of plaque damages the endothelium and, in effect, shuts down the production of the body's natural heart medicine.

Ideally, you want to reduce excess LDL and increase HDL. Movement does both! Exercise causes increased blood flow, which prompts the endothelium to release substances that lower the LDL cholesterol and triglyceride fats in the blood vessels and raise the HDL. Movement has little or no effect on the LDL in some people, but by raising the HDL exercise improves the total cholesterol/HDL ratio, which is a favorable index for cardiovascular risk.

Movement makes more blood vessels. One of the most important heart-healthy effects of exercise is that it increases the vascularization of the heart muscle. The more blood vessels supplying a muscle, the more efficiently it performs. The richer the blood flow to an organ, the healthier it is and the longer it lives. Movement also enables diseased and blocked arteries to get a second chance. As you learned earlier, exercise "opens" the blood vessel pharmacy to release endothelial-derived growth factor, EDGF, a substance that promotes the repair and growth of vessels. Given the right conditions, the body

SCIENCE SAYS: MOVE MORE AND OPEN YOUR ARTERIES

People with more-active lifestyles have larger coronary arteries.

heals itself. If a river is dammed up (main artery blocked), tiny tributaries form to carry the water to the soil. If the main artery to an organ, such as the heart, is compromised, movement helps stimulate the growth of extra blood vessels (collateral circulation). Did you ever try to turn off a congested freeway during rush hour to find a quicker alternative route? That's exactly what exercise does for organs whose blood flow is already partially blocked.

Move more and perk up your fitness genes. Dazzling studies have shown that exercise increases blood flow across the endothelial surface and actually perks up the genes in these cells to release more NO. As the blood vessels pour out more internal medicine in just the right amounts, the vessels become more reactive (open up more) to vasodilating substances and less reactive to vasoconstricting substances, including stress hormones — they are trained to be fit.

Move more and relax your arteries. When those little heart doctors within the endothelial wall hand out extra NO, it reduces the effect of stress hormones, like norepinephrine, on the blood vessel walls. Keeping your arteries relaxed is one of the keys to good health, and that's one way exercise improves cardiovascular health.

Rx FOR PRIME-TIME HEART HEALTH

- ❑ Eat more seafood and omega-3 oils.
- ❑ Eat less animal-based food.
- ❑ Eat more flax, nut, and olive oils.
- ❑ Eat less processed oil.
- ❑ Eat more plant-based food.
- ❑ Eat more potassium and less sodium.
- ❑ Graze instead of gorging.
- ❑ Stay lean.
- ❑ Keep calm.
- ❑ Move more.

CHAPTER 4

Stay Smart and Protect Your Brain

There is merit to the pearl "the wisdom of aging." While the speed at which we think may slow as we age, the *way* we think can actually improve. Our kids may be better at learning new math than we are, and I do have to ask mine to help me decipher the instructions when I'm programming my iPod. Yet we are *wiser* than they are, through precious years of trial and error, countless decisions made, and decades of brain-enriching relationships. Besides, as we get older we have a much larger cerebral library of experiences to replay and to learn from.

And the good news about keeping our brains healthy is that each of the brain-aging insults many prime timers face can be delayed, some even reversed, with this Prime-Time Health program.

DON'T BE A STATISTIC

How much do you know about your brain? Did you know that:

- the average brain loses about 50 percent of its 15 billion brain cells between the ages of twenty and ninety-five?
- the brain, like muscle, shrinks as we age?
- mental ability declines by an average of 20 percent between age forty and seventy?
- almost 360,000 new cases of Alzheimer's disease are reported each year in the United States?

The key word here is *average*. You don't have to be average. Your brain, like muscle, thrives on the "use it or lose it" principle — or, more precisely, "Use it regularly, or lose it to disease."

Another reason not to fret about these statistics is that new research shows that even older folks can *grow* new brain cells. Once upon a time, it was believed that we were born with a finite number of brain cells and that when those deteriorated we couldn't replace or repair them. But we now know that through a marvelous gift called *neuroplasticity,* the brain can suffer stroke, trauma, or plain-old wear and tear, and still regenerate new and vital cells. While brain plasticity is strongest in our younger years, it continues to some degree throughout our lives.

The brain also has ample reserve in its 15 billion cells. Neurologists believe that there is enough spare brain tissue to keep us smart even if we lose some of our brain cells every so often. One reason to start practicing the Prime-Time Health program now is to keep your reserve cells healthy so they'll be ready when you need them.

EIGHT WAYS YOUR BRAIN CAN LOSE ITS PRIME

Here's what happens if you *don't* take care of your brain:

1. Brains shrink. Beginning at around age fifty, the brain can shrink from an average weight of 3.0 pounds to 2.6 pounds fifteen years later. This loss of brain volume is not due to the death of neurons but rather to the shrinkage of individual neurons from loss of connections, especially in the hippocampus and the prefrontal cortex, the areas of the brain involved in memory. Later in this chapter, you will learn how to use and feed your neurons to minimize shrinkage.

2. Brain traffic slows. The brain is composed of trillions of electrical circuits. Thought processes occur through rapid transmissions from one circuit to another. Like the electrical wires in your home, these structures are heavily insulated to keep the current flowing and to prevent it from getting mixed up with other circuits. As we age, two things happen: Myelin, the insulation coating the nerves, wears away or frays, which can cause a short circuit. In addition, the receptors, the receiving antennae between nerves, begin to decline.

To complete a thought or to activate a muscle, one nerve transmits a signal to the next nerve. These impulses travel from nerve to nerve across a gap, or synapse. Chemical messengers called neurotransmitters ferry the messages. But during prime time, the neurotransmitter system begins to slow down. We also produce fewer mood-regulating neurohormones (serotonin and dopamine).

3. Brains rust. Throughout this book, I talk a lot about *oxidation,* a fancy word for rust. Aging is rusting. Think of rust as tissue wear and tear. Rust is also a natural by-product of cellular metabolism. Healthy aging means developing an antirust program.

Two unique features of brain function and structure make it a prime target for oxidation and rust: the fuel it burns and the tissue it contains. Like the combustion and oxidation caused by the mixture of gasoline and air in the carburetor of your car engine, cellular energy generates oxidation or rust. The brain uses proportionately more fuel than any other organ in the body. It burns 25 percent or more of all the carbohydrates we eat and it consumes 20 percent of the oxygen we breathe. Yet, the brain makes up only about 2 percent of our total body weight. Extra fuel burning in the brain produces more oxidation, which produces more rust.

Another reason the brain is such a target for oxidative wear and tear (also known as *oxidative stress*) is that almost 60 percent of the brain is fatty tissue. Just as some metals oxidize more easily than others, so fatty tissue is more vulnerable to the wear and tear of oxidative stress than tissues with high protein content such as muscle.

4. Brains get iBods. The brain is vulnerable to rust but also inflammation. Like a self-cleaning engine, the body constantly tries to repair itself from rust by producing millions of inflammatories, microscopic scavengers that circulate throughout the body and brain; we dub them "iBods." Yet in the process, this immune-boosting army can produce too many iBods and leave behind a lot of waste products that can interfere with nerve function, leading to dementia and even Alzheimer's disease, which is basically brain rust. And the body's production of natural antioxidants — antirust medicines — slows down with aging unless it's reinforced. Because excess iBods prefer to attack fatty tissue, and the brain is mostly fat, the brain is the organ most vulnerable to excessive inflammation. The good news — as you will learn in chapter 18 — is that you can control your iBods.

5. Brains have a repair challenge. As we age, brain tissue becomes less able to repair itself. Production of nerve growth factor (NGF), a neurochemical that helps rebuild worn-out brain cells, declines with age. Our Prime-Time Health plan will help replenish this internal brain-repair medicine.

6. Brain cells become more rigid. My children sometimes jokingly, and sometimes seriously, accuse me of becoming more rigid in my thinking. Perhaps there's a biochemical reason for this. The basis of cellular health, especially in brain cells, is their fluidity. A fluid cell membrane enables the cell to be in constant motion and to adjust its shape to satisfy changing needs. The cell membrane protects a cell's energy mechanisms by allowing healthful nutrients to enter it and by blocking harmful ones. With aging, the cell membrane loses some of its fluidity. This allows a bit of the bad stuff to leak in, which creates more wear and tear at the cellular level.

7. Brains become stressed out. As we age, the cerebral mechanisms that protect brain cells from the effects of stress get weaker. The aging brain simply cannot cope with the biochemical challenges of stress as well as it once did. Perhaps this is one reason optimists live longer, are happier, and show less mental decline than pessimists do.

The body needs a certain level of circulating stress hormones to function optimally — not too little, not too much, just the right amount. Normally, corticotropin-releasing factor (CRF), the brain's stress-hormone sensor, monitors the level of stress hormones circulating throughout the body and brain. When stress hormones get too high, secretion of CRF lessens, in effect telling the adrenal glands to "cool it" and cut back on the stress hormones they secrete. With aging, this protective mechanism becomes less efficient. Also, chronically high levels of stress hormones cause blood cells to stick together, damage the lining of blood vessels, and eventually clog the arteries, leading to stroke.

8. The blood-brain barrier leaks. Because the brain is more susceptible to wear and tear than any other organ, it is protected by a thin layer of cells strategically positioned between the tiny blood vessels and the brain tissue. Called the blood-brain barrier (BBB), this protective wrap screens out *neurotoxins,* chemicals in the bloodstream that may harm brain tissue. But the BBB often weakens with age. In fact, unhealthy aging is often called the leaky-cell syndrome.

So, as you age, the brain gets smaller, slower, and it rusts. But, as you'll soon learn, you *can* protect yourself from the negative effects of aging on the brain — and even turn back the clock. These factors all influence brain health:

- the blood that flows through your brain
- the food you feed your brain
- the thoughts that fill your brain
- how you "exercise" your brain

SIX WAYS TO KEEP YOUR BRAIN HEALTHY

In the previous chapter you learned how to keep your blood vessels open to prevent strokes. Now you will learn six scientifically proven ways to keep your brain healthy.

1. Eat Smart Foods

The brain is the organ most affected by what we eat. It burns about 25 percent of the food energy (mostly carbs) we consume. So, it needs a *right* carb diet. Because the brain is 60 percent fat, it also needs a *right* fat diet. The word *fathead* can be a compliment.

Eat fish and stay smarter. Oceans of research show that omega-3 fats benefit brain health. And since the brain requires more omega-3s than any other organ, it stands to reason that the brain is most affected by an omega-3 deficiency. Not only is seafood the top heart food, it's the top brain food. Here's why it merits the label "smart fat":

Omega-3s help regrow aging brain cells. One reason for the shrinkage of prime-time gray matter is the decline in production of the nutritional building blocks of the brain, mainly the omega-3 fats but also the enzymes the brain uses to metabolize these fats. As a result, the brain is less able to repair itself and grow new tissue. But an old brain is capable of generating new cells, especially if you feed it the right rebuilding food — omega-3s. Omega-3s facilitate the action of *neuroprotectin,* the brain's "youth hormone." Omega-3 DHA fats are the main structural components of the brain cell membrane. (Docosahexaenoic acid [DHA] is the top brain fat.)

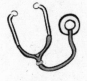

DR. SEARS SAYS...
Omega-3s are to the brain what calcium is to bone.

Omega-3s prevent "stiff" brain cells. The cell membrane is like a bag, and the more flexible the bag is, the healthier the membrane. Omega-3s are "fluid fats" and keep the brain cell membranes supple. A prime function of a healthy brain cell membrane is *chemical selectivity:* it lets in nutrients the cell needs and keeps out harmful toxins.

Omega-3s help you think and act faster. Omega-3s make myelin, the fatty sheath that surrounds nerve cells and helps speed the transmission of nerve impulses throughout the brain. The more omega-3 DHA you have in your myelin, the faster and more efficiently these nerve messages travel, which improves cognitive function. As insulation on electrical wires makes the current travel faster, so does omega-3-enriched

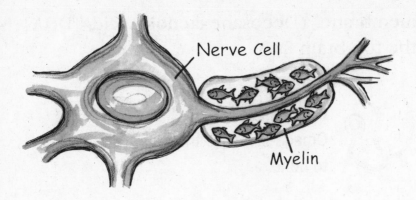

myelin help you think faster. Multiple sclero-
sis is a debilitating disease in which the myelin
insulation on the nerve fibers becomes frayed.
Omega-3s help prevent frayed fibers.

Omega-3s are the fat with the perfect fit.
Nerve cells communicate via neurotransmitters, neurochemical messengers that weaken as
we age. Omega-3 oils provide the food for these
neurotransmitters to function more efficiently.
Neurotransmitters are like sparks flying across
the gap between the nerve cells. On the cell
membrane are microscopic "locks" into which
these neurotransmitter "keys" must fit for communication to be successful. If the cell membrane is
composed of the right fats, the locks and keys
match. Because the DHA molecule is so flexible,

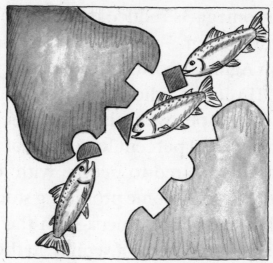

Help your neurotransmitters fit. Go fish!

it can mold itself to fit the incoming key. And DHA can actually promote neurotransmitter function. Yet, if the locks in the cell membrane are clogged with fake fats, such as factory-made hydrogenated oils, the keys won't fit and nerve communication slows. Basically, omega-3s act as the brain's communications director.

Eat fish and reduce your risk of Alzheimer's disease. A diet rich in omega-3 oils is now part of the standard treatment plan for people with Alzheimer's. Neurologists call omega-3s neuroprotective. Even though some studies failed to show that omega-3s reduce dementia, others do show a correlation. A study from Tufts University Center on Aging reported that people with the highest DHA levels, who ate an average of three servings of fish per week, had a reduced risk of dementia and a 39 percent lower risk of Alzheimer's disease compared to people with low DHA levels in their blood. Some promising studies have shown that increasing omega-3s in the diet can even reverse some signs of senility. In the famous Framingham Heart Study, people with the highest blood levels of omega-3 DHA had the lowest levels of dementia. And the risk of Alzheimer's disease increased the more trans fats the people ate. It's the good fat/bad fat story again.

Eat fish and lower your risk of stroke. Studies show that we can lower our risk of stroke by 50 percent by eating at least two servings of salmon per week. In addition, a recent study in the journal *Circulation* revealed that diet *and* lifestyle changes can cut the risk of stroke by 80 percent.

Eat fish and be happy. Omega-3s are not only "smart fats"; they're "happy fats." Research shows that people who eat the highest amount of seafood have the lowest rates of depression. Neuroscientists correlate getting sad with the standard American diet, which contains too much omega-6 (in processed oils) and too little omega-3. Omega-3s seem to act like serotonin-boosting drugs, producing mood-stabilizing and antidepressant effects but without the unpleasant side effects.

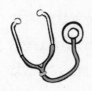

DR. SEARS SAYS...
The prime message for brain health is the same as it is for heart health: *change your oils.*

Have a berry good brain. Blueberries are one of the best examples of the color principle of nutrition: the deeper the color of the food, the better it is for you. The deep blue skin of the blueberry is full of flavonoids, especially antho-cyanin, an antioxidant that keeps brain tissue from rusting. Neuroscientists believe that deep-colored foods, like blueberries and blackberries, contain high levels of antioxidants that keep the blood-brain barrier healthy. What's special about the neuroprotective antioxidants in blueberries is that they cross the BBB and get into the brain tissue. Blueberries also have been shown to *improve memory,* as well as reverse some of the degenerative changes often seen with aging nerve tissue.

Blueberries reduce age-related cognitive decline. While I feel somewhat deflated when my brain is equated with a rat's, there is enough similarity at the cellular level to allow researchers to draw conclusions from rat studies that fit our smarter brains. One famous study compared a group of rats that were fed blueberries with a control group. The blueberry rats showed improved balance and motor coordination. The old rats also acted more youthful, showing a reversal of the effects of mental aging.

Researchers believe that blueberries can reverse age-related decline in nerve-signal transmission, probably by slowing the loss of nerve-growth factors and protecting against the loss of the dopamine receptor cells that normally decrease with aging. Animal studies showed that blueberries increase the concentration of the neurotransmitter dopamine in the brain. Brain researchers generally concluded that the nutrients in blueberries helped facilitate the transmission of messages from one nerve cell to another.

Blueberries also protect nerve tissue from the wear and tear of inflammation. Neuroscientists have shown that there is a difference between how young and old brains react to inflammation. Younger brains are able to generate protective proteins that guard against the damaging effects of oxidation from free radicals (aka rust) and other toxins; older brains do not enjoy as much of this cellular protection. When older experimental animals were supplemented with blueberries, the seniors enjoyed as much inflammation protection from blueberries as the younger animals did.

Blueberries improve brain blood flow. Each organ is only as healthy as the blood flow to it. This principle is especially important for the brain. Blueberries improve blood flow by improving endothelial function, which you learned about in chapter 3. The healthier the endothelium, the better the blood flow — and, like omega-3s, this is where blueberries work their magic.

Blueberries improve blood flow by decreasing excessive blood clotting, reducing inflammation, inhibiting the oxidation of LDL cholesterol (that plaque-building sticky stuff), and helping maintain nitric oxide's vessel-widening effects on blood vessel function. You learned in chapter 3 that NO is like a health tonic that keeps the lining of the blood vessels smooth and the vessels wide open. Experimental animals that suffered stroke and were fed a diet rich in blueberries recovered the blood flow to the area of the stroke much faster and showed less brain damage than animals that received a standard diet.

Go green. Many of the brain-health benefits of blueberries are found in greens, such as bok choy, spinach, collard greens, and asparagus. This is likely because these greens are rich in folate, or folic acid, a vital nutrient for preserving neurotransmitter function. While the best sources of folic acid are green leafy vegetables, other rich sources are lentils, kidney beans, avocados, chickpeas, artichokes, and cereals fortified with folic acid. (For information about the health benefits of spinach, see chapter 16.)

Eat smart carbs often. The brain is called a "carbo hog," meaning that it needs a lot of the right carbohydrates to function. Two brain quirks make it particularly sensitive to getting enough of the right carbs:

- Unlike the muscles, the brain does *not* store glucose. So it needs a steady supply of glucose for steady brain function.
- Unlike other organs that can use fats and even protein for energy in an emergency, the brain is a picky eater. It can only use glucose as its primary fuel.

The brain needs a *right-carb,* not a low-carb, diet.

Here's carb chemistry made simple. The right, or smart, carbs have two or three partners: protein, fiber, and fat. They never travel alone. They hold hands with the carb to keep it from rushing into the brain too fast and getting the brain too excited. (That's why smart carbs are called *slow-release* carbs.) Wrong carbs, or "dumb carbs," have no partners. They travel alone. When you eat dumb carbs, there are no friends to hold the sugar back, so it rushes into the blood and brain and excites the brain too much. Because dumb carbs are *fast-release* carbs, they get used up too fast, leaving the brain hungry and foggy. *The brain likes slow food, not fast food.*

"Smart carbs" are found in nature — in fruits, vegetables, and whole grains. "Dumb carbs" are usually found in packaged foods. For smart brain function, always partner carbs with protein, fiber, or fat. Never eat or drink them alone. Sweetened beverages are the dumbest carbs. Remember, dumb carbs form AGEs, the sticky stuff that clogs brain traffic, which you learned about on page 34. (See the list of lean carbs on page 597.)

In recent years research has shown a correlation between uncontrolled high blood sugar and the risk of developing Alzheimer's disease. In fact, Alzheimer's specialists equate the effects of uncontrolled blood sugar on the brain to smoking on the lungs. Some neurologists have even suggested calling Alzheimer's type 3 diabetes.

Grazing is good for the brain. That's because the two buzzwords for feeding the brain are *slow* and *steady*.

When the brain runs out of fuel, or carbs, it goes into red alert and sends a message to the body: "I need sugar, any type!" And that type is usually the fast-release carbs we tend to grab and impulsively overeat. That's why it's important not to let yourself get so hungry that your blood sugar plummets.

The sugar-craving brain triggers the release of stress hormones that tell the body to quickly release some stored sugar from the liver. Yet, these same hormones stress the brain, which accounts for the uncomfortable mood swings that accompany big shifts in blood and brain sugar levels.

Because the brain can't store glucose, it relies on a steady supply of it from the bloodstream: not too high, not too low. Steady blood sugar results in steady neurotransmitter function and delivery of nutrients that our brains need for repair. Nibbling on nutritious mini-meals throughout the day is more brain friendly than eating fewer big meals. I tell my patients: "Shorten the space between feedings, and you're less likely to feel spacey." (For more grazing guidelines, see pages 86 and 144.)

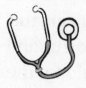

DR. SEARS SAYS...
Keep your blood sugar stable to keep your brain sugar stable.

Go nuts. Nuts are a brain-friendly snack. Walnuts are the top brain nut because they're the richest in omega-3s. (See page 321 for more on the benefits of nuts.)

HOW ALCOHOL BOTHERS THE BRAIN

Because alcohol easily dissolves in fatty tissue, and the brain is mostly fat, it can reach high concentrations in brain tissue. Researchers believe that the power of alcohol to intoxicate is related to its properties as a solvent: it can dissolve the fatty walls of the brain-cell membrane. Of particular concern is research from the National Institutes of Health showing that alcohol decreases the concentration of DHA in brain-cell membranes. The loss of this main structural fat in the brain may be the basic reason why alcoholics suffer various degrees of dementia and is one reason why DHA supplements are prescribed as part of the treatment plan for alcoholics. (See page 671.)

---

2. Exclude Additives

Chemical food additives, or neurotoxins, are bad for prime timers. There's a lot of chemical stuff added to food to make it more tasty, colorful, and to preserve it. Preservatives may prolong the shelf life of packaged foods, but they shorten the cerebral life of your brain. Flavor enhancers may heighten the taste of food (so you eat more), but they rot the tissue of the brain. Food colorings may make food look prettier, but why color the brain? What's more important, preserving your food or preserving your health?

Four reasons to avoid artificial additives. Remember my weak-garbage-disposal-system theory of aging? Chemical food additives are garbage; it's as simple as that. Here's why they're especially dumb for prime-time brains:

Neurotoxins seek out brain tissue. Many chemical food additives are stored mainly in fatty tissue. Since brain tissue is composed mostly of fat, it's likely that this is where most of the molecular mischief occurs.

Neurotoxins create a biochemical imbalance. Chemical additives can damage the brain cell's mitochondria, the tiny packets of energy inside the cell that act like batteries to give the cell energy. They can also throw neurotransmitter activity out of balance. Neurologists believe that these neurotoxins contribute to Parkinson's disease and Alzheimer's disease. Many of the mood disorders affecting prime timers are thought to be chemical imbalances in the brain. So it stands to reason that if you put more artificial chemicals in your brain, you increase your chances of having a chemical imbalance. This is not rocket science.

Food additives have not been proven safe for prime timers. Aren't additives FDA tested and approved? It seems that many chemicals previously approved by the FDA that are added to our food supply and medicines are now believed to be unsafe. And what is considered safe for younger adults may not be so for prime timers.

Neuroscientists are concerned about the cumulative effects of eating too many artificial chemicals. According to neurosurgeon Dr. Russell Blaylock, author of *Excitotoxins: The Taste That Kills*, certain food additives, especially MSG and aspartame (NutraSweet, Equal), can cross the blood-brain barrier and cause a brain-aging effect called *premature pruning.* Normally, the brain grows like a garden and prunes nerve connections that aren't needed to allow for growth of the connections that are needed. Eating too many additives could lead to excessive pruning and a miswired brain.

According to Dr. Blaylock, MSG also increases the absorption of aluminum from foods. Excess aluminum entering the body, especially the brain, has been a subject of recent concern among doctors. In *The Vaccine Book,* our son, Dr. Robert Sears, cites a lot of scientific evidence that suggests that high doses of aluminum (as found in too many vaccines given all at once) could be toxic to the brain.

A DIETARY CAUTION

Could it be that the dramatic increases in autism in the young and Alzheimer's in the old have a common cause? I believe both could result from too much garbage entering the body at a vulnerable stage in life—in the young when the garbage-disposal system is still maturing, and in adults when the garbage-disposal system is weakening. Neurotoxins are easily dissolved in fatty tissue, and the brain is one of the fattiest tissues in the body. Avoid foods with additives. Eat real, pure foods.

"But they don't seem to bother me," you may say. As many of us consume these neurotoxins several times a day for years and years, each day we may lose some brain cells, and some nerve cells may get miswired. Eventually, these neuro-toxic effects add up. The science of common sense says, *When in doubt, leave them out.*

One day while playing golf, neurologist Dr. Vince Fortanasce, author of *The Anti-Alzheimer's Prescription,* and I were discussing the cumula-tive effect of junk food and chemical additives on the brains of growing children. Dr. Vince concluded: "Alzheimer's begins in childhood."

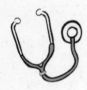

DR. SEARS SAYS...
To be a *keen*ager, don't eat like a teenager.

Prime timers may have a leaky blood-brain barrier. The protective blood-brain barrier may weaken during prime time. How much it weakens is not completely understood, but there seems to be a dose-related effect. Eat high enough doses of chemical additives, and some of them may leak through.

Artificial sweeteners with chemical additives should be in the "when in doubt, leave them out" category. I have thoroughly researched the two most popular sweeteners — aspartame and sucralose (Splenda) — and have concluded that the science attesting to their safety is just not convincing, especially for aspartame.

NDD, nutrition deficit disorder, is a term that I coined to describe the neurotoxic effects of junk food, especially chemical additives, on the developing brains of children. While it's possible that a developing brain may be more vulnerable to the toxic effects of junk food and chemical additives than the prime-time brain, I'm not so sure. And the longer I'm in medical practice, the more I realize that the dietary precaution to just eat real food applies equally to juniors and seniors. For an indepth discussion of why artificial sweeteners and other chemical additives bother the brain, and for healthy alternatives, see AskDrSears.com/NDD.

3. Move

There's that magic word again. Physical exercise is good for our brains as well as for our overall health. Regular exercise can decrease the risk of dementia by 50 percent. The term *active mind-set* has some scientific basis. A 2006 study in the *Journal of Gerontology* showed that at least three hours a week of vigorous walking could

THE DIRTIEST DOZEN

These are the chemical additives that my family avoids and
that science is most skeptical about:

- partially hydrogenated oils
- aspartame (NutraSweet, Equal)
- MSG (monosodium glutamate) and its
  deceiving alias "yeast extract"
- hydrolyzed vegetable protein
- BHA (butylated hydroxyanisole)
- sodium nitrate and sodium nitrite
- propyl gallate
- acesulfame potassium
- sodium benzoate
- potassium bromate
- artificial colors: blue #1, blue #2, green #3,
  red #3, yellow #6, red #40 (i.e., any color with
  a number on it)
- BHT (butylated hydroxytoluene)

help prevent deterioration of memory in people
in their forties. Here are some ways that exercise
makes brains smarter:

Move more and grow brain cells. Researchers have found that the brain loses an average of

15 to 25 percent of its tissue between ages thirty and ninety. Most of the loss is in the areas associated with memory and learning. The good news is that studies also show that the more cardiovascularly fit prime timers are, the less reduction in brain volume they have. Prime-time movers actually have larger brain volumes than sitters. Fitness slows age-related cognitive decline.

LESS BELLY FAT, LESS ALZHEIMER'S

The risk of Alzheimer's goes up in proportion to a person's increase in belly fat. In a recent European study, women whose waists measured more than thirty-five inches and men whose waists were over forty inches had a higher incidence of Alzheimer's disease.

Consider movement another brain food. Movement stimulates nerve growth factors (NGFs), the nutrients that repair worn-out or damaged nerve cells. It also increases blood flow to the brain, which stimulates the release of NGFs, thereby helping to slow down, and even perhaps reverse, the degenerative effects of brain aging. Nerve growth factors are to the brain what fertilizer is to a plant.

Every time you take a brisk morning walk, imagine that you're fertilizing one of the most important "plants" in your body, your brain.

Movement mellows the mind. The increased blood flow during vigorous exercise stimulates the brain to secrete endorphins and other "happy hormones" that have a natural calming effect. I find walking and swimming (or hydrotherapy) the most relaxing. They also help in decision making. Whenever I have an important choice to make, I think, *I'll swim on that*. If I get too tense, I go see my therapist, the pool.

Walk to your therapist! Movement is the most time-tested antidepressant and antianxiety medicine. It's free and without side effects. In fact, studies show that in people with mild to moderate depression, brisk exercise for thirty to forty minutes three times per week produced improvement comparable to that seen with prescription antidepressants — with no side effects.

The mood-elevating effects of exercise are mainly due to the release of the mood-mellowing hormones dopamine, norepinephrine, and serotonin. These are the same neurochemicals that are affected by prescription antianxiety and anti-depressant medications. In our experience, most prime timers who continue their exercise programs do so not only to keep trim but because of the pleasure that movement brings them. They feel that they've got to move to get their daily fix of happy hormones. I suffer from this addiction.

Move more and fall less. Often, our sense of balance diminishes with age. That's because balance requires quick coordination of different muscles, joints, and motor areas of the brain. The slower these messengers are to tell one side of the body to quickly shift weight, the more off balance we become and the more likely we are to fall. Movement keeps your brain-body reaction time quick.

New movements grow young brain cells. Learning new movements, such as a new dance step or a golf or tennis swing, is one of the best therapies to speed up the slower traffic of the brain and lessen the age-related decline in brain tissue. Learning new movements requires developing new nerve pathways in a particular area of the brain. Add some yoga, Pilates, and you can add even more brain tissue. Martha and I took up ballroom dancing in our early fifties. I became an avid golfer at sixty-six. (See "Shall We Dance?" page 618.)

4. Keep Calm

The older the brain, the calmer it needs to be. As we age, the brain's stress-hormone disposal system weakens. A healthy body needs just the right level of circulating stress hormones. A sudden surge of cortisol helps you think clearly and quickly so you can swerve and miss that oncoming car. Yet, if your levels of stress hormones are chronically high, they will damage brain tissue, a prime-time condition called *glucocorticoid neurotoxicity* or GCN. (If you can say it, you probably don't have it.)

The brain's built-in protective mechanism against GCN declines with age. The hippocampus, the area of the brain associated with learning and memory, seems to be most vulnerable to GCN. Prolonged high levels of the stress hormone cortisol not only damage and shrink the brain nerve tissues, they also slow down the ability of glucose to enter your brain cells, so you have less mental energy, which can translate into unstable moods and difficulty with impulse control and focusing. High cortisol can also slow the speed of information processing by causing a drop in the brain's neurotransmitters, especially dopamine. In fact, people suffering from Alzheimer's often have higher levels of stress hormones. The conclusion: the older we get, the calmer we need to be.

Laughter is the best medicine. Laughter musters up your own feel-good neurochemicals. Surround yourself with positive people who perk you up rather than pull you down. Fill your mind with positive thoughts as much as possible. PET scans show that different areas of the brain are activated in response to positive and negative attitudes and thoughts; it's almost as if we have cerebral optimist and pessimist centers. Negative thoughts are like pollution to the mind. An optimal level of the happy hormones dopamine and serotonin are essential for *neuroplasticity* — the ability to repair brain cells and grow new ones. Low levels of these brain-growth hormones, as are found in unresolved, chronic depression, can interfere with the brain's ability to heal itself and can increase the risk of Alzheimer's disease. (See chapter 15 for more about how humor is therapeutic.)

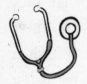

DR. SEARS SAYS...
To become a *keen*ager, sometimes act like a teenager.

5. Exercise the Brain

Use your head. The "use it or lose it" principle is not only good for preserving your muscles, it also helps to preserve your brain. The idle brain may actually shrink. Yet, studies have shown that daily mental gymnastics, such as crossword puzzles and Sudoku, can reduce the risk of dementia and Alzheimer's disease. Neurologists say that "neurons that fire together, wire together." Learn something new, and existing nerves grow more branches that connect with other nerves to form new pathways in the brain that you need for your new activity.

6. Maintain Your Memory

Your memory file is the most useful diary you'll ever carry. Don't lose it. Sometimes I walk upstairs to get something, only to forget what I went for. I'll look up someone's phone number, then quickly forget it and have to look it up again. But, I can remember childhood antics from years ago. That's because we have different storage file cabinets in the brain for short-term and long-term memories. Because different areas of the brain store different memories — a person's name, how to ride a bike, how to dance the tango — aging can affect some memories but not others.

To understand how we forget, consider how we remember. Imagine you just met someone new. How will you remember her name? The first step is *encoding:* the brain changes the audible version of your new acquaintance's name into a neural code, similar to the way a computer translates alphabetic input into code it can store. The next step is *storage.* You store a person's name in your memory file cabinet so the next time you meet her you can greet her by name. Last is *retrieval,* the ability to search through your file cabinet for the right name and to match it to the person walking toward you.

Information may be misplaced or stored in the wrong folder. Perhaps while being introduced, you didn't pay enough attention to her name or were distracted by another conversation at the party. You didn't store the information properly, so you can't retrieve it. Or, maybe you stored the name in a file with other names and associated it with someone else, so when you meet again you greet her by the other person's name.

Even properly stored memories can fade with time. If you haven't seen a person for a few years, you may forget his name at the next meeting. "Use it or lose it" is true of memory too.

Memory maintenance 101. Just as physical exercise enhances muscle strength and builds a strong heart, mental exercise improves memory. Try these techniques:

Visualize. See what you think. First, flash a mental picture of what it is you need to remember, such as your car parked in section A, stall 20. The more outrageous your mental picture of A-20, the more unforgettable it will be. For instance, visualize a giant apple wearing a jersey from your favorite sports team with the number 20 on it. This way, you imprint in your memory "A is for apple" and number 20. Say you forgot your grocery list. Visualize a salad containing the items you're shopping for: greens, salmon, capers, olive oil, and tomatoes.

Replay. As you walk away from the parking lot, put your mind in replay. After you visualize A-20 (a big apple wearing a jersey), rewind your mental recall of the steps you took to the car. Step 1: imagine yourself driving to level A. Step 2: visualize yourself driving into stall 20.

Make a strange association. You meet someone new and would like to remember her name, where she's from, her profession, or some other detail. Suppose her name is Misty Quackenbush and she has six children. Visualize a misty morning and a duck quacking with six little ducklings behind her in a pond. Storing a person's name along with a very picturesque and unique scene will help you retrieve it from your memory file.

Preview. Say you're flying cross-country, and on boarding the plane you hang your garment bag and coat in the closet. If you're concerned you may forget them, during the flight visualize what you'll do to get off the plane: get out of your seat, walk up the aisle, reach into the closet, and retrieve the garment bag and coat. Rehearse this scene several times, and when it actually needs to happen it will already be imprinted in your memory.

Make a reminder. To help you remember to take something with you when leaving home or work (for example, a shopping list or file), place a sticky note on the doorknob or on your coat, or someplace you must pass by.

Take your anti-Alzheimer's medicine. Neurologists are starting to speak the same preventive-medicine language as cardiologists. Both recognize the importance of LEAN (lifestyle, exercise, attitude, and nutrition) in prime-time health. Consider these scary senior statistics: 33 percent of people ages seventy-five to eighty and 50 percent of those over eighty-five may develop Alzheimer's.

Nutrition deficit disorder (NDD; see page 125) may predispose a person for pre-Alzheimer's, or mild cognitive impairment (MCI). MCI means that you often forget where you put your car keys. With full-blown Alzheimer's, you forget where you put your car. One of the biggest steps in Alzheimer's prevention is to identify MCI early and to take measures, as in the Prime-Time Health plan, to prevent it or to keep it from progressing.

There is a growing consensus among experts that although Alzheimer's cannot yet be cured, it *can* be prevented and slowed. While Alzheimer's still remains somewhat of a medical mystery, recent research reveals that it results from chronic inflammation of the brain tissue. *Alzheimer's disease could be another "-itis" illness.* Accumulation of inflammatory chemicals (iBods) called cytokines weakens the synapses, the antennae that help brain cells communicate with each other. Continuous inflammation causes accumulation of sticky stuff called amyloid deposits, which trigger more iBods to try to clean them up, leading to more inflammation and tissue damage. That's why the best preventive medicine for Alzheimer's disease is to slow inflammation — precisely what the Prime-Time Health plan does.

SPICE UP YOUR BRAIN

A study in the *Journal of Alzheimer's Disease* showed that turmeric can stimulate the brain's garbage collectors (cells called *macrophages,* or "big eaters") to begin a plaque attack and dispose of increased beta-amyloid, the garbage (plaque) that collects in brain tissue as we age and seems to cause Alzheimer's disease.

Who is less likely to develop Alzheimer's disease? A survey of scientific studies reveals that certain lifestyle and dietary factors can lessen your chance of developing the disease. The people who improve their odds of avoiding Alzheimer's are:

- movers (runners, walkers, dancers, swimmers, etc.)
- laughers
- brain exercisers
- fish eaters (more seafood, less meat)
- blueberry eaters
- nut eaters
- vegetable eaters (green, leafy veggies)
- grazers
- volunteers
- optimists
- waist watchers
- spiritual folks

Although chromosomal quirks have been found in the gene mutations of some people with Alzheimer's disease, whether the switch on these genetic tendencies is turned on or off can be greatly affected by what you eat and how you live. Genetic tendencies are just that — they increase your risk of developing a certain illness if you don't take the necessary precautions.

Rx FOR PRIME-TIME BRAIN HEALTH

- ❑ Eat more fish and omega-3s.
- ❑ Eat more blueberries.
- ❑ Eat more spinach and other greens.
- ❑ Graze on good carbs.
- ❑ Eat more nuts.
- ❑ Avoid excess alcohol.
- ❑ Avoid neurotoxic food additives.
- ❑ Move your body.
- ❑ Keep calm.
- ❑ Exercise your brain.
- ❑ Enjoy memory-enhancing games.

CHAPTER 5

Be Good to Your Gut

Along with a healthy heart and smart brain, the Prime-Time Health plan promises *good* gut feelings instead of painful ones such as heartburn, indigestion, and constipation that often come more frequently during this stage of life. Pains in the gut are some of the most common reasons prime timers seek medical help (which is why all those ads for laxatives, antacids, and digestive aids are aimed at us). During prime time, the body's need for certain nutrients goes up, and our tolerance for certain foods goes down.

HOW YOUR GUT CHANGES DURING PRIME TIME

The keys to healthy prime-time eating are two words: *smaller* and *slower.* To understand why you need to eat differently, it helps to first appreciate why your gut behaves differently as you age.

The stomach shrinks. With aging, there is a decrease in *gastrointestinal reserve.* This happens for two reasons: the stomach muscle becomes less stretchable, so it can't accommodate as much food; and the intestines lose strength, causing food to move more slowly. Therefore, the prime-time gut is less tolerant of bingeing and gorging. The all-you-can-eat buffet and greasy double cheeseburgers are no longer welcome in your gut.

Acid refluxes. When you eat too much, too quickly, the stomach doesn't expand as much or empty as fast. The muscular valve that keeps food in the stomach and prevents it from being regurgitated back into the esophagus becomes weaker, leading to gastroesophageal reflux (GER). This "burny" pain occurs because some of the undigested food and stomach acids reflux back up and irritate the sensitive lining of the esophagus.

Digestion slows. As we get older, our intestinal function, saliva production, and stomach emptying all slow down as digestive enzymes become a bit more sluggish and intestinal muscle tone gets a little weaker. This gut slowdown can cause problems at both ends: GER, or heartburn, and constipation. Since "slows" sums up what happens to guts in prime time, simply *slow* down when you eat. In fact, your body has been telling you how you should eat all your life, but now you have no choice. Your gut is less forgiving today than it was when you were twenty.

Nutrient absorption slows. The normal folds of the intestine become flatter as we age, which decreases the absorption surface of the intestines. These changes may also cause the intestines to be less able to absorb nutrients, such as vitamin B_{12}, folic acid, calcium, and vitamin D. For years it was thought that older intestines didn't absorb vitamins and minerals as well, so the standard nutritional advice was that every person over fifty should take a daily multivitamin/multimineral pill. New research questions this recommendation. Because our bodies contain so much extra intestinal tissue, we can lose a little function and still absorb enough nutrients from food — provided we have a healthy diet and lifestyle.

Garbage disposal weakens. The intestinal tract serves the rest of the body by processing food, absorbing needed nutrients, and discarding leftover waste. The stomach pulverizes, purifies, and liquefies the food; the small intestine absorbs the nutrients; and the large intestine disposes of the waste. The toxins (chemical additives) that survive this processing and make it into the bloodstream travel to our backup garbage-disposal system, the liver. Like so many organs in our generously designed body, the liver has a lot of reserve. Yet, the liver reserve also decreases as we age, becoming less able to dispose of toxins that sneak into the bloodstream. The solution: put less garbage into your mouth so the rest of your disposal system isn't overwhelmed.

Enzyme secretions from the liver, pancreas, stomach, and small intestine may decrease or work less efficiently as well, so it takes longer to digest foods and eliminate waste. Prime-time intestines may secrete less of certain enzymes, such as lactase, causing lactose intolerance, and wheat-digesting enzymes, causing gluten sensitivity. Many prime timers find they can still enjoy dairy and wheat products, but they have to eat these foods more slowly and in smaller portions.

Metabolism slows. We go from being calorie burners to being calorie storers. As we age, our resting metabolic rate slows. Besides metabolism slowing, muscle mass (muscle is our main calorie-burning organ) decreases if we let it. Less fuel burned means less food is needed. Plus, we're often less active as we get older, although that should not be part of your Prime-Time Health plan. These gut facts translate into a notable change: the older we get, the less junk food we can eat. Quality comes before quantity. The upside to this change: metabolizing healthy food translates into less wear and tear on the body.

The gut is also a giant endocrine organ. In addition to absorbing vital nutrients, the intestines make many hormones. The gut is so richly supplied with nerves that it is called the "gut brain." So, it's no surprise that the prime-time tips for a healthy gut are similar to those for a healthy heart and brain.

SEVEN WAYS TO KEEP YOUR GUT HEALTHY

1. Eat Often

Graze is the watchword for prime-time gut health. Grazing on frequent minimeals keeps the body satisfied — neither hungry nor uncomfortably full. Here's why grazing is especially good for the gut:

Grazing is easier to swallow. Dysphagia, or uncomfortable swallowing, occurs in many older prime timers because the esophagus, the hoselike tube that connects the throat to the stomach, propels the food along more slowly. When less food enters the esophagus, it goes down more easily.

Grazing eases heartburn. How often have you indulged in a big meal, felt lousy afterward, and said, "Oh, that heartburn again!" If there is less volume of food for the stomach to process, there is less chance it will be regurgitated. Filling the stomach with too much, too fast, increases the pressure in the stomach, causing the acid to shoot back up into the esophagus, leading to heartburn.

Grazing increases nutrient absorption. If you present less food to the intestines more frequently, it gives the digestive enzymes more time to do their jobs and to reload for the next

A TALE OF TWO MEALS

Let's follow a gorger and a grazer from their plates to their bloodstreams to see how one is an ager and the other is not. The gorger feasts at an all-you-can-eat steakhouse buffet. First, his gut shouts "overfeeding," and he bloats with heartburn and indigestion. Then, the big helpings rush into the bloodstream, and his arteries get stiff, sticky, and narrower (see postprandial lipemia, page 76). His body then goes into a hypermetabolic state to use up the excess food. This hyperburn generates more oxidative stress and accelerated glycation end products (AGEs) that make the tissues stiff and sticky. Next, the pancreas pours out excess insulin to mop up the excess sugar, and the brain and body go into hormonal disharmony. Finally, because his body doesn't like to waste excess food, it stores his indulgences around his middle.

The grazer, on the other hand, puts real food into his body. By eating smaller amounts more frequently, there is less indigestion, heartburn, oxidative stress (or AGEs), vascular stickiness and narrowing, and brain fog, all of which make for a longer, happier life. The body, in its wisdom, begins to crave quality food instead of quantity and prompts him to keep eating this way. (That's what happened to me, and I trust it will also happen to you.)

small meal. You are not only what you eat; you're what you absorb.

Grazing eases constipation. When you eat twice as often, half as much, and chew twice as long, you're likely to have a bowel movement twice as often, half as large, and twice as soft. This intestinal perk is simple: When the intestines don't need to work as hard at the top end, less effort is needed at the bottom end. The more predigestion that occurs at the top end, the less waste is left over for the bottom end.

2. Enjoy Smoothies

For a *supergrazing* way to eat that will add years to your life and life to your years, try a Prime-Time Smoothie, my sipping solution (see recipe on page 151).

I discovered the sipping solution in 1997 during my postoperative recovery from colon cancer and while undergoing radiation and chemotherapy. Since solid foods were unsettling, every day I'd make a 1,100- to 1,300-calorie smoothie and sip on it throughout the day. Because of the good gut feelings and mental clarity I experienced with this form of grazing, I've continued sipping smoothies an average of four days per week. In my medical practice, I call smoothies "school-ade" for the kids, "prime-ade" for prime timers, "lean-ade" for overfat patients, and a general "health-ade" for everyone else. I sip on my smoothie all day long. It's my breakfast, lunch, and snacks. Then I have a normal, healthy dinner at night. When I'm working at the office or on the go, I take small bottles of it in an insulated container to keep it cool.

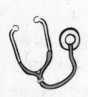

DR. SEARS SAYS...
Make gradual changes to your way of eating. Begin by having the sipping solution one day a week. Instead of shocking your gut and inviting protest (e.g., bloating and diarrhea), ease your gut into a different way of eating.

Why smoothies are smart. Smoothies slide through the twenty-five feet of your intestines. Many prime timers contend with constipation, heartburn, overfatness, diabetes, mood disorders, and depressed immunity. But with a smoothie, the blender does much of the work the intestines would have to do. The sipping solution is good for the gut because it:

Improves absorption. Even science says smoothies are smart. Some prime timers don't absorb vitamins and minerals as well as they did in their younger years. By liquefying the produce, more of the nutrients are absorbed. There is less waste.

Lessens heartburn. Because sipped food enters the stomach slowly and blended food exits quickly from the stomach, there is less left over to reflux.

Is a natural laxative. Liquid food passes more quickly through the intestines, more is absorbed, and the high-fiber liquid is a natural laxative. Expect the sipping solution to increase the number of bowel movements per day, a colon-healthy change.

Helps weight control. The sipping solution trains the gut to enjoy the good gut feelings and not being stretched from gorging.

Boosts immunity. The smoothie is full of phytos, those colorful blue, red, green, and yellow

GUT HEALTH 101: DR. BILL'S RULE OF TWOS

Eat *twice* as often, eat *half* as much, and chew *twice* as long.

foods that are loaded with antioxidants — foods that support the antirust maintenance crew in your body.

Stabilizes blood sugar. The sipping solution rewards your body and blood with stable blood sugar and insulin levels. To avoid speeded-up carbohydrate absorption and spikes in blood sugar from added fruit, be sure your smoothie is high in fiber, protein, and some fat to slow down a sugar rush, as in my recipe on the next page.

Shapes taste. If you are not a veggie lover, adding greens (spinach, Swiss chard, or green vegetable juice) will gradually teach you to enjoy the earthy taste.

I attribute much of my good health, normal blood chemistry, and medication-free living at age seventy to my daily smoothie.

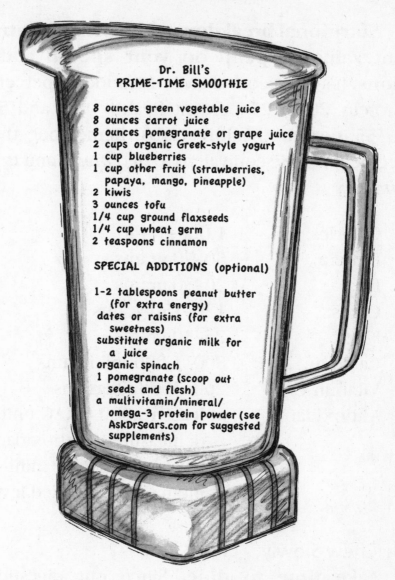

Dr. Bill's
PRIME-TIME SMOOTHIE

8 ounces green vegetable juice
8 ounces carrot juice
8 ounces pomegranate or grape juice
2 cups organic Greek-style yogurt
1 cup blueberries
1 cup other fruit (strawberries,
  papaya, mango, pineapple)
2 kiwis
3 ounces tofu
1/4 cup ground flaxseeds
1/4 cup wheat germ
2 teaspoons cinnamon

SPECIAL ADDITIONS (optional)

1-2 tablespoons peanut butter
  (for extra energy)
dates or raisins (for extra
  sweetness)
substitute organic milk for
  a juice
organic spinach
1 pomegranate (scoop out
  seeds and flesh)
a multivitamin/mineral/
  omega-3 protein powder (see
  AskDrSears.com for suggested
  supplements)

Yield: 8–9 cups

Mix together in a high-power blender. (I use a Vita-Mix Super 5000.) Tastes best when it's fresh and still has that bubbly milkshake consistency.

Nutritional breakdown: The precise nutrient values depend on your special additions. It's a perfect balance of around 25 percent protein, 20 to 25 percent healthy fats, and 50 to 55 percent healthy carbs. Remember, this recipe is calorie equivalent to *two meals* and *two snacks*.

Calories:	1,000–1,400
Protein:	50–70 grams
Fat:	20–30 grams
Carbs:	120–150 grams
Fiber:	25–30 grams
Calcium:	800–1,000 milligrams
Vitamin C:	200–300 milligrams
Antioxidants:	at least 10,000 ORAC units (a measure of antioxidant levels); double the minimum recommended level

3. Chew Slowly

Take time to dine. Since our digestion slows as we age, it makes sense to slow down the volume of food that is presented to those sluggish digestive juices. When we chew slower and longer, we stimulate saliva production so the salivary digestive enzymes can go to work digesting the food even before it reaches the stomach. And, chewing longer stimulates satiety, which means we are less likely to overeat.

Rest your fork. Talk or listen after a few bites. Develop a habit that encourages you to put down your fork, such as using your napkin between bites.

4. Eat Pure and Eat Fresh

Remember, the most vital nutritional tip for healthy aging is just eat *real* foods. The older you get, the fewer packaged foods you should eat. As you age, you *have* to become a food purist. This may mean a total overhaul of your shopping and eating habits, but your body deserves the best. Doesn't healthier food cost more? In the long run, no. While you may pay more at the supermarket, you'll eventually pay less at the doctor's office. If you think health food is expensive, compare that to the costs associated with health care.

Get those good gut feelings. It's like your gut has two types of metabolic switches, an

HEALING HEARTBURN

The stomach has a marvelous design. Gastric acid is produced by glands in the lining of certain areas of the stomach wall. Acid not only helps break up the food, it also kills harmful germs that may be in the food. And the right amount of stomach acid helps maintain the balance of bacteria in the bowels. Lowering stomach acid with antacids can allow some of the bad bacteria to take over and outnumber the good, leading to diarrhea-producing illnesses from bacteria such as *Clostridium difficile* and *Giardia.* Stomach acid is your gut's natural antibiotic. The stomach lining also naturally secretes a thick mucus that bathes the entire lining of the stomach, sort of like a protective paint, to keep the acid from digesting its own tissue. Yet, the very top part of the stomach, especially the lining of the esophagus, doesn't share this protective sealant. So when the stomach is too full of food and acid, some of the acid can be squirted, or refluxed, back up into the lining of the esophagus, irritating or "burning" it. The esophagus is located behind the heart, hence the term *heartburn.*

There is no reason why prime timers should suffer heartburn more than younger folks. While digestion may slow down a bit in prime time, it doesn't have to. The gut, like many other organs, has reserve capacity. We can lose a little bit of its function, and it won't bother us. But if you do suffer from heartburn, try all the eating tips in this chapter, especially these:

Practice the rule of twos. In my medical practice, the top antireflux prescription for all ages is eat twice as often, eat half as much, and chew twice as long.

Drink some meals. A Prime-Time Smoothie can be just what the gut doctor ordered (see page 151).

Don't dine after nine. Eating earlier in the evening allows most of your digestion to take place before you lie down to sleep. Eating too much, too late, literally opens the door for reflux to occur.

Sleep on your left side. This allows gravity to better empty the stomach.

Stay lean. Increased belly fat increases reflux. The extra fat increases pressure on the stomach, which sends some food back up.

Use heartburn medicines wisely. The acid in our stomachs is there for a reason. When we interfere with the natural process of digestion, we often pay an uncomfortable price. Modern heartburn medicines are designed to reduce or to shut off the production of stomach acids, and they have given wonderful relief to serious heartburn sufferers. But it's harmful to take these heartburn medications in doses too high and for too long. Be sure to use the "start low, go slow" method: begin with a low dose, increase the dose slowly as needed, and try to get off the medicine as soon as possible while following the prime-time eating tips included here.

One of the reasons why prime timers seem to suffer more from heartburn is their widespread use of aspirin, ibuprofen, and other anti-inflammatory pain relievers. These medicines are not stomach friendly. They lessen the protective mucus, thus making the stomach lining more vulnerable to attack by its own acids.

"eat right, feel good" switch and an "eat bad, feel bad" switch. After decades of eating the standard American diet, these internal gut voices have been silenced. Now you can turn them back on.

After a few months of eating according to four gut-friendly words — *graze, sip, chew,* and *pure* — your feel-good switch will turn on. And, because your feel-bad switch will also turn on, eating junk food will start to bother you. When you become more aware of how your gut feels, you know your prime-time gut program is working.

5. Go for Quality Over Quantity

Take a tip from the French, well known for their tasty cuisine and lean bodies: eat real, wholesome food. Unprocessed food is naturally more satisfying. Processed, packaged food is purposely fabricated with sweeteners and taste-enhancing chemicals that entice you to overeat, but it's low in the satiety-producing nutrients protein and fiber. In fact, you could call the prime-time diet the *real-food diet*. The longevity benefit of real foods is that they are *nutrient dense*, meaning they pack more nutrition in fewer calories. Processed foods, on the other hand, are calorie dense. I noticed two changes when I traded quantity for quality: I became satisfied with less, and I began craving real food and shunning fake food. I don't do commercial cake mixes anymore. If I'm going to splurge on extra calories, it's got to be real-food calories.

Enjoy fill-up foods. Junk carbs (fast-release sugars) and most processed foods remind me of the beer ad: "Tastes great, *less filling.*" Real food, on the other hand, tastes great and is

LOOK FOR AGING WORDS ON FOOD LABELS

Most food additives add nothing to your health and are likely to shorten your life. In my medical practice, I start teaching kids to look for the "bad words" on food labels (e.g., high-fructose corn syrup, hydrogenated, number symbols, monosodium glutamate [MSG]) and warn them that they are bad for their growth. These bad words are even worse for prime timers.

- As you learned earlier, our garbage-disposal system weakens with age, so the older we get, the more harmful additives in food are to our health.
- Just at the stage in our lives when we need to choose quality over quantity and reshape our tastes so we crave real foods, food additives increase our cravings for junk.

more filling. The gut has a built-in *satiety sensor* that registers, "I'm full." This sensor then sends its signal to the brain, telling it to stop the eating. Normally, there is a delay of around twenty minutes between the gut feeling full and the brain getting the message. Unlike a gasoline

- Remember, when you see additives on a label, it makes the nutritional quality of the whole package suspect. This is especially true of flavor enhancers such as MSG.
- Additives, which are designed by food chemists to make packaged food last longer, are likely to make your body wear out sooner. Jacob, a nine-year-old boy in my practice, triggered this thought as I explained the relationship between junk food and junk health to him. He wisely said: "Dr. Bill, my grandpa ate a lot of junk food, and he died before I was born. I guess the stuff that they put in the food to make it last longer on the shelf doesn't make your body last longer. I wish I had my grandpa."

(See a longer list on page 126.)

pump that automatically shuts off when the tank is full, our feel-full monitoring system can be blunted after decades of overeating. With the Prime-Time Health plan, you will reprogram your satiety center to feel comfortably full after less eating. Your gut will like real foods because

WHY EXCESS ALCOHOL IS NOT GOOD FOR THE GUT

The lining of the stomach is normally protected by a layer of mucus. Yet, alcohol crosses this protective lining and makes its way into the bloodstream and into the liver very fast. (Remember, alcohol is a solvent. You clean stains with it.) Also, alcohol stimulates the glands in the stomach to produce more acid, further aggravating the heartburn that already bothers so many prime timers. Because alcohol passes so quickly in such high concentrations through the lining of the intestines and into the bloodstream and the liver, it can be toxic in high doses. This is one reason why excess alcohol can rot the liver (cirrhosis) and why, if you do drink, it's important to sip alcohol slowly and only with meals and not to drink on an empty stomach. (See Safe-Alcohol-Drinking Tips, page 671.)

they are fill-up foods. Foods with a high satiety factor enable you to eat less of that food and still be satisfied.

Power up with protein. Protein provides satiety more than carbs or fats alone do because it best triggers your satiety hormones. Research shows that people who eat more protein at

---

TOP FILL-UP FOODS

Fill-up foods help you get full before you get fat. The best satiety foods are loaded with lean protein, fiber, healthy (low-glycemic-index) carbs, a few grams of healthy fat, and are bulky with air or water:

Seafood	Milk
Eggs	Yogurt
Lentils	Tofu
Beans	Fruits and veggies
Chili peppers	Nuts
Rice, wild or brown	Steel-cut oatmeal
Potatoes, with skin	Olive oil
Chunky vegetable soup, homemade	Popcorn

---

one meal, such as breakfast or lunch, tend to feel more satisfied and eat less at the next meal. Another protein perk: It's not only uncomfortable to overeat high-protein foods; if you do your body doesn't convert excess protein into excess fat as easily as it does dietary fats and carbs. And, you burn 30 percent of the calories in protein just by digesting it. Try this satiety trick: Eat one hard-boiled egg (seventy-five calories). Notice how satisfied you feel. A few hours later eat a seventy-five-calorie mostly carb snack, such as a sweetened beverage (no fiber or protein). Feel the difference?

Spice down your hunger. Hot, spicy foods help you feel satisfied with less, probably by triggering satiety hormones. Try salsa, jalapeños, cayenne pepper, and chili peppers. Hot foods also rev up your metabolism so you burn more of the calories you just ate.

Fill up with a bit of fat. Enjoying a bit of healthy fat with each snack or meal increases satiety. Besides giving food a more pleasant taste and mouth feel, fat and protein trigger stomach hormones that tell the brain, "You're getting full. Stop eating!"

Fill up with fiber. Fiber is filling without being fattening. Research shows that the higher the fiber content of a carb (high-fiber carbs are also called a low-glycemic-index carb), the greater the satiety. Add fiber and protein, and a carb becomes a *slow-release* carb, and you'll have a meal or snack that's just what the body needs.

Got milk? Milk and yogurt, even nonfat or low-fat, are high-satiety foods. As Barbara Rolls, chair of the Department of Nutritional Sciences at Penn State University, explains in her excellent book *The Volumetrics Weight-Control Plan,* milk turns from a liquid drink into a more filling semisolid food (think curds and whey) in the stomach, and this triggers satiety signals, so you're likely to eat less at that meal. (See "Need Milk?" page 339.)

Air out your eating. Your hunger hormones respond mostly to the *volume* of food hitting the stomach. Airy foods, such as air-popped popcorn, are a great fill-up snack. The calorie-free air fills — and fools — the stomach, which tells the brain that it's full of food when it's partially full of air. Don't worry; increased air in the stomach may cause you to burp a bit, but it doesn't lead to gas at the other end.

Everyone has a satiety set point (SSP), which means the usual amount of food you eat before you feel full. For most, the SSP is too high. After a few months on the Prime-Time Health program, your SSP will automatically reset lower. You will feel just as satisfied with less.

6. Relax Your Gut Brain

The gut has a mind of its own. There are more nerves in the intestines than anywhere else in the body, except for the brain. The gut brain shares many of the mood-altering hormones of the brain, such as serotonin, norepinephrine, and acetylcholine. In fact, it's the main supplier of the "happy hormone" serotonin, the neuro-chemical that is thought to be stimulated by antidepressants.

A disturbance in serotonin levels from depression and anxiety affects the mind, and it also upsets the gut. Digestive disturbances, such as irritable bowel syndrom (IBS), colitis, diverticulitis, and general indigestion, are frequent maladies of prime timers. When your happy hormones are missing, not only will your brain feel depressed, so will your gut. People with IBS tend to have less serotonin in the cells lining the gut. The conclusion: the older we get, the more we need to relax. (See chapter 15 to learn how to relieve stress.)

7. Be Kind to Your Colon

The colon, the last six feet of your twenty-five-foot-long intestinal tract, is often the part of the gut that gets the most upset. Colitis and colon

DON'T ADD IRON TO YOUR COLON

Unless advised that you are anemic and need extra dietary iron by your doctor, men over fifty and postmenopausal women should not take extra iron supplements, such as those often found in multivitamin/multimineral preparations. Excess iron, especially a big dose taken all at once in a supplement, can act as an irritant and pro-oxidant, increasing wear and tear on the intestinal lining. Most prime timers can get all the iron they need by eating real foods, especially the superfoods listed in chapter 13.

---

cancer are two common prime-time illnesses. While the colon is best known as a waste disposal system, it also plays an important role in balancing your immune system.

Medical wisdom teaches us that we're only as healthy as our colon. I paid the price for not listening to this medical truism and got colon cancer, which was diagnosed in 1997.

Colon statistics:
- While colon cancer is the third leading cause of death and disability in prime timers, the good news is that it's one of the *most preventable*.

- Colon cancer is the second leading cause of cancer death after lung cancer, accounting for 10 percent of all cancer deaths.
- Ninety percent of colon cancer cases occur after age fifty.
- Family history increases the risk of colon cancer by 5 to 10 percent.
- The food-cancer correlation (either causative or preventive) is strongest for colon cancer.

The reason for the connection between food and colon cancer seems to be that certain foods scraping against the cancer-vulnerable lining of the intestines gradually cause the cells of the lining to mutate.

Our colon-cancer-prevention program is basically to eat fewer carcinogenic foods and keep the waste flowing faster so it spends less time scraping against the lining of the colon. That's what you will learn to do in chapter 20.

Eat probiotics. One of the best strategies for colon health is putting the best bacteria into your bowels. Billions of bacteria normally reside in your large intestine. In return for a warm place to live, they do good things for the gut. These "bowel bugs" are also called *intestinal flora* because, like plant life, they provide an environment that contributes to colon health, which in turn contributes to the health of the whole body. Healthy bacteria are also known as *probiotics* because they are prolife or add health to life. These probiotics bring health to your gut and your body in several ways.

Probiotics boost intestinal immunity. The intestines are the body's largest immune organ. Probiotics enhance intestinal immune defenses by strengthening the immune barrier of the gut lining. They help increase the germ-fighter immunoglobulin A (IgA) and increase the thickness of intestinal mucus, which acts like a protective shield to keep harmful bacteria from getting into your bloodstream. Probiotics discourage the growth and harmful effects of pathogenic bacteria (bad "bowel bugs"). These good bugs stick to the intestinal lining, effectively crowding out the bad ones and preventing them from getting a foothold in the intestinal lining.

WHY GRILLING ISN'T GOOD FOR YOUR GUT

Grilling over high heat, especially charring, causes some of the proteins in animal meat to produce cancer-causing toxins called heterocyclic amines (HCAs) and other DNA-damaging chemicals called mutagens. Charring can also release AGEs, which promote inflammation. By a genetic quirk called rapid acetylators, some people are more prone to the cancer-causing effects of HCAs. To reduce the HCAs generated from grilling, observe these cooking cautions:

- Instead of grilling, poach, sauté, and bake.
- If you simply can't give up grilling on your barbecue, prebake meat and poultry in the oven to lessen its time on the grill.

They promote a healthy gut environment. Probiotics produce lactic acid. A more acidic environment in the gut favors the growth of good bacteria over bad. Keeping the lower end of the intestinal environment slightly acidic is especially necessary if you are taking antacids at the upper end for heartburn.

They reduce intestinal allergies. Probiotics increase food tolerance. They suppress the

- Flip meat every few minutes to prevent charring.
- Douse flames to prevent flare-ups.
- Don't use pan drippings from charred meat, as they may contain mutagens.
- Wetting meat lowers the surface temperature, decreasing the HCAs. Marinate meat in lime juice (limonene is an antioxidant) and sprinkle with diced veggies or fruit (such as mango salsa), onions, or crushed garlic. Or, make your own marinade with olive oil and spices such as rosemary, thyme, basil, and oregano. These antioxidant-rich marinades reduce HCA production.
- While grilling fruits and vegetables doesn't seem to produce HCAs, avoid charring them.

autoimmune response of the gut and reduce the severity of those "-itis" illnesses, such as gastro-enteritis and colitis. Probiotics also may alleviate inflammatory bowel disease, since people with inflammatory bowel disease tend to have a less-healthy intestinal bacterial balance.

They produce healthful nutrients. Probiotics ferment some of the fiber in food to form short-chain fatty acids (SCFAs), which nourish the cells lining the colon, stimulate healing of these cells, and reduce the likelihood of colon cancer. SCFAs are then absorbed in the bloodstream and travel to the liver where they lessen the liver's production of cholesterol. SCFAs also inhibit the growth of yeast and harmful bacteria in the gut.

To get more probiotics to nourish your intestinal health:

Eat yogurt. Yogurt and other fermented dairy products such as kefir are the main dietary source of probiotics. The two most familiar probiotics added to yogurt during the culturing process are *Lactobacillus bulgaricus* and *Lactobacillus acidophilus.* Be sure to use organic yogurt. My favorite is Stonyfield Oikos Greek yogurt. Besides being organic and higher in protein, Stonyfield yogurts contain inulin, an ingredient often added to high-quality yogurts. It's a *prebiotic,* or a food that feeds the probiotics. (Prebiotics are actually indigestible carbohydrate fibers.)

Take probiotics. In addition to eating yogurt at least several days a week, I take a probiotic called Culturelle, which has been used in most of the scientific medical studies showing the health benefits of probiotics.

Get your bowels going. As you age, waste passes a little more slowly through the intestines, and once it gets to the colon, the waste-management system, it can be even more sluggish. In some prime timers, rectal pressure, also called "squeeze pressure," diminishes with aging, making the rectal muscles less able to do the final push. Correcting constipation simply means improving your waste-management system by keeping the waste softer and moving more freely. All the general tips for gut health, especially grazing on real foods, lessen constipation. In addition, here is a natural laxative I've recommended in my medical practice for years and use myself: add a tablespoon of flax oil to a daily fruit-and-yogurt smoothie. Avoid the popular laxative mineral oil since, unlike flax oil, it has no nutritional value and can lessen the absorption of some valuable vitamins.

Move your body to move your bowels. The more you exercise, the more easily waste passes through your intestines. Be sure to drink extra water following strenuous exercise. The most common cause of constipation is not drinking

GOT GAS?

If you suffer from indigestion, you may produce more gas and be less able to control it. The anal sphincter (the "hold it" muscle) can weaken with age, so you have more difficulty holding gas in. Actually, a little gas is good for us. It's normal to release a bit of intestinal gas (as often as twenty times a day), especially when we eat some of the more powerful gas-producing foods, such as beans and broccoli. Because the most disagreeable intestinal gas is produced by the fermenting of undigested leftovers in the colon, here's how to keep the air fresh around you:

- **Graze.** Grazing lessens bloating from gas. The intestines produce an enzyme called alpha-galactosidase, which breaks down fiber and complex carbohydrates before they get a chance to reach the colon and produce gas. If you eat more food at one time than the intestines are able to break down, the leftover fiber and carbs will remain undigested, ferment, and produce gas.
- **Try ginger.** Ginger is an all-around intestine settler. Grate ginger on your salad, and try ginger tea.
- **Move.** Physical exercise moves the gas through your bowels. Expect to pass more gas during exercise.

- **Try Beano.** Beano is a nonprescription pill that contains alpha-galactosidase, the natural enzyme that helps digest gas-producing foods, such as beans. Take Beano before your first bite. Some people have to take eight pills to notice a difference.

- **Record.** Note your personal fart foods. The stinky smell from flatus comes mainly from sulfur gases, such as hydrogen sulfide. Putting fewer sulfur-containing foods in your mouth can reduce the sulfur gases coming out the other end. Foods with a high sulfur content include: meat, eggs, and cauliflower. Because some of the sugars in beans pass through the small intestine undigested, beans have a reputation for being the most familiar gassy food, but soaking them in water overnight makes them less so. Some people notice that slugging drinks sweetened with high-fructose corn syrup can cause bloating and flatulence because too much fructose enters the intestines too fast. And eating too much of alternative sweeteners, such as sorbitol and xylitol, can cause gas.

enough water. The colon is your body's water conservator. If you don't drink enough water at the top end, the colon extracts water from the waste, hardening the stools.

After a few weeks on this program, expect to comfortably pass at least two to three stools a day. More-frequent bowel movements are not only normal, they are better for intestinal health.

Rx FOR GUT HEALTH

- ❑ Graze! Eat *twice* as often, *half* as much, and chew *twice* as long.
- ❑ Sip on smoothies.
- ❑ Take time to dine. Eat more slowly.
- ❑ Eat more fresh foods, fewer packaged foods, and go organic.
- ❑ Eat pure: omit additives like MSG, artificial sweeteners, and artificial colorings.
- ❑ Eat high-fiber fill-up foods.
- ❑ Power up with proteins.
- ❑ Relax your gut brain.
- ❑ Eat probiotics.
- ❑ Move your body to move your bowels.

CHAPTER 6

Improve Your Eye-Q

Our eyes are our windows to the world. The clearer the window, the more we can see. As with other parts of the body, most age-related vision problems derive from an accumulation of sticky stuff. About 30 percent of prime timers — more than 10 million of us — have some degree of age-related macular degeneration (ARMD), the leading cause of weakening vision. It results from abnormal vessel growth throughout the retina, which eventually leads to scar tissue. To people with ARMD, things look "fuzzy," or they see "dark spots" in the image they are looking at. About 70 percent of Americans over age seventy-five develop cataracts, which cause clouding of the lens of the eye. (The lens is made up of proteins and water. As we age, the proteins in the lens form clumps, so that rays of light, instead of passing easily through a clear lens, are diffused a bit; people with cataracts describe their vision as trying to look through a dirty window.)

Weakening vision is a classic example of our sticky-stuff/weak garbage-disposal theory of aging. Advanced glycation end products (AGEs, explained on page 34) collect in the lens and in the retina. The medical name for this waste is *drusen*.

In presbyopia (aging eyes), the lens of the eye becomes stiff or less elastic, reducing its ability to focus on small print or nearby objects. Visual sharpness diminishes, so that most prime timers require glasses at some point, either for reading or driving. The size of the pupil shrinks, and the eyes accommodate more slowly to changing levels of light. This may decrease visual acuity in the dark and make bright light bothersome. Glare, such as from headlights when driving at night, may also be challenging. As with so many other organs of the body, to maintain vision health we must protect and nourish the eyes.

SHADE YOUR EYES

The pupil, the round window that opens and closes to let more or less light enter the eye, reacts more slowly as we age. I didn't appreciate the damaging effect of sunlight until I noticed our new blue carpet fading badly, after a few short years, from the sunlight coming in through the windows. We eventually had tinted windows installed, sort of like putting on sunglasses, and we replaced the carpet. The same thing happens to our eyes: Sunlight can damage the lens, cause cataracts, and blast the retina, resulting in macular degeneration. Excessive direct sunlight seems to allow free radicals (see explanation of these rascals, page 31) to damage the vital structures of the eye. Besides causing wear and tear on the lens, free radicals can partially clog the tiny blood vessels that pipe into the retina, leading to scar tissue and blurry vision. Shading our eyes can help to preserve these precious structures.

To pick the right sunglasses, make sure the lenses are coated with UV blockers and labeled according to the guidelines for ultraviolet light protection established by the American National Standards Institute (ANSI). If they are labeled "cosmetic," they will block out much less light than those for "general purpose use," which block out much more UV light. Polarized sunglasses have an added protective layer that helps block the glare of light reflected off snow and water.

FEED YOUR EYES

Early in my recovery from cancer, I realized that the eyes, like the brain, are profoundly affected by what we eat. Here's some food for sight. The retina is really part of the brain and is composed mainly of fat nourished by a network of tiny vessels. So, everything you learned about feeding the brain in chapter 4 and caring for your blood vessels in chapter 3 applies to caring for your eyes. The four groups of nutrients that feed the retina are carotenoids (lutein and zeaxanthin), flavonoids, vitamins, and omega-3s. Nourish your eyes.

Eat foods rich in lutein and zeaxanthin. The antioxidants lutein and zeaxanthin are found in both the lens and the macula of the retina, the two areas in older eyes that are most prone to damage. These nutrients, known as *nature's sunglasses,* absorb UVB light, which has the highest energy and therefore the wavelength most potentially damaging to the retina and macula. Lutein absorbs some of the damaging rays from the sunlight and also protects against the wear and tear of free radicals by neutralizing them. Studies show that people who eat more foods that are high in lutein and zeaxanthin are less likely to have cataracts or ARMD. Smokers, postmenopausal women, and adults with light-colored eyes all have half as much of these carotenoids in the macula, so it's particularly important for them to eat foods high in these nutrients. The best sources of lutein and zeaxanthin are kale, spinach, Swiss chard, green peas, corn, and summer squash.

From 6 to 20 milligrams daily of lutein and zeaxanthin improves vision health. You can get the equivalent of this by eating a cup of greens three times a week. Because lutein is a fat-soluble nutrient, small amounts of healthy fat (approximately five grams per meal) can improve absorption. (Think olive oil on spinach salad.) At 0.5 milligrams per 3 ounces, corn has the highest amount of zeaxanthin of any vegetable. A study showed that 10 milligrams of lutein per day from spinach and corn increased macular pigment optical density (MPOD). Doses as low as 2.4 milligrams of lutein per day for six months increased MPOD

"SEE" FOODS

Mix many of these foods together into an eye-opening salad. (See supersalad recipe, page 554.)

- salmon
- blueberries
- spinach
- kale
- Swiss chard
- collard greens
- green peas
- bell peppers
- pumpkin, squash summer squash (zucchini)
- red grapes
- nuts
- yellow corn
- broccoli
- carrots
- egg yolk

by 10 percent. One study showed that eating spinach more than five times a week decreased the risk of cataracts. Plant your own "eye garden." Just outside my writing room grow lush stalks of Swiss chard, one of the easiest eye plants to grow.

Seafood is "see" food. Since omega-3 fat, primarily DHA, is the most important structural component of the brain-cell membrane, it stands to reason that it's also good for the retina. In fact, most of the retina is made up of omega-3 DHA.

DHA improves retinal health by repairing free-radical damage to the retinal cells. It improves circulation in the eye by keeping blood vessels smoother and more open. Cold-water fish, especially Alaskan salmon, are good eye food. Salmon also contains astaxanthin, which accounts for the pink color and is even a more potent antioxidant than lutein, vitamin E, and beta-carotene. Animal studies have shown that astazanthan can protect the retina from the damaging effect of excessive sunlight. While researchers recommend eating around 2 milligrams of astazanthan per day to prevent macular degeneration, in one serving of wild salmon you get five times that amount. Eat like an Eskimo. A study in the *Archives of Ophthalmology* found that people who have a high omega-3 DHA intake cut their risk of ARMD — the leading cause of blindness in people over fifty — in half. Tear production tends to slow with aging, leading to *dry-eye syndrome.* Eating more omega-3 fish fats also can help keep eyes lubricated.

Enjoy berry good eyes. Anthocyanin, the purple pigment in berries (such as bilberries and blueberries), helps strengthen the retina.

This helps the eyes adapt to changing intensities of light so that they can easily adjust when going from a lighted area into a dark room. Berries also help night vision and improve circulation in the blood vessels of the eyes. The healthy purple nutrients found in berries work synergistically with vitamin C, strengthening the capillary walls and the collagen structures of the eyes.

Vitamins and minerals boost eye vitality. Vitamins A, C, and E are particularly good for eye health — again, by putting out the fires caused by free radicals. Zinc is found in high concentrations in the retina, and a deficiency has been shown to decrease vision. Rich sources of zinc are turkey, shrimp, wheat germ, and pumpkin seeds.

Zinc helps strengthen the protective pigment layer of the retina and forms connections between the nerve cells in the retina. (Since copper is inhibited by zinc, if zinc supplements are used, also take 2 milligrams of copper to avoid a copper deficiency.) The Age-Related Eye Disease Study (AREDS) by the National Eye Institute found that taking high levels of anti-oxidants (500 milligrams of vitamin C, 400 IU of E, 15 milligrams of beta-carotene, 80 milligrams of zinc, and 2 milligrams of copper) reduced the risk of developing advanced ARMD by 25 percent in high-risk patients. But, it's best to talk to your doctor before using zinc supplements. For instance, in doses too high, zinc (80 milligrams) can interfere with your immune system. Strive for a minimum of 15 milligrams per day, perhaps going up to 30 milligrams with your doctor's approval.

Keep junk food out of your eyes. Junk food is particularly hazardous to eye health because the retina is mostly fatty tissue, and fat tissue is particularly susceptible to oxidative damage. Omega-3 DHA makes up most of the fat in the retinal tissue, and it is the fat most vulnerable to oxidative damage. Also, eating a diet high in junk carbs more than doubles the risk of ARMD. The junk carbs/junk vision connection seems to be due to the accumulation of AGEs (sticky stuff) in the sensitive tissues and tiny vessels of the eyes.

STAY LEAN FOR GOOD SIGHT

A Harvard study showed that in people who already had the early stages of ARMD, being overweight doubled the risk that it would worsen, and vigorous exercise three times per week reduced the risk by 25 percent. As the people in this study reduced their waist size, they lowered their risk of ARMD. This stands to reason since having less excess body fat (especially around the middle) and moving your body more decreases inflammation and improves blood vessel health, both of which can improve the health of the vital eye structures. Leanness lowers your risk of insulin resistance, which can lead to myopia, or near-sightedness. That's because insulin resistance causes the eyeball to become less sensitive to retinoic acid, a chemical produced by the retina that prevents the eye from growing out of shape, which would in turn cause difficulty focusing.

EXERCISE YOUR EYES

Just like the other muscles of the body, your eyes need exercise. Eye exercises both relax the eyes and strengthen the muscles that surround the eyeball.

Take frequent eye breaks. While reading, working at a computer, or watching TV, give yourself eye breaks. Staring too much and for too long at a screen or book can lead to myopia (nearsightedness).

Strengthen the eye muscles. As you age, you may find that you hold the morning newspaper farther away, almost at arm's length, and that the print looks a bit fuzzy the closer you bring it to your eyes. This is because the eye muscles that focus the lens of the eye weaken with age. Dr. Robert Abel, author of *The Eye Care Revolution,* recommends these exercises:

- To improve your focusing power, hold a pencil at arm's length from your eyes. Focus on the tip of the pencil and gradually bring it toward your eyes until it becomes out of focus.
- To strengthen your eye muscles, extend your arm with your thumb pointed upward and in front of your eyes. Look over your thumb at a distant object, and after twenty seconds look back at your thumb. Repeat this several times.

Rx FOR EYE HEALTH

- ❑ Wear sunglasses.
- ❑ Eat greens.
- ❑ Eat omega-3s.
- ❑ Eat berries.
- ❑ Stay lean.
- ❑ Exercise your eyes.

CHAPTER 7

Tune Up Your Hearing

Many prime timers are turning up the volume on the TV. Do you sometimes miss what your spouse is saying only to hear, "You're not listening, dear!"? By the time they are sixty-five, a third of people experience some degree of hearing loss. Occasionally, this can be hazardous to their health, such as not hearing traffic sounds or their doctor's advice. Many prime timers are reluctant to admit that they don't hear well because that would mean they're old-timers.

Here's a quick lesson on how you hear. Sound waves from your spouse, such as the words, "Please take out the trash," funnel down the ear canal and strike the eardrum, causing it to vibrate. Vibrations of the eardrum are picked up by three tiny bones, which vibrate against a fluid-filled middle-ear structure called the *cochlea*.

The fluid then vibrates against tiny hairlike cells inside the cochlea, which send impulses to the auditory nerves. The auditory nerves connect to the brain, which does all sorts of mental gymnastics to make sense of the sounds.

WHY HEARING LOSS HAPPENS

The middle ear has many tiny moving parts that, like arteries, harden with age. It's that word *stiff* again; just as joints get stiff, all the vibrating structures of the middle ear do too. The less they are able to vibrate, the less accurate they are in reproducing the quality of the sounds. Besides stiffness, inadequate blood supply to these tiny hearing parts can dampen hearing — another reason to keep your blood vessels healthy. Age-related hearing loss (ARHL) usually occurs so gradually that it sneaks up on us. Men tend to have more ARHL than women do. Here are the typical hearing-change nuisances that prime timers experience to varying degrees:

Wax builds up. Increasing buildup of dry, thick wax as we age further dampens the sound. Wax actually does good things for the ear, providing a waterproof seal that protects the ear canal while you swim and bathe, and keeping dust from reaching the eardrum. And it contains natural antibacterial substances that protect the ear canal from infections. Since the ear canal is a marvelous self-cleaner, the buildup of wax is usually naturally swept out of the ear canal or at least moved to the opening where it can be easily removed. If you notice your hearing is suddenly diminished, suspect a buildup of waxy plugs. Here's how to dewax. *Don't use cotton swabs* since all they do is push the wax toward the eardrum and possibly even damage the eardrum.

- First, soften the wax. Take a mixture of one part hydrogen peroxide and one part warm water (or a solution of one part white vinegar and one part warm water) and squirt a dropperful into your ear canal. Lie down on your side with your ear up for ten minutes. Repeat on the other side.
- Next, tilt your head to the side. While leaning your ear toward the floor, grasp your earlobe and pull down. Wiggling your earlobe works the softened wax in the ear canal toward the outer opening

where it can be easily flicked out with your finger.

- If the waxy buildup still bothers you, have your doctor remove the excess wax. Softening it with either the homemade peroxide/water solution or a similar over-the-counter wax softener before your office visit will make it much easier for your doctor to safely remove more of the wax.

Your ears become more sensitive to loud noise and background noise. The middle ear has a built-in mechanism for sounds that overload it. Normally, the middle-ear structures dampen excessively loud noises from being converted to electrical impulses so that they don't bother the brain as much. This built-in monitor also allows us to selectively block out background noises and conversation while attending to our own — known as the *cocktail-party effect.* As we age, this internal monitor also ages and starts to wear out. As a result, noisy restaurants may bother us more, especially kid-frequented family restaurants. High-pitched noises, such as train whistles and the screams of your grandbabies, can be particularly alarming. Even the barking of your beloved Fido may start to bother you. These are normal nuisances to expect and adjust to.

Hearing high-pitched sounds diminishes. Because high-pitched sounds are the first to go, it may be easier to hear male voices than female voices, causing a wife to say, "I hear him, but he doesn't hear me!" At thirty he may have ignored you; at sixty he may really not hear you. Even during normal conversation, you may have increasing difficulty deciphering high-pitched sounds and subtle differences, such as between the letters *s* and *f*.

You may miss, or misinterpret, words. The tiny hair cells in the middle ear that vibrate and transmit sounds work like amplifiers for faint sounds, such as a soft voice, but they begin to get stiff. There is the story of a woman at a cocktail party who responded happily to what she thought the person had said, "My husband is feeling fine." Yet, the speaker had actually said, "My husband is going blind." When in doubt about the gist of a conversation, it's risky to fake it. Either don't respond, or kindly ask the other person to repeat or clarify.

In addition to the usual two causes of aging for the rest of the organs (oxidation and inflammation), *repetitive exposure* to loud noises is the number one cause of age-related hearing loss. Fortunately, it's also the one that you can most easily control.

HOW "SOUND ABUSE" HAPPENS

There's a new disease in our noisy neighborhood. It's called NIHL — noise-induced hearing loss. To appreciate what your ears have to put up with, let's spend a day in the life of an eardrum and its supporting structures. You wake up with the noise of an alarm clock, the ear-piercing whistle of a train, the bark of a dog, the backfire of a car, or the construction sounds next door — and the day has only just begun. Then comes the blow-dryer for your hair, the blender for your breakfast, the traffic noise en route to work, and the iPod in your ear. During the day you have vacuum cleaners, lawn mowers, chain saws, leaf blowers, and loud TV commercials. Throw in a smattering of slamming doors and screaming children. By the end of the day, your eardrums are still shaking.

HOW TO HELP YOUR HEARING
STAY YOUNG

Just as you should protect your joints from getting stiff from too much wear and tear, you can delay the stiffening of all those middle-ear structures by selecting the sounds that strike your eardrum. Since hearing is basically about the vibrations of lots of tiny moving parts, it stands to reason that the best way to prevent ARHL is to soften the sounds that strike the parts.

Muffle loud noises. As much as possible, cover your ears to reduce loud, disturbing sounds. I wear ear protectors (like headphones without the wiring) to dampen the sound of the blender every morning when I make my smoothie. Use the kind of ear protectors that construction workers use (available at hardware stores). Earplugs are also available at pharmacies in a variety of models, from disposable foam plugs to flexible molded plugs. When choosing an earplug, look for the letters NRR (noise-reduction rating) on the package. The higher the NRR, the more the plugs mute sound. Or, you can get custom-molded earplugs that conform to your ear canals;

protecting your hearing is worth it. Forget cotton balls. They can force the ear wax deeper into the canal, and simply don't work.

Cup your hands over your ears when walking by noisy construction sites, at the sound of an oncoming train or a noisemaker at a sports event, and when watching a fireworks display. Just as you avoid a smoke-filled room, avoid loud noises whenever possible; consider them environmental toxins.

Avoid noisy travel. If you're going on a long flight, the constant roar of the engines over a long period of time can cause excessive wear and tear on those moving parts of your inner ear. Use noise-protective earphones. They not only protect your ears, but they allow you to enjoy soothing music. (I use ones by Bose.) The new and annoying train-whistle laws (loud whistle-blowing at most crossings) are hazardous to your ear health. The combination of high pitch and loudness makes train noise even more ear-piercing than plane noise. So, wear your headphones on the train too.

Hear with your eyes. Look at the speaker's lips and facial and body language, and you'll be amazed how much better you hear and understand what the person is saying.

Take a hearing holiday. Every other organ in your body needs a rest, and so do your ears. In fact, periodic noise vacations have been shown to reduce annoying noises in the ears, such as ear ringing, or *tinnitus*. As often as possible, I allow those vibrating structures in my ears to slow down and rest by choosing quiet hobbies and holidays. Golf is ear friendly, especially when you're in the middle of wide-open spaces. Some resorts offer an adult-only pool (no cell phones or loud music allowed). Of course, there's my favorite middle-of-the-ocean solitude of a sailboat powered by the whisper of the wind rather than the roar of an engine.

Can the rock concerts. Since it's not cool to sit in the back row wearing earmuffs when you take your grandson to a rock concert, try a ballgame instead. The worst combination for hearing damage is a noise that is both loud and of high frequency. If you are at a musical performance, or even a worship service, and you see cymbals next to the drums or really big speakers right up front, take that as a cue to sit in the back of the room. Two hours of loud music and clanging cymbals is a recipe for hearing harm.

Have a healthy lifestyle and hear better. The same approach that is good for every other system of the body also saves your hearing. Exercise and nutrition improves arterial health, which improves blood flow to the ear structures. Healthy nutrition, especially the anti-inflammatory foods mentioned in chapter 18, cuts down on the wear and tear to the tiny vibrating structures of the middle ear. And, reducing stress reduces wear and tear on the middle ear for the same reason it does in all the other organs. A resource I have found very helpful is *Save Your Hearing Now: The Revolutionary Program That Can Prevent and May Even Reverse Hearing Loss* by otolaryngologist Michael Seidman. In this resource Dr. Seidman also offers a list of over-the-counter and prescription drugs that can damage hearing if taken in doses too high for too long.

Amplify the sound. If you find your hearing is diminished to the extent that you're missing out on many of the beautiful sounds of life,

besides using the above noise-protecting strategies, discuss hearing aids and telephone amplifiers with your doctor or a hearing specialist.

TAME YOUR TINNITUS

Tinnitus (also called "head noise") comes from
the Latin word *tinnire,* or "to ring." Around
50 million people, including Martha and me,
experience some degree of tinnitus, or ringing
in the ears. Tinnitus and age-related hearing loss
seem to have the same main cause: noise-induced
hearing loss (NIHL). To tame your tinnitus, first
reduce excessive exposure to loud noises, which
seems to be the most common and preventable
cause of tinnitus.

Then, keep a tinnitus diary. On days that your
ears ring more than others, what did you take,
eat, or do differently? Some medications, including antidepressants, anti-inflammatories, and
even aspirin can make tinnitus worse. Caffeine,
high blood pressure, even stress or fatigue, can
trigger it. And certainly nicotine makes it worse
by giving you a bad case of "hardening of the
arteries" in the ear. I find that one of the triggers of my ear ringing is a sudden change in

position, such as hopping out of bed too fast in the morning.

Tinnitus is thought to be caused by the aging structures of the middle ear. Instead of reflecting the sounds from the outside, they produce their own distorted sound. Basically, these damaged inner-ear cells get their sounds and signals mixed up. One of the best ways to reduce the annoyance of tinnitus is to cover it up with soft background music. Your ears and your brain will focus more on the pleasant music than the annoying ringing. This is called *masking*. For more information about ear ringing, see www.tinnitus.org.

Rx FOR HEALTHY HEARING

❑ Remove excess ear wax.
❑ Wear noise-muffling ear protectors when necessary.
❑ Avoid ear-damaging noise when possible.

CHAPTER 8

Enjoy Better Breathing

As the mouth is the entry point for food, so the nose is the entry point for air. A stuffy nose is one of the top nuisances at all ages. Besides causing us to miss the comfort of taking a deep breath through a clear nose, a stuffy nose can compromise breathing and lead to a sinus infection. One of the best ways to keep irritants and germs out of your lungs and sinuses is to keep your nose clear.

KEEP AN OPEN NOSE

The sinuses are small cavities in the bones around your nose. There is a sinus inside the cheekbone on either side of your nose, one right above the nose, and one on each side of it just above the eyes. These cavities are meant to warm and humidify the air going into your lungs. Yet they can gunk up with fluid that, like water in a stagnant pond, gets infected. The body provides a natural drainage system from the sinuses into the nose to keep this from happening. However, the tiny openings between the sinuses and the nose get clogged easily, leading to sinus infections. Also, nasal irritants and allergens can cause swelling of the inside nasal passages that clogs the sinus openings and further contributes to the backup of "snot" into the sinuses. Here's my simple prescription for keeping nasal passages and sinuses clear. I call it "nose hose" and "steam clean."

Enjoy a Nice "Nose Hose"

Make your own saltwater nose drops (½ teaspoon of salt to 8 ounces of water) or buy a ready-made saltwater (saline) solution at your local pharmacy or supermarket. Spritz a few drops of the solution into your clogged nasal passages, and blow or gently suction out the loosened secretions using a *nasal aspirator,* also available at your local pharmacy.

A Neti Pot is nice. *Neti* in Indian or Ayurvedic medicine means *"water cleansing."* I have personally used this handy nasal cleaner and have recommended it in our medical practice as a very effective way to unclog sinuses. My little patients call this nose hose "Aladdin's lamp" because it looks like one. They are available at most pharmacies. The directions are provided. Put warm saltwater in the pot. Stand over your bathroom sink and tilt your head to one side. Put the spout of the pot in the upper nostril and gently tip it. The water flows through one nostril and out the other, flushing gunk out of the nose and sinuses. I believe that the Neti Pot is one of the most underappreciated preventive medicine devices.

THE BEST WAY TO BLOW YOUR NOSE

Do blow gently, one nostril at a time. This allows nasal secretions to get into the handkerchief instead of into the sinuses.

Don't hold both nostrils tightly while you blow, and *don't* blow your nose forcefully. This can jam nasal secretions into the sinus cavities and cause a sinus infection.

Savor a "Steam Clean"

Another way to loosen nasal and sinus secretions is to use a facial steamer (available at pharmacies).

Put the steamer on a table or prop it up with a few books. Add 2 drops of eucalyptus oil to the water. Place your face in the steamer while taking deep breaths of the nasal-flushing warm, moist air. To get your mind off your nose, steam clean while reading a book. A before-bed steam clean (even in a warm shower) is particularly useful.

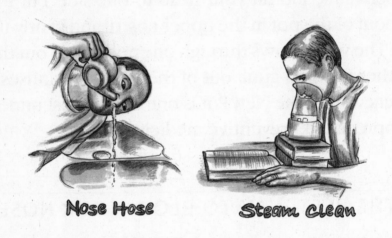

Nose Hose   Steam Clean

Vaporizers are very good. In winter, turn down the heat and put on a vaporizer. Run a warm-mist vaporizer in your bedroom. The dry air caused by central heating can thicken nasal and bronchial secretions, further compromising your airways. Normally, the airways are lined with millions of tiny filaments, or cilia, which flop back and forth like underwater sea plants to move the mucus forward so it can be coughed or sneezed out. Dry air dries out the mucus and slows this cilia action. Vaporizers have a double benefit: Besides adding nasal-friendly humidity to dry winter air, a vaporizer acts as a healthy heat source. Steaming sterilizes the water. And, remember your high-school physics? As steam condenses, heat is released; this can keep a small bedroom comfortably humid and toasty. You not only save fuel costs, but you wake up with a clear nose.

While humidifiers are fine, they are not as effective as vaporizers, especially during colder months. Humidifiers don't put out hot steam, and they are more difficult to keep clean. While the mist does produce humidity, it is not sterile and doesn't act as a heat source nearly as well as a vaporizer.

WHAT HAPPENS TO LUNGS AS WE AGE

The healthier the air that enters your lungs, the healthier you age. Loss of lung capacity does not have to be an inevitable consequence of aging. When you take a deep breath by expanding your rib cage and abdomen, your diaphragm muscles contract and the space inside your rib cage expands. This creates a pressure difference between the inside and outside, which draws air into your lungs. The more you can increase the volume of the lung cavity inside your rib cage, the more air enters your lungs. As you age:

The rib cage becomes stiffer. The muscles and bones of the rib cage become stiffer, and the diaphragm muscles may become weaker. This lessens the amount of air that can enter your airways with each breath.

Less oxygen gets into the blood. Once the air gets through your bronchi, the larger air passages, it navigates its way through smaller air passages (bronchioles), finally ending in millions of tiny balloon-like air sacs (alveoli) that fill and empty as you take a breath. Lining these air sacs are tiny blood vessels that allow the oxygen (and sometimes pollutants) to work its way through the lining of the balloons into the bloodstream, which then delivers the oxygen throughout your body. As we age, these air sacs tend to get stiffer. So it often takes more work to get air in.

Garbage-disposal system weakens. Unfortunately, the air we breathe is less than pure, so the lungs have a built-in waste-disposal system to remove toxic particles that enter with the air. The airways are lined with millions of tiny filaments called cilia, which wave back and forth like underwater sea plants. Also lining the air passages is a protective layer of mucus. This mucus traps the pollutants, and the cilia propel the inhaled pollutants up into the upper airways like a conveyor belt, and we gradually cough them out. With aging, this garbage-disposal system can gradually weaken. The more pollutants the lungs have to reject, the more likely the conveyor belt is to get stuck and the disposal system to become less efficient.

Excess fat restricts breathing. We tend to get fat as we age. Excess abdominal fat can further limit our ability to take a deep breath. Fat that accumulates around the upper airways can restrict the amount of air that gets in, especially while sleeping. This causes a common condition among prime timers called sleep apnea, meaning you don't get enough air when you sleep. (See more about sleep apnea, page 381.)

All this can lead to what pulmonologists call a decrease in maximum oxygen consumption as we age. The ability of the lungs and heart to deliver enough oxygen to the body is called the oxygen capacity, or *aerobic capacity*. By the time many prime timers reach age sixty-five, their oxygen capacity is about 30 percent less than it was when they were in their twenties.

DON'T SMOKE!

I won't belabor the point: People who smoke live shorter and sicker lives. Smoking greatly increases your chance of getting:

Alzheimer's disease   Diabetes

Stroke   Arthritis

Visual deterioration   Cancer

Gum disease   Every other disease

Cardiovascular disease

Enough said!

HOW TO HAVE HEALTHY LUNGS

You can maintain the same high level of oxygen capacity that you had when you were younger by simply being vigilant about the air you breathe and being wise about taking care of your lungs.

Breathe clean air. The less garbage that goes into your lungs, the less wear and tear on the garbage-disposal system. Pollutants in the air damage the cilia, those filaments that line the bronchial passages. Damaged lung tissue becomes scar tissue (called fibrosis), scar tissue becomes stiff, lungs become stiff, and it takes more work to breathe. Do your best to inhale clean air. As much as possible, have a "don't breathe this" mind-set. Little breaths add up. If you take about ten thousand breaths a day, the more clean breaths you take, the healthier your body. Try these tips:

Drive with clean air. A 2008 study from UCLA reported that tiny particles in vehicle emissions may be particularly harmful to the lungs. Put your air-conditioning system on recycle, especially if you are driving in traffic. Go out of your way to avoid driving behind a truck or any other large vehicle that uses clean-air loopholes to escape pollution-emission standards. If you can see exhaust from the vehicle in front of you, change lanes if possible. Avoid traffic-polluted travel.

Purify your bedroom's air. Many people take most of their daily breaths in the bedroom. If you sleep where an open window lets in polluted air, close the window and use a HEPA-type air purifier. These air purifiers are particularly useful if you have allergies and breathing difficulties from asthma. To remove pollutants that may have collected in your carpet, use a HEPA vacuum cleaner.

Enjoy houseplants as air purifiers. Put plants that produce oxygen and remove irritants from the air throughout your house. Proven pollution-reducing (and nonpoisonous) plants are:

- chrysanthemum
- dracaena
- gerbera daisy
- rubber plant
- spider plant
- mother-in-law's tongue
- bamboo palm
- weeping fig

Breathe moist air. Dry air, especially the kind produced by central heating, thickens the protective mucus lining the airways, essentially clogging and slowing cilia movement. You know how dry your skin feels after sleeping in one of those hermetically sealed hotel rooms with unhumidified air. The same thing happens to

AVOID "HOT-TUB LUNG"

The chlorine that kills the germs in the water also kills the protective lining of your airways. Many people with asthma can't use indoor hot tubs because the chlorine triggers an asthma attack. Their lungs are rejecting this polluted air, loud and clear. This is why many European countries have outlawed indoor chlorinators for pools and hot tubs and replaced them with ozone-purification systems.

At a golf resort we visited, I struck up a conversation with an apparently health-conscious prime timer in a steam room. Then I saw him get in the hot tub, turn on the bubbles, and take a short nap. His nose was about two inches above the water. I knew he was at risk for developing what is called "hot-tub lung," the cumulative effects of chlorine gas on the function of the protective cilia that line the airways. This is similar to the harmful effects of cigarette smoke. It's best to enjoy outdoor hot tubs or indoor ones with ozone-purification systems.

Longevity tip: If you can smell it, don't breathe it.

---

your airways. When the nights get cold, turn off the central heating, and turn on a hot-mist vaporizer. If you're confined in one of those hotel rooms where the windows don't open, humidify the room with a hot shower before going to sleep.

Breathe from the belly. I noticed that fitter folks breathe slowly and deeply. Most prime timers take fast, shallow breaths. As a result, much of the valuable lung tissue doesn't get aerated. To expand your lungs more and open up unventilated areas:

- Breathe more slowly.
- Breathe more deeply, from the belly.
- Exhale longer than you inhale.

The belly is like a bellows. The more you expand the bellows, the more oxygen gets into your body. A full deep breath begins from the bottom up: inflate your abdomen, then expand your chest, then lift your upper chest and collarbone. Exhale in the opposite direction: let your chest fall, relax inward, and finally let your belly deflate. Be sure to inhale and exhale through the nose in a *slow, relaxed* manner; don't forcefully tense the muscles. Deep belly breathing gives you a double physiologic benefit: it relaxes the mind and delivers more oxygen to the body. Follow these steps:

1. Inhale deeply through your nose to a count of four. Place your hand across your belly button and inhale from the gut so that you feel your abdomen pressing outward against your hand.

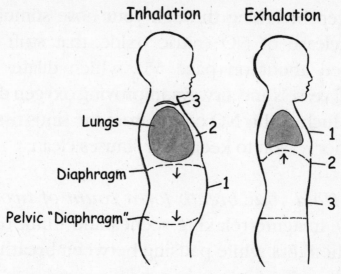

When breathing in, expand your belly balloon while your pelvic muscles descend (1), expand your lower chest (2), and elevate your upper chest and collarbone without shrugging your shoulders (3). When breathing out, let your chest fall (1), feel your diaphragm relax (2), and let your belly balloon deflate.

As you're inhaling through your nose and feeling your abdomen press out against your hand and your diaphragm descending, continue the deep breath by expanding your chest. As you are breathing in, imagine the life- and health-giving air traveling into your lungs and throughout your body. Sometimes it's helpful to concentrate on the whoosh sound of the air. Inhale to a count of four: one is the pot-belly stage, and four is the chest raise.

Deep breathing through your nose stimulates the release of NO (nitric oxide, that stuff you learned about on page 55), which dilates the blood vessels and airways, improving oxygen delivery. Much of this NO comes from the sinus tissues, another reason to keep your sinuses clean.

2. Hold your breath for a count of two (or four). Imagine relaxing scenes and think relaxing thoughts while pausing between breaths.

3. Slowly exhale through your nose for a count of six (or eight). Imagine the toxins leaving your body. (To improve oxygenation, lung doctors often encourage their patients to exhale slowly through the mouth while pursing their lips.)

Make your inhalation and exhalation *slow and rhythmic*, like an elevator going up and down,

---

WINDMILL WALK

When you're walking, periodically stretch your hands high above your head while inhaling deeply. Hold for a count of two, then slowly arc both arms down to your sides. Walking while raising and circling your arms expands your chest and allows more air and oxygen to get into your lungs.

YES FOR YOGA

If you want to get the most bang for your breath (and you're not in the middle of a meeting), do it yoga style: slowly raise your arms over your head while inhaling and slowly bring them back down to your sides while exhaling. Yoga-style deep breathing is believed to give your organs an internal massage of sorts.

not jerky. Don't overbreathe, as it can disturb your body's chemical balance. While expanding your chest, avoid shrugging your shoulders, as this lessens the volume of the rib cage. Watch babies breathe. They do it right: more belly breathing than chest breathing.

While most breathing is an automatic response to oxygen need and not a mathematical exercise, for a few minutes each day, deliberately take your breathing off autopilot and concentrate on deep belly breathing. Eventually, belly breathing will become more of your natural pattern. As I was learning the connection between better breathing and better health, I watched my friends breathe. My fitter friends breathed more slowly and deeply. Breathing rate and depth is a vital sign that deserves more attention.

In this deep-breathing relaxation exercise, you will average around four to five deep breaths per minute, a much slower and deeper rate than you're used to. Do this for a minute when starting out and gradually increase as desired. Doing too much for too long when you first start can cause you to be light-headed, so go slowly. In fact, as a general health tip, any time you do anything different, do it gradually and slowly so that your body gets accustomed to it. (See "Take a Deep Breath," page 410, as a stress buster.)

Rx FOR BETTER BREATHING

- ❑ "Hose" your nose.
- ❑ "Steam clean" your sinuses.
- ❑ Humidify dry air.
- ❑ Breathe clean air.
- ❑ Purify polluted air.
- ❑ Avoid "hot-tub lung."
- ❑ Don't smoke!
- ❑ Enjoy taking deep belly breaths.

CHAPTER 9

Be Good to Your Gums

Dentists say that people with a healthy mouth are likely to live ten years longer. Gum health can influence the overall health of your immune system. For example, heart disease can begin in the mouth. (Don't be surprised if your cardiologist first examines your gums before listening to your heart.)

WHY HEALTHY GUMS BENEFIT HEALTHY BODIES

Unlike a receding hairline, which is only a cosmetic concern, a receding gum line can be hazardous to your health. Periodontal disease is a major factor in compromised wellness and longevity. Bacteria that normally reside in the mouth secrete sticky stuff that enables these "gum bugs" to attach themselves to the teeth and gum tissue. This *biofilm* gradually hardens into plaque, called tartar, which is the stuff you hear and feel the dental hygienist scraping off your teeth.

When plaque builds up on the gum line, it can trap bacteria between the gum and underlying bone and form pockets. The bacteria, in effect, say, "We've got to eat," so they feast on the gum tissue and bone. As a result, the gum tissue and underlying bone recede, exposing the teeth roots to decay. Toxins released from the bacteria inflame the tissue, causing gingivitis, swollen, sore, and eventually receding gums. If gingivitis is not treated properly, it progresses to periodontitis, or inflammation deeper into the gums with deterioration of the root of the teeth and the supporting bone. The result is tender, red, swollen gums that bleed easily, loosening and deterioration of the teeth, and offensive breath.

The sticky stuff that collects along the gum line can trigger sticky stuff, inflammation, in your blood vessels. The pockets of bacteria that get trapped beneath the gums work their way into the bloodstream and settle in other tissues, setting up inflammation. A fascinating study of how those gum bugs can harm the heart prompted me to step up my flossing. Researchers studied plaque from patients who had undergone vascular surgery to scrape out their clogged arteries and found that it contained the *same bacteria* that were scraped out of their gum pockets. All that mischief that goes on in your inflamed gums can cause the body to send out an overzealous repair crew and contribute to inflammation of other organs, such as the cardiovascular system. Studies have shown that people with gum disease tend to have higher blood levels of fibrinogen (a blood-clotting substance) and C-reactive protein, a marker of overall inflammation throughout the body.

THREE STEPS TO GOOD GUM HEALTH

There is a correlation between the health of your gums and the health of the rest of your body, and research shows that people who have healthier gums generally live a longer and healthier life. The three steps to gum health are very simple: rinse them, clean them, and feed them.

1. Rinse your gums. Dry mouth contributes to bacterial breeding. Sip water throughout the day and swish frequently. Enjoy a cup of hot water or herbal tea, especially after eating, and swish those gum lines clean. Research has shown that green or black tea can inhibit the growth of gum-eating bacteria, reduce developing plaque, and contribute to healthier gums. Xylitol-containing chewing gum increases the natural rinsing action of saliva, and it also may reduce decay-causing bacteria. Research has shown that swishing and drinking pomegranate juice can inhibit bacteria from adhering to the teeth.

2. Clean your gums. Gingivitis begins in the *sulcus*, the space between teeth and gum tissue. Bacteria and food debris collect in the sulcus, and this is when the inflammation mischief begins. In a nutshell, to prevent gingivitis, *keep your sulcus clean.* Focus on brushing your teeth and on cleaning your *gum margins.* Here's my good-gums regimen:

- Angle the bristles of a *soft* brush forty-five degrees to the gum line and *gently* brush back and forth ten times across two or three teeth at a time. For the backs of the upper and lower front teeth hold the brush vertically.

- Clean between teeth with a *proxy brush* (a toothpick-like device with bristles on the end), going back and forth a few times just beneath the gum line at the sulcus.
- *Floss* between teeth, scraping away from gum, beginning just beneath the gum line when possible. (Don't force floss too deep between tooth and gum; you don't want to damage the tissue that binds tooth to gum.) While the floss is in a groove, angle it in a C around one tooth and slide it away from gum. Then angle the C against the next tooth and repeat. I use SuperFloss. (Sliding the floss from the gum line up to the top of the tooth prevents stuff from being forced down beneath the gum line.)
- *Scrape* your tongue with a tongue scraper, especially the back of the tongue where food residue tends to collect. Scrape as far back as you can without gagging.
- *Swish* with warm water, not only after the final brushing before bed but also after each meal.

Two to three times a week, *irrigate the sulcus,* especially around problem teeth. This is like flossing with a jet of water. While not all dentists recommend irrigating gum lines with pulsing jets of water (as you would hose junk from crevices in a sidewalk), I believe that flushing out the sulcus beneath the gum line is more effective than flossing too forcefully and jamming the sticky stuff down with floss. Ask your dentist how to use an irrigator. And, have your teeth cleaned by the dental hygienist every six months.

It's best to brush two to three times a day after meals. Do the *big brushing* steps before bed. I carry a proxy brush in my pocket for toothpicking after eating out.

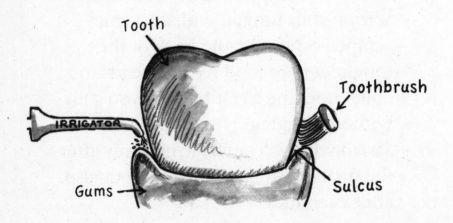

3. Feed your gums. If you eat sticky foods or sweets (such as raisins, caramel, or molasses), rinse your mouth well with warm water immediately afterward and brush as soon as possible.

Important tooth- and gum-protecting nutrients are vitamin D, calcium, folic acid, and vitamin C. (What's good for the bones is good for the teeth. See the next chapter for more on bone health.) *A word of caution:* Don't *chew* vitamin C tablets; vitamin C is ascorbic acid, and overexposure to acid can eat enamel.

Rx FOR PRIME-TIME GUM HEALTH

- ❏ Swish with warm water after eating.
- ❏ Brush efficiently twice daily.
- ❏ Clean between teeth with a proxy brush daily.
- ❏ Floss daily.
- ❏ Scrape tongue once daily.
- ❏ Use a water jet three times a week.
- ❏ Remove sticky stuff thoroughly.
- ❏ Eat gum-health-promoting foods.
- ❏ Seek professional gum and dental care at least twice yearly.

CHAPTER 10

Build Better Bones

Bones don't have to get weaker and softer as we age. Just as old brains can grow new cells, so can old bones get longer and stronger.

HOW'S YOUR BONE HEALTH?

Consider these discouraging bone-breaking statistics:

- Osteoporosis, or thinning of the bones, is the most common bone disorder in the United States, affecting about 10 million prime timers.
- Some women lose 2 to 4 percent of their bone mass per year in the first five years after beginning menopause. Called the *menopausal effect of osteoporosis,* it seems to be due to decreased

estrogen. After menopause the rate of bone loss falls back to less than 1 percent per year in many women. Bone loss tends to begin after age sixty-five in men.

- Prime timers suffer more than 700,000 spinal fractures, more than 300,000 hip fractures, and about 250,000 wrist fractures each year.
- After age fifty, more than 50 percent of American women and 12 percent of American men will suffer at least one fracture due to soft bones.
- By age fifty-five, 33 percent of American women will have had at least one spinal fracture.
- After age fifty, one in six women will suffer a hip fracture, and after age eighty-five, one in three; one in six men will fracture a hip after age ninety.
- In the Baltimore Longitudinal Study of Aging, men lost an average of two inches in height and women three inches in height between ages thirty and eighty. We become shorter as we get older because the gel-like disks between the

vertebrae of the spine become thinner; in effect, our spines shrink.

Encouraging facts. Bones do *not* automatically weaken as we age, despite what you read and hear.

- Just as you can build muscle as you age, so can you build bone.
- For every 1 percent increase in bone strength, the risk of a fracture from osteoporosis decreases by 6 percent.
- The younger you are when you start increasing your bone mass, the stronger your bones will be when you're older. An adolescent whose bone strength increases by 5 to 10 percent may reduce his risk of fractures by 50 percent in later life.
- An exercise program combined with dietary bone builders can improve bone strength and cut in half the risk of fracture for people over sixty-five.

HOW YOUR BODY BUILDS BONES

Bones are the structural steel of our bodies, and inside them a lot of good things go on. Bone marrow is the body's main factory for producing red blood cells, and bones also serve as a giant mineral bank. Ninety-nine percent of the body's calcium, 85 percent of its phosphorus, 65 percent of its magnesium, and 35 percent of its sodium is stored in the bones. These minerals help build up the bones and also are withdrawn from them when they are needed in other parts of the body.

Rebuilding bones. A fascinating give-and-take occurs within the bone bank. Bone is made up of two types of cells: *osteoclasts,* which break down bits of bone and release minerals, such as calcium and phosphorus, into the bloodstream for use throughout the body; and *osteoblasts,* which deposit incoming minerals from the bloodstream into the bone to build it up. These two groups of cells act like a maintenance crew: one cleans up any debris, such as chips of worn-out surface, and the other lays down new bone. If they get out of sync and the new-bone crew doesn't do its job, bones get thinner and weaker, resulting in osteoporosis. (*Osteo* means "bone" and *porosis* means "porous," or thin, bones.)

While bone building can occur at any age, the body builds bones more easily the younger we are. Make bone building part of your prime-time retirement plan for health. The key to healthy bone is a balanced account that contains the optimal amount of minerals. If more minerals are withdrawn than are deposited, our bones eventually go bankrupt, resulting in osteoporosis. The more nutrients we deposit in our bone banks while we are younger, the stronger our prime-time bones will be.

BENT-OVER BONES

An obvious example of osteoporosis, in which the breakdown of bone is greater than the buildup, is the humpback. Weak vertebrae gradually collapse and can no longer support the spine, resulting in a bent-over appearance.

MEASURING BONE STRENGTH

Bone-density measurements are taken to diagnose osteoporosis. The term *bone density* means how much structural stuff you have in your bones, sort of like the amount of concrete and steel in a building. The greater the amount of concrete and steel in a building, the greater its strength and the less likely it is to collapse. Our bone density usually reaches its peak between ages twenty-five and thirty. After that, we gradually lose a bit of bone density. Over a lifetime, a woman might lose up to 38 percent of her peak bone mass, and a man 23 percent. Yet, this is not written in stone. It is possible to lose little or no bone density as we age.

Low bone density does not necessarily mean you have osteoporosis. Rather, it is a sign that you *must* follow the three bone-building tips discussed later in this chapter. Oftentimes, doctors recommend tests such as bone density to motivate patients to take better care of themselves. Remember to make health your hobby.

HOW THE STANDARD AMERICAN DIET AGES BONES

As for many other ailments of aging, osteoporosis seems to be mostly an American ailment because of the standard American diet and a sedentary lifestyle.

Low calcium is not the only culprit. There's more to bone health than calcium. The

WOMEN AND BONE HEALTH

You may wonder why more women than men suffer osteoporosis and fractures as they age, especially in the United States. This is not true for all cultures. Here are some speculations about possible causes:

- American women's obsession with thinness often leads to an inadequate, bone-robbing diet. Losing too much weight too fast and having insufficient body fat can both cause bone loss.

- Nutritional surveys have shown that compared to those of men, the diets of older women are more likely to be lower in calcium. For example, one survey found that one-half of American women over fifty consume less than 1,500 milligrams of calcium a day, the recommended daily allowance of calcium in women that age.

- Strong muscles build strong bones to support them. The fact that most women spend less time than men do on strength-building exercises may account for their weaker bones.

Japanese consume half the recommended daily allowance of calcium, yet their hip and spinal fracture rate is less than half that of Americans. In fact, recent studies have shown that, overall, cultures with a lower calcium intake tend to have fewer fractures. Calcium researchers have found that Japanese women need just 640 milligrams of calcium per day, half the amount required by American women, to maintain adequate calcium levels.

When compared with Japanese women, why do American women need more calcium to maintain bone strength? It seems that American women have more lifestyle and diet-related bone-weakening factors than do women in cultures who consume less calcium. While 80 percent of calcium in American diets comes from dairy sources, in many other parts of the world calcium comes from vegetables and seafood. Could it be that while other cultures take in less calcium, the calcium they do consume is better absorbed? Should we make a change to our dietary source of calcium? Some studies show that the absorption of calcium from nondairy sources may be higher than from dairy sources. So even though people in some other cultures may eat less calcium, a higher percentage of that calcium gets absorbed, which is really what counts. The American mind-set is to take a pill and feel better. But when it comes to osteoporosis, simply taking a daily calcium supplement is not enough to support strong bones.

Other mineral deficiencies. Magnesium is another mineral that helps build bone strength, and low magnesium can contribute to osteo-porosis as well. Since magnesium is the danc-ing partner of calcium, strong bones need both. An imbalance in the calcium-to-magnesium ratio could weaken bones. A diet high in processed foods is low in magnesium. Other bone-building minerals have also been shown to be lacking in the standard American diet: zinc, manganese, copper, and boron. So, there seems to be more to weak bones than simple calcium deficiency. In a nutshell, it's not only how much calcium you eat; it's the balance between calcium and other minerals that builds better bones.

Is vitamin D more important than cal-cium? Recent studies suggest that vitamin D may be an even more important bone-building nutrient than calcium. Vitamin D is the body's regulator of bone-building minerals, especially calcium and phosphorus. Think of vitamin D as a bank teller who keeps an adequate deposit of vital minerals in your bone bank. It helps the intestines absorb more calcium and phosphorus if the bones need it, and prompts the release of vital minerals from the bones if the body needs them. It's also one of the body's most important mineral balancers. It has been found that *80 percent* of people with hip fractures may have had vitamin D deficiencies. If your doctor recommends that you take a vitamin D supplement, be sure it's the most effective form, *vitamin D$_3$.*

Too little sun? Vitamin D is also known as the "sunshine vitamin" because sunlight stimulates the skin to make vitamin D. Dr. Bruce Hollis, professor of biochemistry and molecular biology at the Medical University of South Carolina, recommends that people get their vitamin D from sun exposure rather than from pills. Researchers believe that prime timers need *at least* 2,000 IU of vitamin D daily rather than the standard recommendation of 400 IU. (Fifteen minutes of sun exposure for a person wearing a bathing suit releases 10,000 to 20,000 IU of vitamin D within twenty-four hours.) Vitamin D supplements are particularly necessary during cloudy winter months when sunbathing is impractical. Since the most healthy dose of vitamin D is still being argued, see AskDrSears.com/Prime-TimeHealth for current recommendations. Other vitamins, such as vitamins B, C, K, and folic acid, are also important in bone health.

Go fish. Another reason why Americans are so weak boned and prone to fractures is that we eat less seafood than stronger-boned cultures. Cold-water fish like wild salmon, sardines, and tuna are rich in vitamin D, and the essential fatty acids found in fish are important in forming the protein-collagen structures of the bone, making the bone stronger.

Too much animal protein. Western cultures consume the highest amount of animal protein and also have the highest rates of osteoporosis. Coincidence? Here's how that sixteen-ounce sirloin steak can weaken your bones: Protein is metabolized into acids in the body. The body fights hard to keep the acid-base

SALMON: THE BEST BONE FOOD

Wild sockeye salmon contains nearly 1,200 IU of vitamin D per six-ounce serving, as well as being the richest source of bone-building omega-3 fats. Other kinds of seafood contain less, but seafood is still your best dietary source of vitamin D. Seafood also contains calcium and many other bone-building vitamins and minerals. Nori, a dried seafood vegetable used to wrap sushi, is also rich in bone-building nutrients, such as vitamin K.

---

balance finely tuned (pH regulation). When the body makes excess acid, it needs to buffer this excess. So, it goes to the calcium bank and withdraws calcium. The calcium then binds to the acids and escorts them out of the body via the kidneys. In fact, when people lower their intake of animal protein, less wasted calcium is found in their urine.

The calcium in vegetables — think greens and beans — is often better absorbed than the calcium from animals. With an animal-based diet, we might be taking in more calcium, but we also lose more when we urinate. Also, non-animal foods tend to be rich in potassium, a mineral that helps keep calcium in the bone bank.

CALCIUM ROBBERS

Medications that can steal calcium from your body include:

- corticosteroids
- cholesterol-lowering drugs
- aluminum-containing antacids

Rich sources of potassium are fruits, vegetables, and seafood.

Research shows that vegetarians of all ages tend to have greater bone density than meat eaters. This finding is particularly significant in older people. Researchers believe that vegetarians tend to have more alkaline bodies, so they don't need to rob their calcium bank to buffer excess acids.

Too much phosphorus. Phosphorus combines with calcium like cement mix to give strength to the bone. Calcium and phosphorus partner with each other to build stronger bones, yet theirs is a delicate balance. Too much phosphorus can actually weaken the bone. Ideally, a diet should contain calcium and phosphorus in equal amounts. The standard American diet contains more than twice as much phosphorus as calcium. Meat protein, processed foods, and carbonated soft drinks (high in phosphoric acid, the fizzy stuff) are high in phosphorus. Sodas are really bad for bone health. A twelve-ounce can of cola can rob the body of 100 milligrams of calcium.

Too much salt. Remember, dietary minerals, like sodium and phosphorus, travel to the bones looking for their favorite dance partner, calcium. The calcium bank opens and pairs with salt, and they waltz their way to the kidneys where the excess calcium is excreted with the excess salt.

Too much sugar. Sugar in the diet increases the excretion of bone-building nutrients like calcium and magnesium into the urine. When sugar joins caffeine, as in sweetened beverages, there's a double whammy, causing even more calcium to be lost in the urine. Coffee lovers don't need to worry too much, since research has shown that 300 milligrams of caffeine (the amount in two cups of brewed coffee) prompts the loss of only 15 milligrams of calcium in the urine. That's not much as long as you have adequate calcium in your diet. But if your dietary calcium is marginal, even the loss of a little bit of calcium can add up.

Too much medicine. Certain medicines taken in high doses over long periods of time can rob the bones of calcium. Excessive and prolonged use of aluminum-containing antacids, for example, such as those taken for reflux or heartburn, can increase calcium loss. If you already have osteoporosis, be sure to check with your doctor about whether the medications you

---

WEAK GUT, WEAK BONES

The older we get, the less calcium we absorb. While babies can absorb 50 to 80 percent of the calcium they eat, older folks may absorb less than 30 percent. As we age, our stomach makes less acid. While that may be good for heartburn, it's not good for nutrient absorption. Adequate stomach acid is necessary to help the intestines absorb the many nutrients we need more of as we age, such as calcium, folic acid, vitamin B_6, and vitamin B_{12}. Some calcium supplements, especially calcium carbonate, are poorly digested without the help of stomach acid. As you can see, there is more to osteoporosis than simply downing more calcium.

---

are taking can increase calcium loss. Also, anti-depressants and sedatives have been linked to a higher risk of hip fractures because they increase the likelihood of falling.

HOW THE AMERICAN LIFESTYLE WEAKENS BONES

As the standard American diet weakens bones, so too does a sit-too-much, sedentary lifestyle. Exercise is the best preventive medicine for osteoporosis. Like muscle, bone strength follows the "use it or lose it" principle. Even injured athletes who need to rest their bones for a prolonged period of time — in a leg cast after a fracture, for example — lose a significant amount of bone during that period. When you build muscle, you also build bone, since these two depend on each other for strength. By some built-in body talk, the stronger muscles tell the bones, "I need you to be stronger to support me," and the bones cooperate.

Here's how exercise makes the bones stronger. Movement increases blood flow, which also brings nutrients to the bone-building cells. It stimulates the parathyroid gland to secrete hormones that promote calcium absorption in the intestines and buildup of calcium in the bones. Part of the bone structure, called spongy bone, is actually softer and acts somewhat like a shock absorber when weight is applied. When you stand, the weight slightly compresses the softer parts of the leg bones. This compression

WORRY WEAKENS BONES

You may have heard the term *stress fracture*, which really means tiny fractures, usually in the bones of the feet, caused by overuse of certain bones and joints. But there is another type of stress fracture: weak bones caused by mental stress.

A recent finding showing that women with depression tended to have lower bone densities called attention to the stress/bone-loss relationship. Depression decreases bone-strengthening hormones. Anxiety increases the stress hormone cortisol, which increases calcium loss in the urine. Factor in the general poor nutrition and inactivity that often accompanies prolonged depression, and you have a recipe for weaker bones. Relaxation and meditation lower stress hormones and increase the bone growth hormone DHEA-S, dubbed the "youth hormone."

triggers a signal in the bone to grow and repair the wear and tear, similar to the way muscles grow when they are exercised.

The effect of movement on bone health has been shown in tennis players, whose bones in the dominant arm can be 20 percent stronger than the bones in the other arm. Weight lifters often have the strongest bones. It stands to reason then that walking would build stronger leg bones than swimming. Although all movement is good for the bones, weight-bearing exercises, where the bones actually strike or push against a weight, such as walking, weight lifting, dancing, jogging, and tennis, are best; they build stronger bones.

THREE WAYS TO BUILD BETTER BONES

Now that you know what causes bones to stay strong or get weak, build your own bone-strengthening program by following these helpful guidelines:

1. Be Good to Your Gut

As you've learned, you can swallow all the bone-building vitamins and minerals you want, but if they don't get through your gut and into your blood, they will just wind up in the toilet. To build up your gut health to better absorb these nutrients:

Follow the rule of twos. Eat twice as often, eat half as much, and chew twice as long.

Drink hot beverages, such as water or herbal tea, with your meals. Cold beverages or ice water with meals can weaken digestion. Ask for water at room temperature — specify that you want it with no ice and not chilled.

2. Feed Your Bones

It helps to compare bone-building to bone-breaking foods in your body's nutrient bank (see next page). Think of these bone-building foods as deposits in your bone bank and as insurance against excess withdrawal.

Reduce processed foods. The fresher the food, the higher the nutrients. Eat lots of fresh fruits and vegetables, whole grains, and seafood, and you're unlikely to have a nutrient problem in your bones.

BONE BUILDERS AND BONE BREAKERS

As long as the deposits exceed the withdrawals, your bones and body are healthy. If the reverse occurs, bone health deteriorates. Here are the nutrients your bones need and the foods that best supply these nutrients.

Bone Builders	Bone Breakers
Vitamin D	Phosphorus (excess)
Calcium	Animal protein (excess)
Magnesium	Sodium (excess)
Seafood	Carbonated beverages
Omega-3s	Sweetened beverages
Vitamin C	Caffeine (excess)
Vitamin B	Some medications
Vitamin K	Stress (unresolved)
Folic acid	Sunlight (too little)
Zinc	Sitting (too much)
Sunlight, appropriate for your skin type	
Weight-bearing exercises	

Calcium supplement guidelines. As you learned earlier, simply popping a calcium pill will not prevent osteoporosis. The reason that

BEST CALCIUM-CONTAINING FOODS

Food	Calcium (milligrams)
Yogurt, nonfat, 1 cup	450
Sardines, 3 ounces	370
Parmesan cheese, 1 ounce	336
Orange juice, calcium-fortified, 1 cup	300
Tofu, 3 ounces	190
Salmon, 3 ounces, canned	180
Collard greens, ½ cup	180
Rhubarb, ½ cup	174
Spinach, ½ cup	136
Cereal, calcium-fortified, ½ cup	100–200

the recommended daily allowance for prime timers over sixty-five has recently been raised to 1,500 milligrams of calcium is because of all the other calcium-robbing factors mentioned above. Chances are that most of us could get by with eating less calcium, and no or fewer calcium supplements, if we minimized the mineral-robbing effects of our diets and lifestyles. If, after following our dietary and lifestyle guidelines, your health-care provider still recommends that you take a calcium supplement, consider these guidelines:

- Calcium is best absorbed when taken in *smaller amounts more frequently* and with meals. You're better off taking a 500 milligram tablet twice a day than taking two tablets all at once.
- Most doctors recommend the calcium citrate form of supplement because this is better absorbed by the intestines and is not dependent on stomach acid (which can be diminished in some prime timers) for absorption.

3. Move

Don't be a lazy bones. Lazy bones tend to be weaker bones. The more weight-bearing exercises you do, the stronger your bones will stay. When your weight pushes on bones and your muscles pull on bones, this push-pull effect stimulates the bone-building cells to start growing more bone. See chapter 22 for how to develop your personal strength-building program.

So, as is true for all the other systems in the

body, it seems that diet and exercise are the two best medicines for bone health.

Rx FOR PRIME-TIME BONE HEALTH

- ❏ Eat more bone-building foods.
- ❏ Eat fewer bone-weakening foods.
- ❏ Be careful with calcium-depleting medicines.
- ❏ Take calcium, magnesium, and vitamin supplements, if necessary.
- ❏ Enjoy weight-bearing exercises to strengthen bones.

CHAPTER 11

Rejuvenate Your Joints

My golf friend Mark became an iBod. Soreness and stiffness in his knee and shoulder joints limited his enjoyment of golf, so he preferred to sit and watch TV rather than to move and play. As a result, he put on more belly fat, which increased the severity of his arthritis and made it even more uncomfortable for him to walk, which further increased his belly fat, and the painful cycle escalated.

Each year, millions of prime timers limp into doctors' offices seeking treatment for their sore joints. Joints, particularly the ones that bear the most weight, such as our knees, can slow us down as we age. Taking care of our joints is especially important because pain and limitation of movement can keep us from exercising, which in turn can cause us to suffer even more infirmities. The less we move, the more we get sick — it's as simple as that. Since knee, back, and shoulder problems top the list of aging-joint nuisances, we will focus on these, though the same principles apply to all the other joints in the body. (For example, what is good for the knee is also good for the hip joint.) Consider this joint-health program *"prehab"* for prime timers — getting your joints conditioned to avoid injury and rehabilitation. We can improve the health of our joints by:

- strengthening the muscles that support the joints;
- feeding the joints the right nutrients; and
- keeping the joints moving and well lubricated.

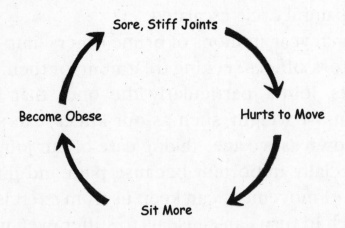

KNOW HOW YOUR KNEE WORKS

Since the knee joint is the one that seems to slow us down most as we age, we'll begin with some knee knowledge.

The knee seems like a simple hinge joint, but its design is marvelous and complex. The knee bends, straightens, and rotates. By understanding what the parts of the knee do to choreograph these movements, we can better appreciate how to take care of them.

Muscles that support and move the knee. Two major muscle groups run from the femur (thigh bone) across the knee joint, and their tendons attach to the tibia, the major lower leg bone. The muscles on the front of the thigh are the quadriceps, or "quads." The quads cause the knee to straighten after you bend it and are the most important muscle group for the knee. The muscles behind the thigh bone that run down the back and sides of the knee to the tibia are called hamstrings. When hamstrings contract, the knee flexes, or bends. The hip muscles and buttocks muscles also play a role in walking and running and help to stabilize the knee and hip joints.

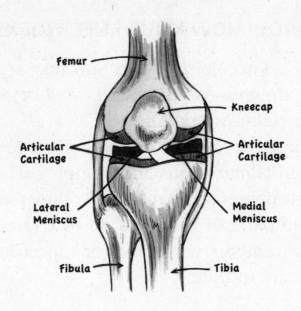

Lateral and medial meniscus. Menisci are like rubber doughnuts made of fibrous cartilage and collagen bundles, thick structures that are attached to the tops of the tibia and fibula, the lower leg bones. They serve as cushions, or shock absorbers, protecting the knee from excess force. Menisci also lubricate and feed the joint by producing synovial fluid, an egg-white-like substance. They add support to the knee by keeping the leg and thigh bones properly aligned with cartilaginous cups (see illustration). As we age, these collagen bundles loosen and the menisci soften, in much the same way that collagen breaks down in the skin, allowing it to wrinkle. The once-strong surfaces of the menisci become filled with fat deposits rather than dense fibrous tissue. Because of their limited blood supply, the menisci heal very slowly when torn or damaged. They are particularly susceptible to twisting injuries. I actually tore my meniscus while doing the twist.

Articular cartilage (AC). This smooth, slippery surface lining the ends of the thigh and lower leg bones is so named because when bones move against each other, they are said to articulate. Next time you're preparing a chicken or a turkey, separate the thigh from the drumstick and notice the shiny, smooth articular cartilage on the ends of the bones. That's what young cartilage is supposed to look and feel like. The AC helps your joints work in three ways: It provides a smooth surface for the upper and lower leg bones to glide over each other as the knee bends; the smoother the surface, the more efficiently the ends of the bones glide. Like menisci, the AC functions as a shock absorber and is able to sustain loads of up to ten times our body weight during daily activities such as walking and running. Last, it protects the underlying bone. Wear and tear and roughening of the AC happen with aging and osteoarthritis.

The AC does not have its own blood or fluid supply, so it has to rely on the underlying bone for nourishment. The area where the cartilage joins the bone acts like a slightly wet sponge. The constant compression and release during normal walking, for example, causes synovial fluid, carrying nourishment and repair nutrients, to move in and out of the layers of the cartilage. When we take a step and bear weight on the knee, the joint fluid is squeezed out. When we lift our foot to take another step, the joint fluid rushes back into the cartilage and is ready to cushion the next step. This nourishing fluid moves in and out as our cartilage responds to changing forces exerted on the knee.

Healthy AC reduces stress on the underlying bone. Following an injury, the cartilage has diminished resilience, and with increased wear and tear, arthritis or inflammation of the cartilage and underlying bone can develop. While the cells within the cartilage (called chondrocytes) are able to regenerate themselves and repair damaged cartilage, with age the ability of chondrocytes to regenerate lessens. Movement nourishes the cartilage and keeps it younger.

Knee ligaments. As you can see in the illustration of the knee, the ends of the thigh and lower leg bones are connected to each other with strong, fibrous bands called ligaments. These ligaments can be torn during high-impact or twisting sports injuries, such as might occur during football, basketball, soccer, or tennis.

FIVE WAYS TO BE NICE TO YOUR KNEES

By now you have learned that "move more" is a key to prime-time health. If you can't move much because your knees hurt, the health of your whole body suffers.

1. Stay Lean
Being overweight harms the joints in four ways:
- It increases the weight the joint has to bear.
- It limits the ability of the joint to move.
- It throws the body out of balance when you walk, which puts further strain on your hips, knees, and ankle joints.

- Excess body fat (especially abdominal fat) spews inflammatory chemicals into the bloodstream that can settle in the joints, increasing wear and tear and leading to arthritis.

Excess weight is especially aggravating to hip and knee joints. For every extra pound of body weight you carry, you put over *three times* as much load on your hips and knees. So, if you're carrying an extra twenty pounds, your knees have to bear an extra sixty pounds every time you take a step.

Here's the typical knee scenario for many prime timers: At forty, your knees are fine. Then you put on a pound a year, and by age sixty, your knees start bothering you. Remember, that extra twenty pounds of weight translates to an extra *sixty* pounds of pressure your knees have to bear. Also, carrying more weight around the middle triggers an off-balance posture when walking, which causes more stress on the knee, back, and hip joints.

When you see an obese person do a waddle walk, it's a sign that the hip joints are already arthritic. The waddle walk leads to a more

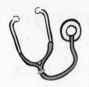

DR. SEARS SAYS...
Lean equals less wear and tear everywhere.

bowlegged stance and puts uneven pressure on the knees, resulting in more arthritis. Finally, the increased load on the feet causes the arches to fall, which is why so many obese people suffer from painful flat feet. Staying lean is Joint Health 101.

2. Strengthen the Muscles That Support the Knee Joint

The knee joint is only as strong as the muscles around it. We all know that muscles move our joints, but we forget that they also protect them. This is especially true of the knees and is why strengthening exercises are so important when recovering from knee injuries. Strong muscles also take some of the load off the knee joint and can prevent injuries. To get a feel for the importance of your leg muscles (especially the quads and the hamstrings), while walking place your palm against the side of your thigh with the thumb on the quads and the fingers on the hams. Notice that every time you take a step and bear weight, your thigh muscles contract and get hard. Without help from these strong muscles, your knee joint would have to bear all the weight, leading to more wear and tear and arthritis. The quads are the key muscles supporting the knee. Strong quads protect the knee by absorbing some of the weight as your heel strikes the ground.

3. Tread Lightly

Prior to tearing my medial meniscus (the shock absorber that lines the knee joint), I was a heel pounder. Like most men, I was a heavy walker — clomp, clomp, clomp! Now I walk much more softly. Develop a less heel-pounding gait that takes much of the pressure off your heels and therefore your knees. Some sports medicine clinics will do a gait analysis and then show you how to improve your walk so that you put less pressure on your knee joints.

Cushion your heels. To further minimize joint jarring while walking, get a running shoe with shock-absorbing heels. Also, use heel cushions, sponge-rubber inserts available at most pharmacies and sporting goods stores. Routinely wear heel cushions *before* your knees and ankles start to hurt.

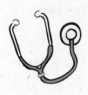

DR. SEARS SAYS...
When a body part talks, listen to it. Pain is a signal that some change is needed in how you are using your joints.

Lower your heels. Since legs are often "the last to go," some women are tempted to continue showcasing them with high heels. Say so long to the spikes and save your knees and back. Legs don't look very lovely wrapped in a cast while you recover from a fall.

4. Feed Your Joints

The better you nourish your knee joints, the better they work. The healthier your diet, the less the inflammation and wear and tear. The two main inflammatory problems of the knee joint are *arthritis* (wear and tear and roughening of the articular cartilage and underlying bone) and *synovitis* (where inflammatory cells get into the synovial fluid). When inflammatory stuff gets into the synovial fluid, it's like bathing the cylinders

OIL YOUR JOINTS

Fish oil gets our vote as the top superfood for the joints. Fish oils help rebuild damaged articular cartilage, mainly through their anti-inflammatory properties. The body is constantly in a state of breakdown and repair. The omega-3 fatty acids in fish oil deactivate the enzymes that cause cartilage to break down, which enables the repair process to speed up. In a Danish study, people with arthritis who ate an average of four ounces of fish daily had less joint swelling, morning stiffness, and pain than those who did not.

---

of your car engine with dirty oil. Eventually, it can damage the moving parts of the knee joint. The sixteen superfoods in chapter 13 are super for joint health.

5. Move

Movement helps you stay lean and therefore keeps excess weight off your joints. It also strengthens the muscles that support the joints and bathes the structures of the knee with synovial fluid. Just as a well-traveled highway needs periodic resurfacing, so does the knee joint. Movement mobilizes the repair crew. The repetitive loading and unloading of the knee joint, such as occurs during weight bearing and rest when walking, draws nourishment into the cartilage from the underlying bone.

Studies show that a healthy low-impact activity such as walking not only helps repair worn-out cartilage in the knee joint but also builds new cartilage.

Unlock your knees. Avoid standing for long periods of time with your knees locked. Locking the knees causes the joints of the knees and the back to bear most of the weight, instead of sharing the load with the muscles, and increases the wear and tear on the knee joints.

Pump your synovial fluid. Just as oil doesn't move in your car engine when the engine is shut off, neither does synovial fluid move through the knee joint when you rest. Movement, especially flexion and extension (called pumping — the same motion you use when cycling), causes the synovial fluid to lubricate the knee joint. I noticed during recovery from my knee injuries that I instinctively pumped my knee joints, even while standing in line. This both takes the weight

Rx FOR A KNEE INJURY: ICE OR HEAT?

Both. Ice relieves pain and swelling, which is why it's good to use it for a day or two immediately after an injury, especially if there is swelling or tenderness around the knee joint. Once the swelling subsides, alternate cold and heat, which increases the blood supply and delivers healing nutrients to the joint. Don't use heat right away. If the knee starts to swell, heat will increase the swelling, and even bleeding, into the knee joint.

off the knee for a while and allows the synovial fluid to heal the irritation and soften the pain. Knee pumping is one of my anytime, anywhere exercises (for more see page 622).

HAVE A NICE KNEE WORKOUT

The purpose of the knee exercise program is to strengthen the muscles supporting the knee, improve the shock-absorbing structures that protect the knee, and replenish the synovial fluid and articular cartilage that nourish the knee. See chapter 22 for a list of additional leg exercises that strengthen the hip and knee joints.

Walk Well

Walking is a great workout for the knees. As much as possible, walk on flat surfaces, which mainly involves compression of the knee joint with minimal twisting or sliding. With hill walking, there is a sliding and possibly abrasive motion that can stress the knee. (Knee joints are like a ball and socket. When walking downhill, the top half of the body moves the weight forward and *slides* the thigh bones [the ball] forward.) Running or walking downhill is harder on the knee joint than going uphill. Your stride lengthens, and the weight and impact on the knee can easily double going downhill. Sustained downhill walking also creates a lot of pressure on the knee joint because of the forward sliding of the joint on the downhill knee. Try zigzagging downhill to lessen the stress on the knee. (See also related back-care tips, page 263. These are also nice to the knees.)

Land Exercises

The more you strengthen your hip, thigh, and leg muscles, the better they support your knee joints. Try these:
- Quad curl
- Hamstring curl

DOES GOLF HELP OR HURT THE KNEES?

Both. Walking and other movements associated with golf help keep you lean, which decreases the wear and tear on all the weight-bearing joints. Yet, if you play golf you need to be particularly diligent in following this whole knee-health program. Walking downhill is hard on the knees. The sudden torque or twisting toward the end of a golf swing can do a number on the knees, particularly the left knee for a right-handed golfer. That's how Tiger Woods injured his left knee; he needed a surgical repair and missed six months on tour. The cleats on golf shoes can contribute to meniscus injuries by anchoring the lower leg and preventing it from moving with the knees, causing a twisting tear.

If you are an avid golfer, especially if you already have knee issues, consult a golf pro. Have a video analysis of your swing done and learn how to modify your technique to take some of the final torque off your forward knee.

- Toe raises (this is really a partial squat): Bend your knees slightly (don't lock them), flex slowly up on your toes, hold for 10 seconds, descend.

- *Careful* squats (prime timers need to be careful with squats, as squatting too forcefully and deeply can damage the knee; don't attempt squats with free weights without the supervision of a trainer)
- Cycling (one of the best knee exercises because it pumps the knee joint without putting any rotational forces on it)
- Elliptical trainer (my favorite — I believe the elliptical trainer gives a more effective workout than a stair-stepper because it also moves the upper body)

Pool Therapy

Water works well because it offers three-dimensional resistance. Water is also wonderful for the joints because there is no pounding or twisting. Last, water relaxes.

- Water walk: Walk forward, backward, and sideways in chest-deep water with as normal a gait as you can.
- March in water: Lift your knees to ninety degrees or as high as you can without feeling knee pain.

- Standing leg swings: Stand erect and hold on to the side of the pool for stability. Swing your leg straight forward, then swing it down and to the rear. This stretches and strengthens your quads and hamstrings. Next, lift your leg out to the side as far as possible to stretch your groin muscles, then bring it back across your body to the other side to stretch your hip muscles. Repeat this sequence with your other leg.

- Flutter kick: While holding on to the side of the pool with both hands, kick your feet.

- Dolphin kick: If you have had a previous medial meniscus injury, avoid the frog kick, as this can further injure the tissues of the medial aspect of the knee. Instead, enjoy the dolphin kick (pumping both knees).

- Scissor kick: As a daily breast-stroke swimmer, I often use the scissor kick (the one used in the side stroke) instead of the less-knee-friendly frog kick; the scissor kick stretches and strengthens the hip muscles.

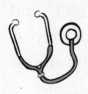

DR. SEARS SAYS...
Don't jerk the joints. Sudden twisting can tear tight muscles and the menisci in the knee joint. Stretch to warm and loosen muscles before engaging in twisting movements such as dancing and golf.

TEN TIPS FOR A BETTER BACK

What often makes prime timers look young or old is their posture. Remember your mother and grandmother lovingly poking your back and saying, "Stand up straight. Don't slump over"? They were right. Yet, the older we get, the more slumped we tend to become. In fact, the older we get, the better our posture needs to be because our bones and muscles aren't as resilient as they were when we were younger. Preserving the natural S curve in the spine is the key to back comfort. Unfortunately, many of the ways we use our backs (sitting, bending, lifting) misshape that natural curve. To save your S curve:

1. Head Ahead
Good head posture means keeping the chin parallel to the ground, the neck long, the shoulders

relaxed downward, and the pelvis tilted slightly forward. If your posture is poor, the neck and upper back are bent forward (kyphosis), or there is swayback (lordosis). Try these posture pointers:

- **Center your head over your body; don't flex it forward.** While standing or walking, imagine that a string is attached to the top of your head, pulling you toward the sky. Ask a friend to videotape you standing and walking and watch to see what posture adjustments you need to make. Or take a pole, yardstick, or golf club, place it behind your head and back, and walk around while keeping the pole in contact with your head and lower back and perpendicular to the floor. Stand in front of a mirror and get a feel for proper posture. When your head is held correctly, your whole spine is more likely to be in proper alignment.

- **Look up to the sky.** Think about it: You spend most of your day looking down — using the computer, reading a book, and watching where you walk. It's no wonder that years and years of looking down causes the neck muscles to weaken and backbones to bend, eventually giving the typical stooped-over appearance of old age. To give the neck muscles and backbones a lift, periodically look up. This stretches your neck muscles and straightens your backbone. As often as possible, try to keep your head up, even while walking. Look down with your eyes, not your head.

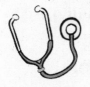

DR. SEARS SAYS...
Preserve your lumbar curve.

2. Stand Smart

Stand straight but not too straight. Standing strains the back. The key to standing smart is to divert some of the weight bearing from the lower back to the muscles of the hips and thighs. "Stand short" (knees slightly bent) instead of "standing tall." (Don't lock your knees and rigidly straighten your back.) Feel your thigh muscles flex. To help strengthen the structures of your back:

- *Bend your knees* slightly instead of locking them, which transfers some of the weight to your thigh muscles from the knee and back joints.

- *Tilt hips* and pelvis slightly forward, tucking in your buttocks. This often requires tightening the buttock and abdominal muscles. This is in contrast to arching your back and letting your abdomen protrude when you stand.
- To lessen the strain on your back, stand with your hips flexed by *placing one foot on a stool or step.* This will keep your lower back from sliding forward when you have to stand for any length of time. (Did you ever notice that bars have foot rails to help patrons stand more comfortably for longer periods?)

3. Sit Smart

Sitting too much can stress the back. Contrary to popular belief, the chair is *not* a back's best friend. Here are some sit tips:

Sit straight. Instead of slumping over, keep your head in line with your back (remember that

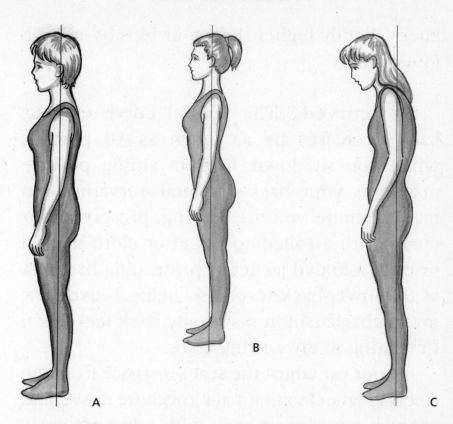

Healthy posture showing proper alignment between head, shoulders, hips, and ankles (A); more rigid posture with a swayback and locked or hyperextended knees (B); typical stooped-over posture caused by the habitual head-down position (C).

string), and your neck perpendicular to the seat of the chair. When sitting, put as much weight as possible onto your feet, and keep one or both knees slightly higher than your hips by using a footstool.

Sit "curved." The natural curve of your back decreases by as much as 30 percent when you sit down. Correct sitting posture maintains your back's natural curvature. No matter where you are sitting, preserve your curve with a rolled-up towel or cloth napkin or even a folded jacket. A protruding backrest at the lower-back level also helps. I love how my lumbar cushion makes my back feel when I'm sitting in my writing chair.

In your car, adjust the seat's distance from the steering wheel so that your knees are raised, and support your lower back with a lumbar cushion. Putting the seat too far back and extending your legs causes your lower back to bend forward, yet placing it too far forward puts you too close to the air bag if it deploys. Try to get it just right.

Sit for a shorter period of time. Avoid sitting for a long period of time and then suddenly springing up. Many back injuries are due to sudden twists or a sudden stretch of stiff ligaments.

Sit comfortably. Use a chair that adjusts in height. (I use the Steno chair from Staples.com.)

- Sitting in a chair that is too high increases swayback, but one too low flattens the lumbar spine. It's best to keep your feet flat on the floor or on a footstool and the knees level with or slightly higher than hips.
- Swivel the chair to get up to avoid twisting your back.
- Have an adjustable backrest that conforms to the natural curvature of the spine.

Sit slow and soft. Descending butt first onto a hard chair is tough on the disks between the lumbar bones. Ease slowly into a cushioned seat. While riding in hard-seated vehicles, like a bus, on bumpy roads, cushion your seat if possible. Your coat can serve as a cushion in a pinch. Sitting on a hard seat when driving on a bumpy road or jumping onto a hard surface constitutes lumbar-bone bashing. Picture blocks (your lumbar spine) compressing a gelatinous cushion in between.

Dr. Stuart McGill, director of the Spine Biomechanics Laboratory at the University of Waterloo, Canada, teaches that prolonged sitting is hard on the lumbar disks and is a major contributor to low-back pain. He recommends taking standing breaks: stand and while inhaling deeply, slowly stretch your hands to the ceiling. This lumbar extension exercise relieves the prolonged pressure on the lumbar disks that occurs while sitting. If you're sitting at your desk and the phone rings, get into the habit of standing while talking.

Stand up correctly. Here's how to lessen the strain on your lower back when going from a seated to a standing position. Instead of leaning forward with your shoulders (which is lousy for your lumbar spine), keep your spine straight, hinge forward at your hips, and with your hands on your knees or on the armrests push up.

4. Lift Smart
   • To avoid lower back strain — and pain — *use your legs.* Don't use your back as a lever. Bending at the waist

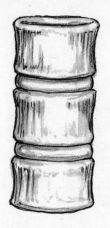 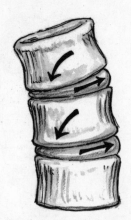

Intervertebral disks are like fluid-filled doughnuts that act as shock absorbers for the spine. Repeated compression from bending, and wear and tear from twisting, can lead to weakening and rupture.

and lifting puts too much strain on the lower back muscles. When preparing to lift a heavy object:

1. Bend your knees and keep your back straight.
2. Pull the object onto or close to your thighs.
3. Gradually stand up, allowing the legs to bear most of the weight.

- When moving a heavy object off a table, don't bend at the waist toward the object. Instead, keep your upper body perpendicular to the floor, and the

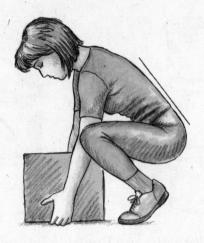

heavy object as close to your body as possible.

- Try to avoid lifting heavy objects above the level of your elbows. Doing so arches and strains your back.
- If your back is sensitive, be careful when reaching or stretching upward, such as when you need something out of a high cupboard. Instead, stand on a stool. Be especially careful when reaching up to change a lightbulb, since your back tends to arch in this position. If you do need to reach up, do not twist or rotate your body, and stand straight up.
- When using a broom or raking, stand up straight rather than bending over.

THE BIGGER THE BELLY, THE WEAKER THE BACK

A heavy belly tilts the pelvis forward and downward, and the belt line moves down. This extra weight in the front exaggerates the curve in the back (swayback), eventually wearing out the lumbar spine. In addition to causing back pain, a protuberant front weighs down the hip and knee joints, leading to arthritis. The best way to avoid a knee or hip replacement is to reduce your excess belly fat! (See page 280 for exercises to strengthen your back.)

5. Carry Smart

Carrying heavy bags can be bad for the back. To distribute the weight onto the other muscles of your body rather than solely on the back:

- Carry heavy objects as close as possible to your chest and abdomen. This helps your lower body bear much of the weight. If you extend a heavy object in front of you, most of the weight is borne by the back muscles.
- When holding grocery bags, try to distribute the weight evenly on both sides, in the same way you would hold barbells of equal weight in each hand.

6. Stoop Smart

When possible, squat instead of bending over. When bending over, keep your back straight and your knees bent. Never bend over without first bending your knees. Contrary to popular belief, the spine is not really a joint in the way that shoulders, arms, hips, and knees are. While the spine will bend to accommodate the usual daily movements, the more you can preserve its normal S curvature and use the other joints, the better your back's health will be.

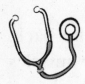

DR. SEARS SAYS...
Hinge your hips—don't bend your back.

7. Sleep Smart

Sleeping on your abdomen or on your back with your feet straight out is bad for the back. Try to preserve the natural curvature of your spine. Because sleeping flat stresses the lower spine, it may not be smart. These are the best sleeping positions for back health:

- Sleep on your side with a pillow between your flexed legs (A).

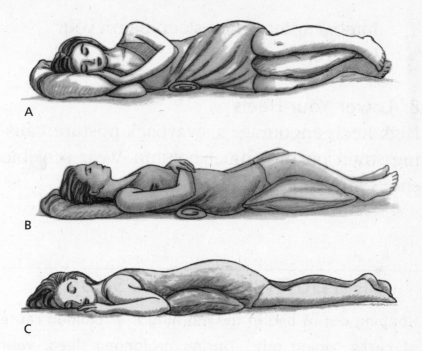

A

B

C

- If you prefer sleeping on your back, place a large pillow under your bent knees, which lessens pressure on the back (B).
- If tummy sleeping, place a small pillow under your abdomen to prevent overarching your back (C). Prolonged tummy sleeping forces you to twist and strains your upper spine.
- Try placing a folded towel between your waist and the mattress when sleeping on your side, and under your

lumbar spine when sleeping on your back (optional).

8. Lower Your Heels

High heels encourage a swayback posture, causing strain on the spinal column. Wear sensible shoes, and your back will thank you.

IF YOU TWIST, YOU'LL SHOUT

Hopping out of bed in the morning is a common cause of backs "going out." During prolonged sleep, your lumbar disks swell, making them prone to injury from sudden torques. Avoid sudden twisting. Instead, roll over on your side, use your hands to push your upper body up into a sitting position, place your feet on the floor, and then stand. Slinging your feet over the side of the bed torques the back—ouch! Follow a similar back-friendly procedure when getting into and out of a car. When getting into a car, ease yourself into the seat backside first. When exiting a car, open the door, turn your whole body to plant your feet on the ground, then hold on to the door for support as you slowly stand up. Don't twist as you enter or exit a vehicle.

---

9. Strengthen Your Front Muscles

To have a strong back, you need a strong front. Strong abdominal muscles support the curved part of the lower spine. Weak abdominal muscles allow the spinal column to sag forward, causing swayback. With swayback, the vertebrae tend to bulge forward, putting pressure on the cartilaginous disks between them and on the nerves that branch out between the bones (see illustration on page 271). This can cause pain and muscle spasms. If a disk becomes displaced or ruptured, the pain can be intense and disabling. Sometimes a weak or ruptured disk can cause *lumbago,* painful catches in the lower back, or *sciatica*, a sharp pain along the leg and buttocks. Strong muscles are like guy wires that anchor the spine, protecting its natural curvature. Fit bodies and fit backs go together. As back surgeon Arthur White says, "The flag looks good if the pole is straight."

10. Strengthen Your Back Muscles

Like any joint, the backbone is only as strong as the muscles supporting it. The stronger and more balanced the back muscles, the better they support the bone. Exercise regularly.

EXERCISE DON'TS

Before we get to exercises for building back strength, familiarize yourself with the don'ts of exercise:

- **Avoid sudden, jerky, bending-over movements.** Backs often "go out" when you drop something and reflexively bend over or twist to pick it up. Mentally program yourself to stop *before* you stoop. (See "Stoop Smart," page 274.)

- **Don't speed up sit-ups.** Avoid *full* sit-ups in which you place your hands behind your head and pull your neck and back all the way up to a sitting position. This is too hard on the neck joints and the lower back. Instead, do a partial sit-up or crunch by lying with your lower back flat on the floor, bending your knees, and lifting your head and shoulders up only about a quarter of the way, with your arms crossed over your chest.

- **Twist the hips, not the back.** Twisting the top half of the body independently of the lower half with those soft-gel lumbar disks caught in the middle is—ouch! Rotate wisely. If you're doing rotation warm-ups, say with a golf club or a baseball bat, be gentle and don't jerk quickly or rotate too far. The older the back, the more careful you have to be about jerky, rotating motions. When doing rotating motions, I imagine that my shoulders and hips are connected. Practice by putting your hands flat against your outer thighs, and turn your hips and shoulders together as a unit. Your lumbar spine will love you!

- **Don't bear too much weight on your back.** As we get older, we have to be increasingly careful when lifting weights to strengthen our back muscles. Do this with the supervision of a knowledgeable trainer. Be especially wary of barbell presses in which you place the bar behind your neck and lift. Simple walking is always good for the back, since the back-bones have to share the weight bearing.

GREAT BACK BUILDERS

The Superman exercise. Also known as the airplane, this is one of my favorites. Lie across a large exercise ball on your chest. Spread your legs for stability, and keep your toes on the floor. Raise your back and arms. Hold for 10 seconds. Repeat three times.

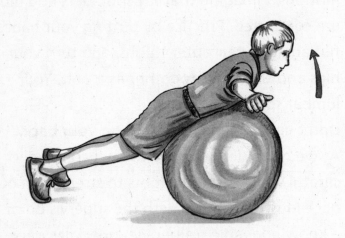

The shoulder and leg raise. Here's a more strenuous version of the Superman. Lie flat on your stomach (with a small pillow under your abdomen) with your hands at your sides and lift your upper body off the ground. Hold for 10 seconds. You'll feel the muscles in your back working to keep your chest up. Next, add one leg raise, toes pointed to the floor, then raise both legs. While your legs are raised, keep your head raised only slightly. Be sure to keep your toes pointed to the floor when doing this exercise, as twisting the legs can strain the hips and lower back.

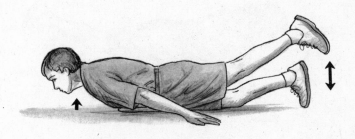

The head lift. Lie on your back with your knees bent and your hands under your lumbar spine. Tighten your abdominal muscles, and lift your head straight up. Hold for 10 seconds. Relax and repeat five to ten times.

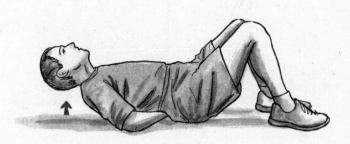

The bird dog. Get on all fours. Extend your right arm and left leg. Tighten your abdominal muscles, and keep your head down and in line with your back. Hold 10 seconds. Repeat three times using opposite arm and leg.

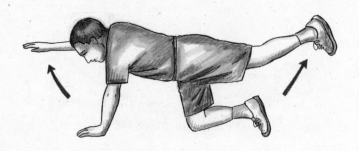

The back press. Another yoga favorite. Lie on your back with your knees bent. Take a deep breath, then exhale, contracting abdominal muscles and pressing lumbar spine against the floor. Don't arch your back during this exercise. Hold for 5 seconds and repeat five times.

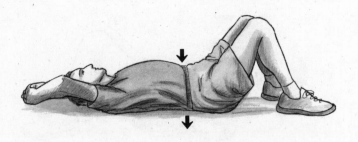

SAVE YOUR SHOULDER

The shoulder enjoys the greatest range of motion of any joint in the body. We use it to throw a ball, comb our hair, and scratch our backs, among other things.

Like the hip joint, the shoulder joint has a ball-and-socket design. The ball end of the arm fits into the rounded socket area of the shoulder, and these bones are held in place by the *rotator cuff,* four muscles that encircle the joint. If healthy, these cuff muscles allow the bone to freely and painlessly rotate in all sorts of directions. To help cushion this movement, a *bursa,* a fluid-filled sac, is strategically located between the arm bone and the top of the shoulder bone.

With the wear and tear of aging, two things can happen: the muscles of the rotator cuff can weaken, and the joint surfaces can get inflamed, or roughened, both of which lead to painful limitation of motion. Because the muscles surrounding the shoulder joint weaken with age, they are more prone to injury when you fall on an outstretched arm, wrench your shoulder lifting a heavy object, or, as happened to me, wrestle with your teenage son.

The sliding surfaces of the joint are also prone to inflammation (tendinitis) from simple overuse. Rotator cuff tendinitis is particularly common in overhead sports, such as swimming and tennis. This is one of the main reasons major-league baseball pitchers need to rest their shoulders frequently and are discouraged from throwing too many pitches per game.

SIX WAYS TO SAVE YOUR SHOULDER

Because this joint is one of the slowest to heal, I can't emphasize enough the importance of strengthening rotator cuff muscles and tendons to prevent injuries. The stronger these supporting structures are, the less prone the shoulder is to injury.

1. Feed your shoulder joint. Stick to an anti-inflammatory diet. If you strain your shoulder, load up on anti-inflammatory foods, especially higher doses of phytonutrients and omega-3s. (For a list of anti-inflammatory and healing foods, see page 476.)

2. Think before you move. Many shoulder injuries occur when you move hastily, such as grabbing a heavy suitcase from the overhead compartment on a plane or hauling a heavy object with one arm when you're in a hurry. (Both of these movements are also bad for the back.) Before you lift anything heavy, first think about how you can safeguard your shoulder — or even wait until you have help.

3. Rest your shoulder. Wear and tear from overuse can lead to tendinitis of the rotator cuff structures. If you do a lot of overhead sports, such as tennis, take an occasional day off to rest the shoulder joint. Taking a long rhythmic walk is not just good for the legs, it's good for the shoulder joint. The natural swinging motion of the arms while walking keeps rotator cuff muscles fine-tuned.

4. Warm up cold muscles. Rushing into swimming, sprints, or a tennis match with cold muscles and tendons is a recipe for tears and tendinitis. Always warm up muscles first with M&Ms — movement and massage. Do a minute of windmill rotations and a minute of self-massage to get the blood moving. Deep heat massage, such as from a Jacuzzi jet, gives a double benefit: it warms the muscles and increases blood flow; and, if you've had a recent injury or strain, it decreases the formation of scar tissue.

5. Stretch your shoulder. (For more on stretching, see page 656.) After you have done the windmill warm-up, try these stretches:

- *Hands behind back.* Clasp hands behind your back and slowly lift them up. Hold stretch for 20 seconds. Repeat three times.
- *Pull against rail.* Grasp a countertop or railing and gently pull. Hold for 20 seconds. Repeat three times.
- *Push against doorjamb.* Stand in an open doorway and push against it. Hold for 10 seconds.
- *Arms above head.* Extend arms overhead with palms touching. Stretch arms up and back.
- *Arms out in front.* Lock your fingers together and extend your arms in front of you. Turn your palms outward and gently rotate arms in a circle.

- *Shoulder shrug.* Shrug your shoulders up to your ears. Hold for 10 seconds then relax.

6. Move your shoulders. Remember the golden rule of healthy joints: joints are as healthy as the muscles supporting them. The stronger

---

EASY ON YOUR ELBOWS

The elbow has the dubious distinction of being the only joint to have sports injuries named after it: tennis elbow (pain on the inside of the elbow) and golfer's elbow (pain on the outside). Tennis elbow is an inflammation caused by overuse and just requires rest. Golfer's elbow is due to *abuse* and is a sign that you need to correct your swing.

To prevent elbow tendinitis, try these elbow-strengthening exercises, both shown on pages 648–49:

- Finger flex
- Squeeze-ball finger flex

Also, try wraparound elbow pads (available at tennis shops) to remind yourself to use your elbow joints properly during sports that involve swinging a racquet or club.

---

your shoulder muscles are, the better they are able to protect your rotator cuff. Try these exercises to strengthen your rotator cuff muscles:

- *Swimming.* The breaststroke and overhand stroke are two of the best movements for strengthening rotator cuff structures. Swimming is easier on the shoulder joint than stop-and-start sports like tennis and volleyball.
- *Stretch bands.* Stretch bands are safer and easier on the rotator cuff muscles than free weights. Free weights require more concentration to avoid jerky movements that can damage the muscles or tendons. While anything is possible, it's hard to overdo it with stretch bands. (See "Strike Up the Bands," page 648.)

Rx FOR PRIME-TIME JOINT HEALTH

❑ Stay lean.

❑ Strengthen the muscles that support the joints.

❑ Don't pound your heels while walking.

❑ Use heel cushions.

❑ Eat an anti-inflammatory diet.

❑ Move the joints.

❑ Enjoy water movements—pool therapy.

❑ Don't jerk the joints.

❑ Stand and sit with proper posture.

❑ Preserve the natural lumbar curve while sitting and sleeping.

❑ Stoop, lift, and carry smart.

CHAPTER 12

Keep Your Skin Looking Younger

We all know about the effects of sun and wind on skin. Yet, there is more to skin health than what's on the surface. Keeping your skin healthy means not only protecting it from the elements but also nourishing it from the *inside*.

HOW SKIN CHANGES DURING PRIME TIME

Your skin weathers with age just like anything else; for example, the covers on your patio furniture or the paint on your car. By learning about the stages of wear and tear that normal skin goes through during prime time, you can take preventive measures to keep your skin more youthful.

Skin gets thinner. Over the years, the skin's built-in repair system slows. Normally, the old cells on the surface of the skin slough off and are replaced by new cells, but as we age old cells aren't replaced as readily by new ones. As a result, the outer layer of the skin gets thinner. Declining estrogen during menopause also contributes to drier, thinner skin. Thinner skin is more vulnerable to environmental irritants such as clothing, soaps, and especially the sun.

Skin gets drier. The sebaceous glands of the skin — called *natural moisturizing factors* — slow down in their production of natural oils and so trap less of the skin's natural water. The drier the skin, the more sensitive it is to further drying by environmental irritants, prompting a vicious cycle.

Skin has less bounce. The underlying fibers of tissue, called elastin and collagen, weaken, leading to lines and wrinkles, especially around the eyes, the forehead, and the corners of the mouth. Expression lines deepen, revealing years of frowning and laughter. While young skin bounces back like a trampoline, older skin loses its elasticity so laughter lines gradually become etched in the skin. Since hair, skin, and nails come from similar cell lines and have a similar cellular regulatory mechanism, the same aging mechanism that causes hair to thin and nails to become more brittle also causes the skin to become weaker, thinner, and drier.

Skin gets stretched. The typical increase in body fat during prime time stretches the skin unevenly, causing dimply areas.

Skin gets darker. The sun stimulates natural pigment-producing cells called melanocytes, which darken the skin. As we age, pigment production occurs unevenly, resulting in the telltale age spots that all prime timers eventually get.

Skin gets stressed. We often forget that what bothers the brain also bothers the skin. Stress stimulates an inflammatory response — or wear and tear — which is reflected in the skin.

Skin gets less "productive." Normally, skin that is exposed to sunshine produces vitamin D. As skin ages, it produces not only less natural moisturizer but also less vitamin D, prompting some researchers to advise that as we age we need *more* sun exposure, not less.

SIX WAYS TO KEEP YOUR SKIN LOOKING AND FEELING YOUNGER

Skin health is more than just skin deep. It is not only about what you put *onto* your skin; it is also about the nutrients you put *into* the underlying tissue that supports your skin. As we were writing this section on skin health, we were building an extension onto our patio. First we laid down a bed of sand over the soil, over which we placed a layer of bricks. I realized that skin health is much like patio construction. The outermost layer is what we see: the bricks, layers of thick skin cells. Yet, underlying those layers is the supporting structure of subcutaneous tissue, which is composed of fibrous tissue, fat, and then muscle. If the sand and soil underneath the bricks are not supportive, the bricks will sag.

These skin-health tips will help keep your skin looking good and help prevent undue aging and weakening of the muscles and tissues underneath.

1. Water it. Much of the normal water loss from your body is due to evaporation from the skin. Since water is the primary component of skin and its underlying tissues, it makes sense to keep the skin well hydrated. Aging skin becomes thinner and drier, especially if it's been sun damaged. Thinner skin doesn't retain moisture well, and the natural moisturizing oil-producing glands become less productive. You need to moisturize your skin the right way. Here's how:

- Drink eight to ten glasses of caffeine-free fluids daily. Even though you may have read lately that the "eight glasses a day" recommendation was downgraded to an "unproven myth," that's only because the purists decided that there were no scientific studies to support it. Despite what science doesn't say, I believe it makes good sense to hydrate your body well. Foods high in water content, like soups and fruits and vegetables, contribute to overall fluid intake.

DON'T SMOKE!

Besides excessive sun exposure, the most common cause of premature aging and wrinkling is smoking.

- Moisturize the air with a humidifier, a vaporizer, or a pan of water on your radiator. This is especially important when your central heating is on. Try to keep the humidity in your bedroom to at least 50 percent; higher can cause mildew. (You can buy an inexpensive humidity-measuring device called a hygrometer at your local hardware store.) Cut down on central heating during the winter months by running one or two hot-mist vaporizers in the bedrooms. The steam not only humidifies the air but provides a cleaner and healthier source of heat.

SOAK AND SEAL!

After bathing or showering, gently *pat* your skin dry rather than vigorously rubbing it. Apply a moisturizer to help seal in the water while your skin is still a little damp.

2. Wash it—lightly. Thinner skin is more easily irritated by soaps and scrubs. Use mild soaps (preferably those with built-in moisturizers) and don't scrub. The purpose of cleansing is to remove the worn-out, superficial skin cells, which prompts the underlying skin to replace them with more youthful cells. Scrubbing with harsh cleansers can remove some of the natural moisturizing factors in the skin and make it drier. Vigorous cleansing can also remove natural skin proteins, called aquaphorines, which control moisture retention. If you have dry skin, don't use soap on it every time. Use warm water rather than hot water for bathing, since hot water can rob the skin of some of its natural oils.

3. Cover it. How do you recognize a man over forty? When outside, he wears a baseball cap — or should. The older we get, the more we need to cover our skin, especially the face. Excessive, intense exposure to the sun damages collagen, the elastic tissues that weaken with age. Dermatologists refer to sun damage as "chewing of the skin." Sun damage is a vicious cycle: repeated, intense sun exposure thins the skin and damages its self-protective mechanisms, and over time this makes the skin even more vulnerable to sun damage.

To lessen photo aging, use a *sunblock* rather than sunscreen. Sunblocks (which contain zinc oxide or titanium dioxide) reflect the sun's damaging rays away from the skin. In contrast, sunscreens absorb the damaging rays. While some sunblocks may be less visually attractive (some look like a dab of diaper paste on the nose), others are clearer and less opaque. If you do use sunscreen, use one with an SPF (sun protection factor) of at least 15. (I've been using the same sunscreen on my face for the past ten years:Aloe-Kote, an emollient with an SPF of 25.) Be sure to apply sunscreen at least twenty minutes prior to sun exposure since it takes a while to sink into the skin. Sunblocks can be applied immediately before exposure. Here are other ways to protect your skin:

- As much as possible, avoid direct midday sun exposure between 12 a.m. and 2 p.m.
- Wear a wide-brimmed hat.
- Wear protective clothing. There are whole lines of summer-wear clothing that use tight-weave fabrics and are treated to shield you from sunlight.

4. Feed it. Junk food grows junk skin. In my medical practice, the look and feel of a person's skin often gives a clue to the quality of their nutrition. Remember the AGEs (or stiff and sticky stuff) you read about on page 34? AGEs infiltrate collagen, the protein structural fibers of the skin, and weaken its elasticity, causing skin to sag. All the superfoods listed in chapter 13 are super for the skin. In particular, I recommend the following:

Fish. Seafood is the top skin food. I first discovered the health effects of omega-3s on the skin in 1999 when I began prescribing omega-3 supplements and a diet higher in seafood to infants and children with all kinds of dermatitis — from eczema to dry, scaly skin. I still remember one of my first "experiments" with a newborn who had congenital icthyosis, a hereditary condition in which the skin is thick and scaly, almost like that of a fish (the Greek word for fish is *icthyos*). I advised the breastfeeding mother to eat large portions of wild Alaskan salmon and to take omega-3 supplements. Within a month the baby's skin improved markedly, compelling the university dermatologist to remark, "What on earth are you doing? We've never seen a

IS OUR SKIN UNDEREXPOSED TO THE SUN?

There's an ongoing battle between vitamin D researchers and dermatologists about the optimal amount of sun exposure. Researchers believe that vitamin D deficiency from underexposure to the sun is a prime factor in cardiovascular disease, colon cancer, and especially osteoporosis, and that vitamin D is a natural skin anti-inflammatory. Dermatologists argue that sun overexposure causes skin cancer. I consider sun exposure like a health food, an essential vitamin, that needs to be dosed appropriately for your skin type. Fair-skinned people need less sun exposure to get adequate vitamin D than dark-skinned people do. Again, *balance* is the key. (Please read *The UV Advantage* by Michael Holick.)

baby improve so fast before!" High doses of omega-3s were the answer. I then started using omega-3 therapy for children with eczema and dry, scaly, or unhealthy-looking skin. Again, remarkable results. The skin, like all the other organs of the body, is only as healthy as each cell. Omega-3s work their magic by increasing the fluidity of the cell membrane and strengthening it to keep the good stuff in and the toxic stuff out. Try to eat seafood, preferably wild Alaskan salmon, three times a week, or take an omega-3 supplement of 1 to 2 grams daily, or as advised by your health-care provider. (See recommended dosages of omega-3s, page 310.)

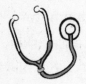

DR. SEARS SAYS...
If you don't want your skin to feel scaly like a fish, eat more fish.

Eat antioxidant, anti-inflammatory foods. Because the skin is exposed to environmental damage, it needs high doses of dietary antiaging "medicines" to protect it from inflammation. So, add lots of fruits and vegetables to your seafood diet, particularly green and yellow ones.

Spice up your skin. We sprinkle turmeric on salad and in salsas at least several times a week. Spices are healthy anti-inflammatories for the skin. (See "Spice Up Your Life," page 360.)

5. Relax it. The skin and the brain are intimately connected. Witness your goose bumps when you are nervous or excited. Unresolved stress releases inflammation-producing chemicals into the skin, which accelerates aging, not to mention more frown lines. Keep stress to a minimum (see chapter 15).

6. Move it. Increasing blood circulation to the skin through exercise not only helps remove waste products that may accumulate there but also increases the delivery of antioxidants from seafood, fruits, and vegetables. Also, strengthening the underlying muscles makes the skin more taut and less dimpled, which helps to diminish cellulite.

In a nutshell, your skin will stay healthy longer if you do just what your mother always told you: eat more fruits, vegetables, and fish, and go outside and play.

Rx FOR PRIME-TIME SKIN HEALTH

❑ Drink lots of liquids.

❑ Don't smoke.

❑ Humidify the air.

❑ Use *mild* soap.

❑ Don't scrub harshly.

❑ Get the right amount of sun for your skin type.

❑ Eat fish.

❑ Eat fruits, vegetables, and spices.

❑ Strengthen underlying muscles.

PART III

Prime-Time Well-Being

Well-being and being well! That's the goal of every prime timer. In part III you will learn the four *S*s of prime-time well-being: superfoods, sound sleep, subdued stress, and satisfying sex. These four account for much of the "peace of mind" component of the Prime-Time Health plan. Much of your prime time will be spent eating and sleeping, so you might as well enjoy it. And, science says that people who sleep better, manage their stress better, and enjoy more satisfying sex live longer and healthier. Let's start with the sixteen superfoods that can most influence prime-time wellness.

CHAPTER 13

Eat Well with the Sixteen Superfoods

Hippocrates famously pronounced, "Let food be thy medicine and medicine be thy food." When the good doctor said this more than two thousand years ago, all food was real. But today there is good medicine and bad medicine. A modern Hippocrates might say, "Think *nutraceutical* instead of pharmaceutical." A simple fact of prime-time life is that those who *eat* better *live* better.

To qualify for our superfood list, a food must:
- be nutrient dense (packing the most nutrition for the calories)
- contain nutrients that have proven benefits
- be nature made rather than factory made
- taste good and be satisfying

- be able to be prepared in a variety of ways
- contain no ingredients that are harmful to health

While the following foods are healthy for all ages, they are ideal for prime timers. Each contains one or more nutrients that research has shown promote healthy aging. Most of these superfoods have what I call the AAA effect: anti-inflammatory, anticancer, and anti-Alzheimer's.

Foods That Lengthen Prime Time	Foods That Shorten Prime Time
These foods contain the healthiest nutrients.	*These foods have little or no nutrient value and can be harmful to your health. That's why we call them antinutrients.*
Seafood, especially salmon	Hydrogenated oils, trans fats
Berries, especially blueberries	
Spinach	

Foods That Lengthen Prime Time	Foods That Shorten Prime Time
Nuts	High-fructose corn syrup
Olive oil	Highly processed oils (e.g., cottonseed oil)
Broccoli	
Oatmeal	
Flaxseed meal	
Avocados	Most processed French fries
Pomegranate juice	Charred meats
Tomatoes	Sweetened beverages
Tofu	Artificial colorings
Yogurt	Preservatives
Red onions	Gelatin desserts
Garlic	Nitrite-preserved meats
Beans and lentils	Artificial sweeteners (sucralose, aspartame)
	Flavor enhancers (e.g., MSG)
	Foods with numbers on the label (e.g., red #40)

GO FISH

Suppose you are preparing for prime time, and you don't want to be a metabolic mess. You make a list of all the ailments you don't want to get: Alzheimer's, depression, poor vision, cardiovascular disease, and all the "-itises" — gingivitis, colitis, bronchitis, dermatitis, and arthritis. Or, suppose you are already a metabolic mess. Yet, you're a "show me the science" type of patient, concluding, "I'm only going to put pills in my body if they are backed by solid science done by university professors in white coats." So, you do your research and select the top doc in the world for your head-to-toe metabolic makeover. You hop on a plane to visit the top doc. You say, "Doctor, I'm here to get the most scientifically proven medicine for my metabolic mess." Top doc hears your history, but instead of reaching for a pad and scribbling out a prescription, she surprises you and reaches in the bottom drawer and hands you a fish. Surprised, you say, "Doctor, I want medicine!" The doctor replies, "You asked me for the preventive medicine that is backed by the most scientific research. I'm giving you the medicine that is backed by more than ten thousand published medical journal articles."

In part II, you learned why seafood is the top superfood. Fish high in omega-3s acts like an all-purpose medicine, or *polypill*. Here's an overview of what science says about the health benefits of omega-3. It:

- **builds better brains:** lowers the incidence of Alzheimer's disease; lessens age-related cognitive decline; acts like a mood stabilizer to relieve aggression, anxiety, and depression; prevents strokes; alleviates attention deficit disorder
- **helps hearts be healthy:** lowers high blood pressure, lowers high blood cholesterol, prevents the heart from misfiring, prevents blood clots, prevents heart attacks
- **is good for the gut and endocrine system:** lessens inflammatory bowel disease, reduces the risk of colon cancer, lessens diabetes
- **enriches eyesight:** lessens age-related macular degeneration, improves visual acuity, moistens dry eyes

- **builds better bones:** lessens osteoporosis, "oils" squeaky joints (antiarthritic)
- **improves immunity:** prevents those "-itis" illnesses: arthritis, bronchitis, cognitivitis (Alzheimer's disease), colitis, dermatitis
- **alleviates asthma:** potent anti-inflammatory against bronchitis
- **reduces cancer:** especially colorectal and prostate cancers
- **softens skin:** prevents dermatitis, eczema
- **helps with weight control:** fills you up with more nutrition in fewer calories

How much omega-3 should you eat each day? I base my own omega-3 consumption on the recommendations of the International Society for the Study of Fatty Acids and Lipids (ISSFAL) and the U.S. National Institutes of Health: at least *600 milligrams* of omega-3s (DHA and EPA total) per day.

ISSFAL and NIH base their recommendation on pure science, unlike the USDA, which is swayed by special-interest groups and, at this writing, still has not published a daily recommended value for

GO FISH, AND STAY YOUNG

Here's where science really shines. A 2008 study published in the *American Journal of Clinical Nutrition* showed that in 254 patients with an average age of eighty-two, those who had the highest level of the omega-3 eicosapentaenoic acid (EPA) lived the longest. A medical truism for healthy aging is "You're only as young as each cell in your body." Why? Here's the cellular basis of omega-3s and healthy aging in a nutshell: Omega-3s are biochemically known as the "flexible fat." They are just the opposite of stiff and sticky animal fats. Lipid chemists (fat experts) dub them "cell conditioners" because they soften cell membranes. With aging, cell membranes, like joints, become stiffer. Omega-3s help cell membranes retain their fluidity so they can let in the nutrients the cell needs and screen out toxins.

omega-3s. In its revised food pyramid, the USDA does recommend two four-ounce servings of fatty fish per week, which would provide about 3,500 milligrams of DHA plus EPA per week, or 500 milligrams per day. Also consider:

- Eating 6 ounces of *wild salmon twice a week* would give you the equivalent of 600 milligrams of omega-3s (DHA and EPA) daily.

- Or, take *at least 2 grams of omega-3 oils per day* (which should equate with getting at least a total of 600 milligrams of DHA and EPA). For best results, be sure the omega-3 oils contain the two most important fatty acids: DHA and EPA in a 1:1 to 2:1 ratio, the ratio that naturally occurs in wild salmon.
- If you need to take omega-3s for therapeutic reasons, for example as an anti-inflammatory for arthritis or if you are at high risk for cardiovascular disease, consider taking at least *3 grams of omega-3 fish-oil supplements per day.* For neurological problems or mood disorders, your doctor may recommend taking *5 to 6 grams per day.*
- The source we recommend in our medical practice is Sockeye Salmon Oil from vitalchoice.com.

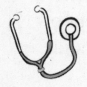

DR. SEARS SAYS...
For optimal prime-time health, eat 6 ounces of wild salmon at least twice a week.

SOS: NO SHARK OR SWORDFISH FOR SENIORS

As a general guide, the bigger the fish, the longer it lives; and the more predatory the species, the more mercury and other pollutants it is likely to contain. Shark and swordfish usually top the list for pollutants, so it would be wise for prime timers not to eat these two fish.

What kind of fish is best? Our favorite is wild Alaskan salmon (preferably king or sockeye) because it has the heart-healthiest oil profile, and it's tasty. Be sure it is wild and not farmed, which is less expensive but contains more pollutants and fewer healthy fats. Too expensive? What's your health worth? We order our salmon directly from Alaska, as do many of the patients in our medical practice. Try vitalchoice.com. (For other fish, see "Traffic-Light Seafood," page 315.)

Does eating too much processed vegetable oil lessen the healthful effects of omega-3 oils from seafood? Yes! To get the best results from your dietary "oil change," it's not enough just to eat more fish and fish-oil omega-3s. You also must *decrease* how many omega-6 foods you eat (see "Prime-Time Oil Changes," page 80). The same enzymes metabolize omega-3 and omega-6 oils into nutrients for body tissues. A diet high in omega-6s hogs the enzymes so not enough are left to utilize the omega-3s. Cultures that enjoy the longest and healthiest prime time, such as the Japanese, eat around a 1:1 to 1:3 balance of omega-3s and omega-6s. Studies show that people who eat more omega-3s and less omega-6s enjoy many more years of prime-time health — a powerful motivator that helped me change my oils!

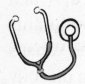

DR. SEARS SAYS...
For more years of prime-time health, eat *more* omega-3 oils and *less* omega-6 oils.

What about the mercury in seafood or fish-oil supplements? The good news is that the richest source of omega-3 oils — wild salmon and other seafood from the pristine waters of Alaska — is also the safest. Always ask the source of the fish. Farm-raised seafood, such as salmon, has much greater concentrations of industrial chemical contaminants — biopollutants such as PCBs (polychlorinated biphenyls) — than wild

TRAFFIC-LIGHT SEAFOOD

Green-Light Fish (enjoy without worry)[*]	Yellow-Light Fish (eat in moderation)[†]	Red-Light Fish (don't eat!)[‡]
Salmon, wild Alaskan/ Canadian (canned or fresh)	Salmon, Atlantic	Shark
	Mahi-mahi	Swordfish
Artic char	Tuna, albacore	Tilefish
Tuna, Pacific[§]	Lobster	King mackerel
Tuna, canned light	Halibut, Atlantic	Marlin
Halibut, Alaskan	Orange roughy	
Anchovies	Sea bass	
Sardines	Shrimp, Atlantic	
Catfish (U.S.)		
Rainbow trout		
Shrimp, Pacific		

Green-Light Fish (enjoy without worry)*	Yellow-Light Fish (eat in moderation)†	Red-Light Fish (don't eat!)‡
Sablefish, Alaskan Cod, Pacific		

Note: For the most current cautions about risky fish, see AskDrSears.com.

* For easy-to-understand advisories on seafood safety, see www.vitalchoice .com.

†The Environmental Protection Agency (EPA) recommends limiting intake of these fish to no more than 12 ounces per week.

‡These large, predatory fish are most likely to be contaminated.

§ Know the source. Troll- and pole-caught tuna tend to be smaller and contain fewer contaminants than long-line, deep-water tuna that tend to be larger and therefore more contaminated.

fish, mainly because of the pollutants in the fish feed. Until the government starts setting higher standards for fish-farming safety, we recommend sticking with wild seafood, especially salmon. Canned salmon also tends to be wild and is usually labeled as such. Mercury and PCBs are more likely to be found in large, fatty predatory fish, such as shark and swordfish, and also in industrially contaminated lake fish. It's wise to avoid them. Fish-oil supplements are purified of possible pollutants. For the omega-3 supplements and safe seafood we recommend, see AskDrSears.com.

At this writing, most experts who have reviewed the studies have concluded that the medical benefits of eating seafood far outweigh the risks. I agree!

PICK BLUEBERRIES

Blueberries could rightly be called the body's "repair berry." Blueberries contain more anti-inflammatory nutrients than most other fruits. Most of these nutrients are found in the dark blue skin of the blueberry, which is full of phytos called *flavonoids,* specifically anthocyanin, an antirust antioxidant that helps keep the brain healthy. Although most of the studies thus far have been done in the laboratory on experimental animals, researchers have shown that blueberries can reverse the effects of mental aging and improve balance and motor coordination. Here's a summary of their health benefits. Blueberries:

- improve neurotransmitter function of the brain
- reduce inflammation throughout the body

SUPPLEMENT YOUR DEFICIENCIES WITH REAL FOODS

We have listed the nutrients that science says prime timers tend to be deficient in as well as the best food sources of these nutrients.

Nutrients You Need	Best Food Sources
Vitamin C	Guava, papaya, cantaloupe, kiwi, strawberries, orange juice, chili peppers, sweet yellow peppers, broccoli
Vitamin D	Sunshine and salmon (see full discussion of vitamin D needs, page 230)
Vitamin E	Raw sunflower seeds, raw almonds, peanut butter, wheat germ, avocados, fortified cereals

- improve blood flow and cardiovascular health
- lessen the risk of cancer
- help you see better
- decrease belly fat

Nutrients You Need	Best Food Sources
Folic acid	Think green, leafy vegetables, asparagus, lentils, pinto beans, spinach, kidney beans, avocados, papaya, wheat germ, fortified cereals
B_{12}	Sardines, salmon, wild game, wild shrimp, lean beef, lamb, yogurt, milk, eggs
Zinc	Lean beef, lamb, wild game, shellfish, pumpkin seeds, yogurt, sesame seeds, green peas, spinach, tofu
Magnesium	See page 526.
Selenium	Brazil nuts, seafood, eggs, shiitake mushrooms
Omega-3s	Wild salmon, sardines, tuna, trout

Blueberries are also dubbed the "belly berry." A study from Japan suggests that the anthocyanins in blueberries somehow "talk" to preadipocytes (cells, especially in belly fat, that turn into fat cells) and convince them not to become fat cells. (To learn more about this brainy berry, see "Have a Berry Good Brain," page 113.)

GO GREEN

You learned why green is good for the brain in chapter 4, but eating greens is so important that we want to elaborate a bit more here. While I was growing up, my mother, like all mothers in our neighborhood, used Popeye's muscles to get me to eat greens. And, like most kids, I resisted. Now, after researching how good greens are for us, we have our own garden of spinach, collard greens, kale, and Swiss chard. Greens are a rich source of vitamins A, B, C, E, and K. Spinach and asparagus are high in the brain-vitality vitamin folate. Folate, also called folic acid, is a critical repair nutrient that helps maintain genetic codes for tissue health. Greens are also high in calcium, potassium, and magnesium. Spinach, collard greens, Swiss chard, bok choy, and broccoli are some of the best nondairy sources of calcium. Broccoli is one of the best vegetable sources of vitamin C. And, greens are loaded with fiber.

Greens are great for the eyes, and this is where their nutrient profile really shines. Spinach, Swiss

VEGGIE TIPS

- Cook vegetables *lightly* with minimum water (for example, steam or stir-fry) so they maintain their bright color and are still crunchy. A pale, mushy veggie is a less nutritious one.
- Choose smaller fruits and vegetables, such as cherry tomatoes, which have a higher skin-to-pulp ratio, because the colorful skin is high in antioxidants.
- Enjoy a *colorful* plate. Phytonutrients give fruits and vegetables their rich color. Health is where the color is.
- Eat as many *raw* veggies as you can.
- Eat organic produce to keep the "garbage" (pesticides) out of your body and, as recent studies reveal, to receive more nutrients. (Organically grown vegetables are higher in nutrients than conventional produce.)

chard, collard greens, and kale are the top sources of the vision-saving carotenoids lutein and zeaxanthin. (For more about eye nutrients, see chapter 6.) A good green rule to remember when you're shopping: the greener the veggie, the greater the nutrition. Eat spinach and romaine lettuce; forget iceberg (we call it "see-through" lettuce).

BE NUTTY

Raw nuts are one of the most nutrient-dense foods you can eat. They are rich sources of protein, healthy fats, fiber, vitamin E, calcium, and many other vitamins and minerals. Yes, nuts are high in calories and fat, but they are *healthy* calories and healthy, cholesterol-free mono-unsaturated fats. Because of nature's perfect balance of healthy fats, protein, and fiber with a minimum of carbs, nuts enjoy one of the highest satiety factors — filling you up with less — of any food. Because of this appetite-taming perk, people who snack on a palmful of nuts (instead of and not in addition to chips) tend to eat less at the next meal. Those skinny little nuts, unless you mindlessly overeat them, are unlikely to make you fat.

My jungle story. In 2006 I volunteered to serve as a doctor after the tsunami in Indonesia. As I was packing for the trip, one of my friends

SCIENCE SAYS . . .

Nut eaters tend to:

- have less heart disease
- have lower blood levels of cholesterol and triglycerides
- be leaner
- suffer fewer gallstones

sent over packages of homemade trail mix. I almost didn't take them along since I thought we'd have plenty of food over there, as I was scheduled to stay at an existing medical facility. The day our plane landed was the day a devastating earthquake hit the nearby island of Nias. Our team was immediately diverted to the jungle area of this devastated island. We worked from dawn until dusk setting broken bones, repairing wounds, and helping with many other injuries. I would nibble on a palmful of trail mix every couple of hours. I noticed how comfortable, yet energetic, I felt by grazing all day on nutty snacks. As soon as I returned home, I delved into my nutrition library, and, sure enough, there were lots of studies validating my gut feelings.

A NUT-BY-NUT CASE

Different nuts offer different nutrients. That's why it's smart to combine the nuts in a homemade trail mix. Here is how each nut shines in the top nutrients.

Nut	Nutrient
Almonds	Top heart nut; highest in calcium, vitamin E, and lowest in saturated fats
Walnuts	Top brain nut (even looks like a brain); most omega-3s and melatonin
Peanuts	Botanically a legume, not a nut; highest in protein and arginine, a vital nutrient for a healthy endothelium; go organic
Hazelnuts	Sleep-inducing nutrient tryptophan

Nuts are the perfect snack. What makes a snack perfect?
- at least *5 grams of protein* per serving
- at least *3 grams of fiber*
- healthy fats

Nut	Nutrient
Pistachios	Vision-enhancing lutein and zeaxanthin, vitamin E
Brazil nuts	Anticancer, antioxidant selenium; one or two a day gives you all the selenium you need
Macadamia	Dessert nut, highest in fat, but most of the fat is the heart-healthy monounsaturated type
Pecans	Top in vitamin E
Chestnuts	Lowest-fat nut
Cashews	Highest percentage of saturated fat; highest in copper

- healthy carbs
- high satiety factor
- good taste

Nuts score high in all categories.

MIX UP YOUR NUTS

Make a trail mix of dried fruit and a half dozen of your favorite raw nuts. By mixing nuts, you capitalize on the nutritional principle of *synergy:* eating a lot of nutrients together from different sources helps the nutrients become more biochemically beneficial to the body. Take a zip-seal bag full of trail mix with you when you travel; it's especially good to have on planes.

If I'm going to have a particularly strenuous day and know I'll need more energy, I'll pack a baggie full of raw nuts or add a tablespoon or two of peanut butter to my smoothie (see "Dr. Bill's Prime-Time Smoothie," page 151). And, I still love an occasional peanut butter and jelly on whole-wheat sandwich.

Butter It Up!

Nut butters make a tasty and filling addition to spreads, sauces, and smoothies. The two most popular nut butters are peanut butter and almond butter (which is a good alternative for those who are allergic to peanuts). Each has its special something. Peanut butter is higher in protein, fiber, niacin, and folate, and slightly higher in saturated fats. Almond butter is higher in calcium and slightly lower in saturated fats. Also, raw almond butter is a better choice than roasted.

Buyer beware! Healthy nut butters should contain only nuts. Don't buy peanut butter that lists the word *hydrogenated* on the label.

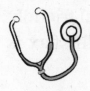

DR. SEARS SAYS…
Go raw! Why ruin good nuts by roasting them? Roasting adds fat and destroys some of the nutrients.

SAVOR SUPERSEEDS

Seeds are not only for birds; they're also super for humans. Like nuts, seeds are nutrient dense, packing a lot of nutritional power. Seeds are rich sources of healthy fats.

Fabulous Flaxseeds
Each morning I put a quarter cup of flaxseeds in a coffee grinder and pour the ground meal into

my smoothie. Martha adds two tablespoons of flax meal to her waffle recipe. We also sprinkle ground flaxseeds on our salads and oatmeal and mix them into muffins and cookie batter. Flax is chock-full of nutrition, especially healthy fat, protein, and fiber. My recommended daily amount is 2 tablespoons, which is a good nutritional deal. In 2 tablespoons, you get 100 calories, 7 grams of fat (half are the healthy omega-3 fats), 4 grams of protein, and 6 grams of fiber. As a protein perk, flax, like other seeds, is gluten free. And, the few carbs that are in flax are mostly intestinal-friendly fibers. Here are some health reasons why flax is so fabulous:

Flax helps boost the immune system. Besides lignans, flax contains other phytochemicals, such as phenolic acid and flavonoids, phytos that have anti-inflammatory actions that essentially feed the "soldiers" of your immune-system army. Flaxseeds also contain other vitamins, minerals, and phytos, such as calcium, zinc, potassium, magnesium, and folic acid.

Flax promotes heart health. The oil in flaxseeds is an omega-3 fatty acid called alpha-linolenic acid, which has similar, but weaker effects than the omega-3s found in seafood. Adding flaxseeds to the diet has been found to lower cholesterol. Also, research has shown that giving experimental animals a diet high in flaxseeds results in less hardening of the arteries in the animals. Veterinarians have long appreciated the benefits of flaxseeds, which is why these ground-up seeds are commonly added to animal feed. In a study in the *British Journal of Nutrition,* women who took 2 tablespoons of flax a day lowered their LDL cholesterol by 18 percent.

Flax lowers cancer risk. Flax is full of antioxidants called *lignans,* a phytoestrogen nutrient that, at least in experimental animals, competes with the effects of the body's own estrogen on breast tissue and has been shown to reduce the rate of breast cancer in the animals studied. Lignans are thought to act in a way similar to anti-breast-cancer drugs. Because lignans resemble estrogen, they compete with the estrogen receptors on breast cells, thereby possibly lowering the risk of breast cancer. In a pilot study at Duke University Medical Center, men with prostate cancer were given a diet that included 3 tablespoons of flaxseeds a day. The flax-fed men enjoyed a slower rate of tumor growth.

Flax contributes to colon health. The fiber in flax is fabulous for colon health. A tablespoon of flax oil is a nutritious and effective stool softener. Flax researchers believe that flaxseed may prevent colon cancer. In fact, colon-cancer-prone experimental animals who were fed flax meal as preventive medicine developed fewer tumors.

Flax helps stabilize blood sugar. Not only is the high fiber in flax good for the gut, but the endocrine system likes it too. An interesting study at the University of Toronto showed that people who ate breads made with ground flaxseeds had lower blood sugar levels than those who ate flaxseed-free bread. Diabetes researchers suspect that the high fiber in flax may be one of the reasons why flax is helpful for diabetics.

Is flax oil as healthy as flaxseeds? While flax oil is certainly healthy and a natural laxative, with ground flaxseeds you get the health benefits of *both* the oil and the seeds. Use a coffee grinder or a spice grinder reserved only for flaxseed, or your flax meal will smell like coffee and your coffee will have little floating flax particles.

The healthier the oil, the quicker it can spoil. Because flax oil is predominantly a healthy fat, it spoils easily. It should be refrigerated and has a shelf life of six to eight weeks. You'll find it in the refrigerated section in the health-food store. If it smells mildly like paint thinner (linseed oil comes from flax), you'll know the oil has gone rancid. Buy flaxseeds in bulk and store them indefinitely. You can grind them fresh as needed or grind a cupful at a time and then store the flaxseed meal in your refrigerator.

Home-ground flaxseeds are slightly healthier than the flaxseed meal that comes in bags at your local health-food store. In the factory processing of flaxseed meal, much of the oil is removed; this prolongs the shelf life but eliminates some of the most nutritious part of the seed.

DR. SEARS SAYS...

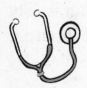

Grinding is good! Since flax is now a fashionable nutrient, you'll see whole flaxseeds sprinkled on top of muffins and cookies and as an ingredient in breads. The problem is that if these tiny seeds make it to the gut without getting stuck in your teeth, they pass mostly *undigested*. That's why ground flaxseeds are preferable, especially in baked goods.

Is flax oil as good as fish oil? Not necessarily. Plant foods contain a different omega-3 fat. Bear with me for a quick biochemistry lesson. Omega fats are called long-chain fatty acids. The longer the chain, the healthier the oil, and the more good biochemical stuff it does for the body and brain. DHA is the longest (twenty-two carbons), and EPA is the next (twenty carbons) — I call them the "tall guys." The omega-3s in flax oil, alpha-linolenic acid, are only eighteen carbons long (the "short guys"). The body must then go through a series of complex biochemical steps to add two or four carbon atoms to the short guys to upgrade them to the tall guys that the body and brain prefer. People's bodies vary widely in their ability to make this conversion. Research has shown that some people convert as little as 1 percent of the alpha-linolenic acid in flax oil to the longer-chain omega-3s the body needs. Diets high in omega-6 oils (see list, page 80) reduce this conversion because these oils use up the enzymes needed to add carbon atoms to the short guys.

We recommend taking flax oil *in addition* to fish oil, not instead of fish oil. A tablespoon of flaxseed oil daily or, better, 2 tablespoons of flax-seed meal (ground flaxseeds) is very healthful. They both mix well in smoothies, sauces, and soups. While flax oil is not as nutritious as fish oil, it's still very nutritious. So give your body a double break. Eat the two *F*s: fish and flax.

More Superseeds

Besides flaxseeds, there are three other seeds that are perfect for prime timers: sunflower, sesame, and pumpkin seeds. Only 10 percent of the fat is saturated; the rest is the heart-healthy, unsaturated type that has been shown to lower LDL cholesterol. While all three of these seeds are packed with vitamins and minerals, each one shines in a different way nutritionally.

Sunflower seeds. Sunflower seeds are high in heart-healthy polyunsaturated fats. They contain more nutrients than the other two popular seeds, sesame and pumpkin. A quarter cup of *raw* sunflower seeds is a rich source of these nutrients (given in percent of recommended daily value):

- vitamin E: 90 percent
- vitamin B_1 (thiamine): 55 percent
- magnesium: 33 percent
- selenium: 30 percent
- folic acid: 22 percent
- fiber (4 grams): 20 percent
- tryptophan (the relaxing and sleep-inducing amino acid): 33 percent

Sesame seeds. Sesame seeds are highest in calcium, 35 percent of the recommended daily value, which make them a rich nondairy source of calcium. A quarter cup of sesame seeds contains 350 milligrams of calcium. They're also high in omega-3s and contain 20 percent of the recommended daily value for zinc, slightly more than sunflower seeds.

Pumpkin seeds. They contain 25 percent of the recommended daily value for vitamin K.

HAVE A YEN FOR YOGURT

Yogurt in Middle Eastern languages is derived from the root word for "life." Even in biblical times, yogurt was associated with longevity. I eat an average of 1 to 2 cups of nonfat Stonyfield Farms Greek yogurt daily. While yogurt is a superfood for all ages, here's why it's especially good for prime timers:

Yogurt is good for the gut. Because prime timers have more-sensitive intestines and more indigestion, yogurt is just what the gut doctor ordered. The culturing of yogurt predigests the protein and lactose sugars (healthy carbs in milk), so that many milk-allergic or lactose-intolerant people can comfortably enjoy yogurt. The *probiotics* in yogurt contribute to colon health.

Because of its intestinal-healing properties, it is now standard for doctors to treat people suffering from diarrheal illnesses or inflammatory bowel diseases with daily doses of yogurt. Also, your doctor is likely to recommend a daily cup of yogurt (or probiotic capsules) if you are taking antibiotics. This replenishes the healthy intestinal bacteria that are killed by the antibiotics.

A TALE OF TWO YOGURTS

Yogurt is a great example of why prime timers should preview what they buy. Here's a label-reading lesson comparing a nutrient-dense yogurt—that is, a nonfat, organic, plain yogurt—to a "lite" or "fit" brand of yogurt.

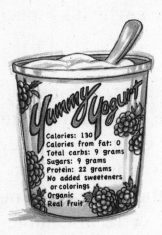

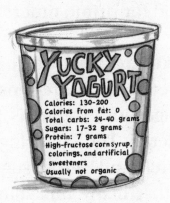

Yogurt is a yummy carb. Yogurt is high in good carbs; the partnering with protein makes these *slow-release* carbs.

Yogurt is calcium rich. A cup of yogurt contains an average of 450 milligrams of calcium compared to 300 milligrams in a cup of milk; this is nearly one-third of your total daily calcium requirements. Since prime timers tend

Notice how much more nutrition you get from the Yummy Yogurt for roughly the same number of calories. That's what we mean by choosing nutrient-dense foods. Notice also that in the Yummy Yogurt, the sugars and total carbs are the same. This is because the sugars are naturally occurring lactose. In the Yucky Yogurt, the total carbs are higher than the sugars, which usually means that sugars were added to the sugars already present in the food. The 9 grams of sugars in the Yummy Yogurt are healthy lactose. The extra grams of sugar in the Yucky Yogurt are added high-fructose corn syrup or fruit sweeteners. Also notice that in the Yummy Yogurt, you get three times as much protein. That's because it's Greek-style yogurt. The lower protein in the Yucky Yogurt results from the dilution effect of all those fillers. Last, Yummy Yogurts often contain a lot more probiotic cultures.

to become calcium deficient anyway, yogurt is just what the bone doctor ordered.

Yogurt is packed with protein. Few foods give you as much protein per calorie as yogurt. We use what I dub the "protein number" in selecting yogurt at the supermarket. The higher the number of grams of protein per calories, the healthier that brand of yogurt tends to be.

(A high-protein yogurt indicates that it's nearly all dairy products, and there is no room left for junk fillers.)

Enjoy yogurt's versatility:

- Buy plain yogurt and add your own fruit, such as blueberries. Add a dab of honey.
- Enjoy it on top of oatmeal with blueberries.
- Put some yogurt in a fruit smoothie. (See "Dr. Bill's Prime-Time Smoothie," page 151.)
- Substitute yogurt for ice cream. One or two nights a week, we enjoy my homemade yogurt gelato: I partially freeze an 8-ounce carton of Greek-style (full fat for a real treat) yogurt, add honey or blueberries, and enjoy.
- Use yogurt instead of mayonnaise in dips and salads.
- Dab a dollop of yogurt (healthier than sour cream) on fajitas or on baked potatoes. (Greek-style yogurt, even nonfat, has a consistency and taste similar to sour cream.)

NEED MILK?

Not if you eat yogurt. Ounce for ounce, yogurt gives you the same (or more) nutrients as a glass of milk. And, the added probiotics, cultured proteins, and predigested lactose make yogurt more gut friendly than milk. But if you and your gut like milk, remember "you are what you eat": the cow's milk contains what the cow eats, so be sure to *go organic!* A 2006 study in the *Journal of Dairy Science* comparing the fat composition of the milk from organic-fed, free-roaming cows to conventional milk from feedlot-fed cows showed that the organic-fed cows produced milk that had a much healthier omega-3 to omega-6 ratio than did that of the cows that were fed food not designed for cows. Low-fat milk is preferable to skim since a bit of fat helps the absorption of the fat-soluble vitamins A, D, E, and K. Nature put fat in milk for a reason.

Go organic. While organic yogurt is good for all ages, it is essential for prime timers, as our bodies' ability to eliminate pollutants and environmental toxins is reduced. Because of the hormones, antibiotics, and other yucky stuff fed to non-organically-raised dairy cows, we strongly believe prime timers should eat *only* organic dairy products.

Go Greek. Greek-style yogurt often contains twice the protein of regular yogurt, a nutritional perk that helps even the nonfat variety taste almost like full-fat yogurt.

Read the fine print. Generally, the longer the ingredient list, the yuckier the yogurt. It's best to get plain yogurt and to add your own fruit, such as blueberries.

ASK FOR AVOCADO

Reasons why avocados are awesome:
- Avocados are the most nutrient-dense fruit, rich in vitamins A, B, E, and folic acid, as well as heart-healthy monounsaturated fats.
- They're a versatile food. Enjoy as a guacamole dip, alone as a snack, as an accompaniment to an omelet or scrambled eggs, or in a sandwich or salad. One of my favorite breakfasts is Eggs Florentine (like Eggs Benedict, but substitute spinach for Canadian bacon), and a side of guacamole. And one of my favorite dinners is fajitas with guacamole.

- Avocados have a high satiety value. It's a perfect partnership of healthy fats, proteins, fiber, and healthy carbs.
- Avocados are a nutritious example of food synergy. Adding avocados to a salad or salsa increases the absorption of antioxidants, carotenoids, lycopene, and lutein. They may be high in fat, but it's *healthy* fat.
- Avocados have the highest levels of the eye-enhancing nutrients lutein and zeaxanthin of any fruit.
- Want to shine as a nutrition-savvy grandparent? Avocados are a top baby food.

To get the most enjoyment and nutritional value from avocados, buy them when they're slightly underripe — firm, but not hard, so squeezing doesn't leave a dent. Then store them at room temperature until they're slightly soft. If you use only half of an avocado, leave the seed in the other half and sprinkle it with lemon juice to prolong freshness. Store avocados and guacamole in airtight containers.

ENJOY EGGS

What a nutritional deal that little egg is.

- Eggs are nutrient dense. For a mere 75 calories, you get 6 grams of protein and a bunch of vitamins and minerals, namely vitamin B_{12}, vitamin E, riboflavin, folic acid, calcium, and zinc.
- Second to whey, the protein in egg white has the highest biological value (how well the body uses the protein) of any food.
- Like nuts, eggs have a high satiety factor, meaning that you feel fuller and are satisfied longer after eating an egg than most other foods that contain the same number of calories.
- Eggs contain more choline, the nutrient that is an important component of the neurotransmitter acetylcholine, than any other food.
- Eggs are eye food. Egg yolks contain a bit of the retinal antioxidants lutein and zeaxanthin.
- Eggs help you sleep. They're high in the sleep-inducing amino acid tryptophan.

- Eggs are versatile: poached, soft- or hard-boiled, in egg salad, in pie crust, or for Easter egg hunts!

Egg yolk has gotten an unfair rap for being "high in cholesterol." It's disheartening to hear prime timers order "egg whites only, please." This unwarranted and scientifically incorrect cholesterol fear has scared folks away from a very nutritious part of the egg — the yolk. (The healthy fats, omega-3s, and the yellow nutrients from the corn fed to the hens, lutein and zeaxanthin, are all found in the yolk, as is half the protein.)

The only people who need to eat less egg yolk are those who have a familial or genetic tendency toward high cholesterol, which is probably less than 5 percent of the prime-time population. There's a blood test to find out if this is true for you. Also, while egg yolk is high in cholesterol, it is lower in saturated fat than most cuts of meat. This is why the American Heart Association has exonerated the egg as an okay food for most people. An egg a day is okay! Try to buy free-range, organic eggs and those that advertise "omega-3 DHA-enriched" on the label. (*Note:* Read the fine print to be sure the omega-3s are from a marine source, not flaxseed, which is cheaper.)

There is a sunny side to the egg-cholesterol concern. Even though an egg contains 200 milligrams of cholesterol, for most people dietary cholesterol doesn't raise blood cholesterol. Also, studies show that the type of LDL that goes up tends to be the large particle rather than the heart-harming small particle LDL, called very-low-density lipoprotein (VLDL), which seeps into the arterial lining. Recent population studies found no link between eating an egg a day and cardiovascular disease. I've always suspected that the fatty bacon and sausage that often accompany the eggs are the culprits.

A chicken and egg story. You know that you are what you eat. Well, you're also what the animal you eat eats. Eggs with thinner and more fragile shells and paler yolks are from chickens fed a junky diet. I noticed the difference one day when I cracked open an egg from a farm-raised, free-range chicken whose feed was supplemented with omega-3s. The shell was harder, and the yolk was a deeper orange-yellow.

POWER UP WITH PROTEIN

Studies have shown that as we get older we tend to eat less protein, just the *opposite* of what we should be doing to maintain nutritional health and muscle mass. According to the American College of Sports Medicine, eating a bit of extra protein a day is especially important for very physically active persons. To maintain your muscle, you need to maintain enough protein in your diet. As a general guide, eat *at least* three-fourths your body weight in grams of protein daily. For example, if you weigh 160 pounds, eat at least 120 grams of daily protein. Try to get 20 to 25 percent of your daily calories from protein. With nutrient-dense food choices, this is easily achievable.

Protein-Rich Foods	Protein (in grams)
Seafood, salmon or tuna, 6 ounces	40
Greek yogurt, 10 ounces	30
Beef, lean, 4 ounces	25–30
Poultry, breast, no skin, 4 ounces	25–30
Cottage cheese, nonfat, ½ cup	15
Cereal with milk	10–15
Tofu, 3 ounces	8
Nuts or sunflower seeds, 1 ounce	7
Kidney beans or lentils, ½ cup	7
Egg, 1 whole	6

GO BIG ON BEANS AND LENTILS

These legumes are loaded with nutrients. Beans and lentils make our superfood list for two reasons: they're nutrient dense, and they have a high satiety factor. They are so satisfying because they are very high in protein and fiber. In fact, beans and lentils are higher in protein and fiber than any other vegetable. Beans are also high in the brain-building nutrient folic acid and the brain-relaxing nutrient tryptophan, and are a good source of B vitamins, calcium, and many minerals, especially potassium and magnesium — the blood-pressure-regulating nutrients. Lentils are the legumes with the most protein, fiber, and folic acid. Beans and lentils are also a nutritious and tasty accompaniment in other foods, such as hummus (garbanzo beans) and chili and salads (kidney and black beans). The slow-release carbs in these legumes are one reason the Mediterranean diet is one of the healthiest in the world. I sleep better after a lentil meal, probably because of the excellent balance of protein and carbs.

TRY TOFU

Tofu is basically soy cheese, fermented from the curd of soybeans. It is a nutrient-rich source of protein, calcium, vitamins and minerals, and cancer-preventing phytonutrients, and has cholesterol-lowering properties. Tofu is a versatile food that can blend undetectably into smoothies or add meatiness to a vegetable stir-fry. And it's a great nutritional deal: for a mere 60 calories you get 8 grams of protein and 200 milligrams of calcium. Tofu comes in two types: soft (or "silken") and firm. While firm tofu is more nutrient dense, it is also higher in iron, a mineral that prime-time men and postmenopausal women should avoid in excess. Too much iron can act as a proinflammatory intestinal irritant. So go for the soft tofu.

LOVE TOMATOES

The tomato is one of the top foods for phytos, those healthy antioxidants that are "anti-" every disease you don't want to get. The phytonutrient that gives a tomato its red color, *lycopene,*

GO ORGANIC!

We are often asked, "Are organic foods worth the extra cost?" Answer: Definitely yes! An important prime-time economic lesson you have learned throughout this book is that illness costs more than wellness. Prime timers must go organic for two main reasons:

- Remember our weak-garbage-disposal explanation of aging on page 28? Because your ability to eliminate toxic food chemicals lessens with age, doesn't it make sense to put less garbage into your system?

- As we age, most of us put on some extra body fat. Toxic chemicals tend to be stored in fat, so these agers are more likely to hang around longer and pollute your body. Actress Bette Davis once quipped, "The older I get, the more preservatives I need." Actually, the older we get, the less chemical food additives we should eat.

As an added nutritional perk, new studies reveal that organic fruits and vegetables tend to be higher in vitamins and minerals. The explanation: if growing plants aren't tainted with commercial pesticides, they have to muster up their own natural ones.

Go organic produce. When selecting produce, try to go organic for those fruits and vegetables whose peels you eat or whose surfaces are hard to clean. Definitely buy the organic "dirty dozen":

Apples	Nectarines
Apricots	Peaches
Blackberries	Pears
Cantaloupe	Raspberries
Cherries	Spinach
Grapes	Strawberries

Go organic meat, poultry, and dairy products. Free-range grazing, organically fed livestock, besides being free of chemical pollutants like synthetic hormones and anti-biotics, have meat and milk that are more nutritious. On page 80 you learned the nutritional importance of getting an oil change: eating more omega-3 and less omega-6 fats. New studies reveal that free-foraging livestock, like wild game, have a healthier fat profile of more omega-3s and less omega-6s. This more nutritious fatty-acid pattern is also seen in the milk from organically fed cows. One of the reasons we urge you to eat organic animal products is that agricultural researchers believe that animals tend to discard chemicals in their milk and eggs.

(continued)

If on occasion you are not able to buy organic meats and dairy products, at least choose lean and low-fat varieties since pesticides tend to concentrate in fatty tissue. For this reason, always buy organic butter, cheese, and cream.

Not yet convinced? Try the taste test. Not only are organic foods healthier and safer, they tend to taste better. I noticed that organically grown vegetables taste sweeter, and I wondered why. After delving into agricultural studies, I discovered that organic produce tends to be higher in natural sugars. Food chemists believe that pesticides interfere with a plant's ability to make its own sugars. And, there is no comparison between the delicious taste and texture of the meat from wild game and free-foraging livestock and that of feedlot-fed animals that sat around in a pen and ate junk food all day.

Spend the extra money to go organic. Your body and your medical insurance company will thank you.

---

belongs to the family of carotenoids that have cancer-preventing and heart-healthy properties. Lycopene is reported to lessen the stickiness of blood cells, so it's also preventive for blood clots and strokes. Tomato is one of the few foods that actually release more of their nutrients, especially lycopene, when cooked. Also, oils increase intestinal absorption of lycopene (think tomatoes sautéed in olive oil). Dr. David Snowdon, researcher of the Nun Study, found that people with the highest blood levels of lycopene tended to live the healthiest and longest. Remember, lycopene for longevity. Other rich sources of lycopene to load up on are watermelon and pink grapefruit.

BET ON BROCCOLI

Broccoli is one of the most nutrient-dense foods. For a mere 44 calories a cup, you get lots of nutritional perks:

- As the top anticancer (especially colon cancer) vegetable, broccoli is loaded with tumor-taming phytonutrients called sulforaphane and indoles. These phytos in broccoli help the garbage-disposal system and the liver work better.
- Broccoli is a rich source of many of the vitamins and minerals prime timers need more of: folic acid, vitamins A and C,

WHY "WHITE" CAN BE WRONG
FOR PRIME TIMERS

One day I took a group of schoolchildren on a field trip to a supermarket and was teaching them how to shop for "grow foods," which is how I refer to the sixteen super-foods when speaking with kids. We came to the bread rack. I had the students hold a loaf of white bread in one hand and a loaf of 100 percent whole-wheat bread in the other and compare the feel of each. These sharp kids got it right, describing the white bread as "squishy" and "not so heavy." I asked, "Do you want your muscles to get weak and squishy like the 'air bread' or strong like the one hundred percent whole-grain bread?"

Wonderful wheat becomes airy white bread because the most nutritious parts of the wheat kernel, the wheat bran and the wheat germ, have been removed, leaving a lousy loaf of bread with a longer shelf life. Just look at the ingredients list, and you'll notice how much more nutritious the whole-grain bread is. It is packed with protein, fiber, vitamins, and minerals. Don't be swayed by the term *enriched*, which is a cover-up for the impoverished nature of white bread. White-bread makers don't put back nearly as many of the nutrients as they take out.

Wild rice is more nutritious than white rice. While both are good for us, pink fish (such as arctic char, some trout, and salmon) is more nutritious than white fish because of the powerful antioxidant astaxanthin. Dark chocolate contains more antioxidants than milk chocolate. Sweet potatoes have more nutrients than white potatoes. In general, colorful foods get the nutritional nod over white foods.

Still, it's nutritionally incorrect to put white potatoes in the same category as white bread. Many nutritionists believe that white potatoes should be in the vegetable category rather than being downgraded as a starch, because white potatoes have a nutrient profile similar to many other vegetables, especially if you eat the skin. (If you eat the skin, be sure to choose organic potatoes.) The carbs in a baked potato become slower-release carbs when you add a dollop of yogurt or olive oil. Whipping pureed vegetables into potatoes—we call them "veggietators"—is a way to get our grandkids to eat more vegetables. One of our tastiest combos is a fillet of wild salmon over mashed potatoes, skin and all.

calcium, and carotenoids (especially the eye-enhancing lutein and zeaxanthin).
- This colorful vegetable contains more fiber and protein (4.7 grams of each per cup) than most other vegetables.

To preserve the rich nutrients in broccoli, steam it just enough so that it is crisp-tender and retains its bright green color.

GO FOR OATMEAL

Oatmeal is rich in protein, fiber, vitamins, and minerals. Because it lowers blood cholesterol, it is listed as a heart-healthy food by the American Heart Association. The fiber in oatmeal, beta-glucans, is particularly effective in slowing the absorption of carbs and steadying blood sugar fluctuations. Use real oatmeal, not the instant stuff, which has some of the fiber and the vitamin-mineral-rich bran layer removed. One of our favorite breakfasts is crockpot oatmeal. Prepare steel-cut oatmeal in a crockpot, and let it cook slowly overnight. Awaken to the aroma of fresh oatmeal. Add a handful of blueberries, a dollop of yogurt, a sprinkle of cinnamon, and enjoy!

Besides oatmeal, three other supergrains (especially if you are sensitive to the gluten in wheat) are quinoa, amaranth, and buckwheat. And enjoy wild rice; it's more tasty and nutritious than brown rice and white rice.

DRIZZLE OLIVE OIL

This tasty and nutritious oil is a staple in the Sears family. Olives and their oil have been revered since the early days of Mediterranean cuisine more than five thousand years ago when the olive was regarded as a tasty food and valued for its medicinal properties. Olive oil is a top salad oil because:

It's less processed. Unlike other vegetable oils, such as sunflower, safflower, and cottonseed oil, olive oil is made from the *flesh* of olives rather than from seeds. Less pressure and lower temperatures during the pressing process preserve more of olive oil's nutritional value.

It's rich in heart-healthy fats. Ninety percent of the fats in olive oil are the heart-healthy, cholesterol-lowering monounsaturated type, which acts like a sponge to suck up LDL cholesterol. Unlike most processed, commercial vegetable oils (such as corn, safflower, and sun-flower), olive oil is dubbed a "neutral fat," as it doesn't compete with heart-healthy omega-3s. To get the best of both heart-healthy worlds, I mix my two favorite oils, flax oil and olive oil, in my supersalad (see page 554).

It spoils more slowly. Generally, the healthier the oil, the faster it turns rancid and the less versatile it is when cooking (such as flax oil and fish oil). Yet, the fat quirks in olive oil — high oleic acid and low linolenic fatty acid — make it spoil less quickly.

It's tasty and versatile. Olive oil is delicious in salads, dips, sauces, and stir-fries, and is a healthy alternative to butter. Early on in my prime-time program, I replaced the bread and butter of my younger and less-healthy years with bread dipped in olive oil (I like to add some balsamic vinegar). Request that alternative when eating out. As an added perk, even the white bread that is served in most restaurants causes a lower carb spike when it is dipped in olive oil.

It has more antioxidants. Olive oil is a rich source of vitamin E and has more antioxidants, mainly polyphenols, than other oils.

It helps nutrient absorption. Olive oil is a top synergy food, meaning that when it's added to other foods, especially vegetables, it increases the absorption of nutrients, allowing antioxidants, such as the lycopene in tomatoes and the beta-carotene in carrots, to be more easily absorbed by the body. Mamma Mia knew best when she served tomatoes soaked in olive oil.

For the healthiest oil, choose "organic" *and* **"extra-virgin."** That way you'll avoid the risk that the olive plant may have been sprayed with pesticides. And extra-virgin olive oil (that is, the oil that comes from the first pressing of the olives) is not only the most flavorful and least acidic but also the richest in antioxidants.

Cook with it carefully. Extra-virgin olive oil has a low smoke point (the temperature at which the oil starts to smoke and disintegrate), so you need to be careful about overheating

WHERE'S THE BEEF?

You may notice that you're nearing the end of the chapter on superfoods, and there has been no mention of meat. No, the authors are not vegetarians. We eat *real, free-range, organic meat,* not the feedlot pork, beef, and poultry that is served in fast-food restaurants and sold in most supermarkets. In fact, researchers who study how humans have adapted over time believe that the human body was designed to thrive on meat, especially in regions where seafood was not available.

Not only are we as a nation eating more junk food and getting junky health, we're also feeding junk foods to the animals that produce our food. It's not the beef that's bad for you; it's what the beef cattle eat that make it bad.

When humans started feeding animals what they were never supposed to eat, animals started getting diseases they were never supposed to get. Any correlation? If you analyzed the nutrient profile of a steak from a farm-raised, free-range animal and that from a feedlot animal that sat around in a pen and ate junk food all day, you would notice that the two steaks are, shall we say, different animals, especially the fat profile. Feedlot beef has a double fault: it is low in good fats and high in bad fats. In contrast, wild game is higher in healthy omega-3 fats and lower in artery-clogging, saturated fats. In 2002 researchers proved that what's in an animal's feed affects the nutrient profile in the blood of the people who eat that animal. One group of volunteers ate the meat from feedlot animals fed a corn diet high in omega-6 and low in omega-3 oils. The group who ate meat from these animals showed an "oil change" in their blood: higher omega-6s and lower omega-3s. In contrast, the group who ate meat from grass-fed animals showed a higher omega-3/omega-6 ratio in their blood. (See why this oil change makes a difference, page 76.)

I look forward to the fall hunting season when, like a small-town doc of decades ago, I am given select cuts of venison by my hunter-friends and patients. It's worth the extra trouble, and the extra price, to insist on farm-raised instead of feedlot-fed livestock. (See AskDr. Sears.com for a list of sources we recommend for farm-raised beef and poultry.)

it. In general, the healthier the oil, the lower the smoke point. Even though olive oil is only mildly heat sensitive, it shouldn't be used for deep-frying. In fact, deep-frying is a no-no in the Prime-Time Health plan. Olive oil is one of the preferred oils for sautéing — especially wet sautéing. Pour around a quarter cup of water in the skillet or pan and heat just below the boiling point. Then add the food and cook it a bit before adding the oil. This shortens the time the oil is in contact with the hot pan. Stir the food frequently to further reduce the time the oil is in contact with the hot metal.

Not too much! While olive oil is healthy, it's also high in calories. Depending on the recipe, try to limit to one tablespoon, 125 calories, per day.

SPICE UP YOUR LIFE

Unless your gut says otherwise, the older you get, the healthier spicy food is for you.

- We need the high levels of antioxidants and immune-boosting nutrients that are found in spicy and pungent foods, such as chili peppers, garlic, and onions. Each of the foods and spices mentioned in this section benefits the immune system by decreasing inflammation, or wear and tear, on the tissues.

- Nutrition researchers dub spices "molecular mimics," because they act like the body's own chemical regulators, for example, insulin and anti-inflammatories.
- Spices have AAA effects: anticancer, anti-inflammatory, and anti–Alzheimer's disease.
- Spices can preoccupy the attention of your taste buds and curb your appetite.

Turmeric. There is more scientific evidence for the positive health effects of turmeric than for any other spice.

- Studies show turmeric can lower artery-clogging LDL cholesterol.
- It's a good gut food, increasing the flow of bile that breaks down fats, so it helps digestion.
- It lessens excessive stomach acid production, so it can be used as a

heartburn (reflux) remedy. Some people may find spices make reflux worse; others find they help digestion.

- It can relieve the inflammatory soreness of people with rheumatoid arthritis and improve how insulin regulates blood sugar.

- Because of its neuroprotective properties, turmeric is dubbed the "smart spice" by Alzheimer's disease researchers. Curry-loving cultures, such as India, have the lowest rates of Alzheimer's disease. A 2001 study at UCLA showed that when fed curcumin (the active ingredient in turmeric), experimental animals genetically engineered to develop Alzheimer's disease had 43 percent fewer brain amyloid plaques.

- Turmeric is a top anticancer spice that enhances the ability of the body's natural immune system to kill cancer cells.

Several times a week, I sprinkle a tablespoon of turmeric on my salad (see recipe, page 554).

TURMERIC TIP: COMBINE
WITH BLACK PEPPER

One day I was touting my love of turmeric to one of my patients from India. She advised me that to get the most healing power from terrific turmeric, I should always combine it with ground black pepper. Indian folklore, I presumed, until I pursued one of my "what does science say" inquiries. Sure enough, science said she was right. Turmeric eaten alone is very poorly absorbed. Yet, combine it with black pepper, and the absorption of turmeric is enhanced over a thousand times. That's why in my supersalad (see page 554), I sprinkle ½ to 1 teaspoon of turmeric, ¼ teaspoon black pepper, and 1 tablespoon of olive oil, which further enhances absorption.

Cinnamon. This spice is one of the few sweet nutrients that may do good things to blood sugar and blood lipid levels. Fascinating new research reveals that people with type 2 diabetes who consumed 1 to 2 teaspoons of cinnamon daily had lower levels of blood sugar, triglycerides, LDL cholesterol, and total cholesterol. Experiments at the USDA's Human Nutrition Research Center revealed that an ingredient in cinnamon called methylhydroxy-chalcone polymer (MHCP) mimics insulin and increases the sensitivity of the receptors on the cells to the action of insulin. The researchers found these beneficial metabolic effects with as little as ½ teaspoon of cinnamon per day. A 2007 study in the *American Journal of Clinical Nutrition* showed that adding a teaspoon of cinnamon to rice pudding blunted the usual high-blood-sugar response following dessert. Besides helping to stabilize blood sugar, cinnamon has anti-inflammatory qualities. As an added nutritional perk, 2 teaspoons of cinnamon contain 57 milligrams of calcium. Enjoy swirling cinnamon sticks in hot tea and a sprinkle on oatmeal. Each morning I add 2 teaspoons of cinnamon to my smoothie.

Ginger. Long valued as a seasickness remedy, ginger is good for relaxing the gut and relieving heartburn and is also helpful as an anti-inflammatory for arthritis.

Cayenne. Several nights a week just before dinner, I walk out to our garden and pick a red-hot chili pepper to dice into my supersalad. It seems that the hotter the spice, the more potent its anti-inflammatory effects. Capsaicin, the active ingredient in cayenne pepper and chili peppers, is a potent anti-inflammatory, anticoagulant, and analgesic. In fact, capsaicin is the main ingredient in potent pain-relieving skin creams. Apparently, it works by blocking the pain-signaling chemicals in the skin from traveling to the brain. And chili peppers are very high in vitamin C. Cayenne pepper is a potent flavor mask for people who don't like the taste of fish.

Garlic. As soon as you chop or press that innocent-looking little clove, out comes the smelly stuff that's good for you. To get the most health (anti-inflammatory, anticoagulant, and anticancer) benefits from garlic, eat it when the odor is strongest, usually ten to fifteen minutes after pressing. The longer you cook garlic, the less healthful it is. Garlic is like a time-release capsule of medicine. Picture the clove of garlic as having two compartments containing different chemicals: the enzyme alliinase and a substance called allicin. Pressing or chopping allows the garlic to release the allicin, the health-promoting active nutrient and sulfur-containing substance that gives garlic its odor. Letting garlic sit for a short while after pressing allows more of the active compound to be formed. (Onions also contain allium compounds, which probably have health-promoting effects similar to garlic, though the science behind this is not as strong for onions as for garlic.)

HOW TO EAT MORE GARLIC BUT NOT EXUDE IT

How much the odor of garlic whiffs from your breath or oozes from your skin varies greatly from person to person. A quirk among male members of the Sears family is that, to put it bluntly, we really stink after eating uncooked garlic. Perhaps it's helpful I didn't discover the health-promoting effects of garlic until after I had fathered so many kids. (Martha says, "It's that bad!") Try these tips to lessen garlic breath and garlic body odor:

- Chew fresh parsley, orange peel, grapefruit, mint, or fennel seed.
- Rinse out your mouth with lemon water.
- To get rid of garlic odor from your skin, take a soapy bath after your high garlic meal.

Garlic may also have a cholesterol-lowering effect. Scientific opinions are mixed about the degree. More and more studies show that garlic does indeed have an anticancer effect, especially for colon cancer. And research is cropping up suggesting that garlic may also protect against Alzheimer's disease.

For some prime timers, garlic upsets the gut by aggravating reflux. Because high amounts of garlic can reduce blood clotting — generally a beneficial effect — people taking prescription anticoagulants should check with their doctor before having lots of garlic.

POUR POMEGRANATE JUICE

This deep burgundy, delicious juice is a new addition to our list of superfoods. I want to thank Dr. David Heber, founding director of the UCLA Center for Human Nutrition, for calling my attention to the new and exciting research on the health benefits of pomegranate juice. It's rich in the antioxidant polyphenol and contains nutrients called *ellagitannins,* which have the ability to suppress cancer cells, especially those of colon and prostate cancer.

Pomegranate juice has also been shown to slow the progression of atherosclerosis in experimental animals with high blood cholesterol. A 2003 study that followed ten patients who drank pomegranate juice for one to three years showed a reduction of atherosclerosis and blood pressure in those with cardiovascular

---

FOOD SYNERGY FOR PRIME TIMERS

Savor the principle of nutritional synergy. When eaten together, many nutrients help each other work better in the body. Combining foods helps you get more bang for your nutritional buck because it allows some foods to bring out the nutritional best in the others.

- Mix it up in salads, stews, and smoothies. For example, add a few cubes of meat to vegetables in a stew. The vitamin C in the vegetables increases the absorption of the iron from the meat.
- Drizzle olive oil on vegetables to enhance the absorption of fat-soluble vitamins and minerals. The healthy fats in olive oil and nuts in salads increase the absorption of vitamins A, D, E, and K. Olive oil increases the

---

disease. Simply put, pomegranate juice seems to decrease the accumulation of sticky stuff in the endothelium of blood vessels.

This is why I choose pomegranate juice as one of the juices in my smoothie (see recipe, page 151). When shopping for pomegranate juice, be sure to check the label. Dr. Heber

---

absorption of the antioxidant lycopene in tomatoes.

- Juice it up! Besides enhancing taste, a little acidic addition, such as lemon or lime juice or vinegar, increases the absorption of many vitamins and minerals. This is why I sprinkle lemon and lime juice and balsamic vinegar on my supersalad, and add a twist of lemon or lime to water. Lemon and lime juice are also fabulous antirust protectors for the body. Some studies suggest that these juices can also lower and slow down glucose absorption from a meal and therefore help stabilize blood sugar. Because they are seedless, limes are easier to juice than lemons.

also revealed that in studying brands of pomegranate juice, many of them are weak in the actual pomegranate fruit and diluted with other juices. From his experiments, he recommended POM Wonderful.

YOU CAN RESHAPE YOUR TASTES

In formulating my own eating plan for prime-time health, I realized that it was absolutely necessary to *reshape my tastes* to favor real foods. First, I researched how nutritious and longevity enhancing these sixteen superfoods were. That motivated me to like eating them. After a few months, my body craved all sixteen of these foods, even though I wasn't initially fond of a few of them. That's what you can expect too. It's like your gut brain says, "Finally, you're feeding me what's right for me. And I like it!"

Rx FOR PRIME-TIME NUTRITION

❑ Make the sixteen superfoods your prime foods.

❑ Graze: eat twice as often, half as much, and chew twice as long.

❑ Eat more seafood.

❑ Eat less meat.

❑ Eat more greens.

❑ Put more color on your plate.

❑ Change your oils.

❑ Eat more whole grains; eat less white bread.

❑ Go organic.

❑ Avoid the "four bad words" on food labels (high-fructose corn syrup, hydrogenated, numbers [e.g., red #40, yellow #5, etc.], flavor enhancers [MSG])

❑ In a nutshell: eat real foods!

CHAPTER 14

Get More Restful Sleep

The older we get, the more quality sleep we need. Sleep is a holiday for the body, a time when every system has a chance to relax and repair itself. Doctors who run sleep laboratories tell me that when people come to them for help, they are amazed at how much time the doctors spend scrutinizing what they do during the day. What you do with your body and brain throughout the day influences how well your body and brain sleep at night. If you put a lot of junk food and junk thoughts into your body during the day, don't expect the resulting neurochemicals to become nicer at night. The vicious cycle begins: Suboptimal sleep throws the sleep-inducing neurochemicals out of whack, and this in turn leads to more suboptimal sleep. Inadequate sleep amps up the inflammatory system and causes you to store excess body fat, both of which increase your chances of getting sick and sleeping less.

HOW SLEEP REJUVENATES YOUR BODY

When you snuggle down with your head in the pillow, your muscles relax, your respiratory and heart rates slow, and blood pressure and body temperature drop slightly. These physiologic changes signal the release of the sleep hormone *melatonin,* which prompts the brain to slow down and rest.

Then around every ninety minutes throughout the night, your body cycles through *light sleep,* the state in which you dream, and *deep sleep,* the state in which you repair and rejuvenate. You may have heard that the older you get, the less you sleep. While this is often true, it's not optimal. We are naturally programmed to enjoy the physiologic ideal of sleeping eight to nine hours. Studies show that there is decreased blood flow to the brain (temporal lobes) of people who get less than six hours of sleep a night. Chronic sleep deprivation leads to many health problems. You can tell if you are sleep deprived: you nod off any time you sit down to read, at a movie or a concert, or at the wheel of your car.

You snooze, you heal. Many of the tips you will learn in this chapter are aimed at giving your night-repair crew enough time and the right working conditions to shore up your body's garbage-disposal system, which, as you know, is important for healthy aging. One of the keys to quality sleep is to let the body ease into the deepest level, or slow-wave sleep, in which the most rejuvenating and healing takes place. It's the stage of sleep when the immune system is most active. It calls on the body's maintenance crew to get to work, sort of like a healing night shift reporting for duty while there is less traffic on the road. Melatonin, mostly secreted at the beginning of the night, not only promotes restful sleep but also detoxifies wear-and-tear substances (inflammatories). That's why sleep-deprived people are likely to have more infections: insufficient sleep inhibits the production of the body's natural immune substances. During slow-wave sleep, the production of other rejuvenating substances, such as growth hormone and the hormone dehydroepiandrosterone (DHEA), also increases, and worn-out cells are replaced with new ones. While you sleep, your brain repairs and reorganizes, just as your computer does when the defragment and antivirus software clicks on at night.

You snooze, you lose. Excess body fat, that is. Obesity researchers have long noticed the correlation between poor sleep and excessive weight gain. Restless sleepers have a higher level of the hormone ghrelin, which stimulates the appetite and encourages overeating, and a lower level of leptin, the appetite-controlling hormone that has the opposite effect of curbing the appetite. People with poor-quality sleep tend to suffer from this hormonal imbalance and crave more calorie- and sugar-rich foods.

PRIME-TIME NIGHT QUIRKS YOU MAY EXPERIENCE

As we age, nighttime sleep depressors can deprive us of adequate rest:
- Our hormonal symphony orchestra is designed to play perk-up music (more cortisol, less melatonin) during the

day and to switch to softer wind-down music at night (more melatonin, less cortisol). As we age, this hormonal harmony becomes less sleep-inducing: cortisol stays higher at night, and melatonin stays lower.

- We enjoy less slow-wave, or deep, sleep. This is the state of sleep in which our immune and repair systems are most active.

- The amount of melatonin that the brain makes during sleep declines with age. Since melatonin is primarily secreted during the stage of deep sleep, the aging brain does not enjoy as much of this sleep aid. Many of our sleep-tight tips, especially mellowing your mind with meditation as you get into bed, will help your body make more melatonin. Melatonin is not only the body's own natural sleep aid; it is also a powerful antioxidant that shifts your body's repair system into high gear.

- We tend to put on more belly fat, which itself contributes to hormonal imbalances that disturb sleep.

- Hormone fluctuations during menopause can keep women awake. An enlarged prostate, and the consequent full-bladder sensation, makes men get up to go.
- Quirks in the gut, such as heartburn and indigestion, are also more common as we age and can contribute to sleeplessness.

FIFTEEN SLEEP-TIGHT TIPS THAT WORK

As we get older, we typically need to go to bed earlier and awake earlier, but not necessarily sleep fewer hours. Here's how to get your body to produce more of its own natural "sleeping pills."

1. Get enough daytime exercise. Daytime exercise sets up the brain for a more restful sleep at night. Exercise increases the percentage of time you spend in the deep stages of sleep. Some people find that exercising near bedtime can rev them up so much that they have more difficulty falling asleep. Morning exercise seems to be best for restful sleep. If you exercise in the evening, try to do so at least three hours before bedtime.

2. Eat for sleep. The brain is highly affected, for better or for worse, by nutrition. So it stands to reason that sleep can also be highly affected, for better or for worse, by what you eat. Some foods help you sleep restfully; others have the opposite

SNOOZE FOODS

Sleep-inducing foods are rich in tryptophan and healthy carbohydrates (foods that naturally contain fiber, protein, and fat in addition to sugars). Good carbs help more tryptophan get into the brain tissue to make sleep-inducing substances, such as melatonin and serotonin. (High-protein meals are also good for breakfast, since protein tends to perk up the brain.) For a restful night's sleep, shoot for an early evening meal and before-bed snack that in total contain at least 300 milligrams of tryptophan.

Snooze Foods	Tryptophan (in milligrams)
Wild game, elk, 6 ounces	900
Turkey, 6 ounces	600
Chicken, 6 ounces	600
Beef, 6 ounces	600
Lamb, 6 ounces	600

effect. "Sleepers" are foods that contain trypto-phan, the amino acid that the body uses to make serotonin, the neurotransmitter that slows down nerve traffic so your brain isn't so busy. The body also uses tryptophan to help make melatonin.

Snooze Foods	Tryptophan (in milligrams)
Salmon, 6 ounces	400–500
Tuna, 6 ounces	400–500
Bean burrito with cheese	200
Cottage cheese, ½ cup	175
Hazelnuts, 1 ounce	167
Pumpkin seeds, 1 ounce	164
Eggs, 2 large	150
Tofu, 3 ounces	125
Milk, 8 ounces	115
Sesame seeds, 1 ounce	105
Almonds, 1 ounce	100
Cheese, cheddar, 1 ounce	91
Beans, ½ cup	90
Sunflower seeds, 1 ounce	84
Oatmeal, 1 cup	84

"Wakers" are foods that do the opposite; they stimulate neurochemicals that perk up the brain.

In the chart on page 378, you can see that it is not difficult to get 300 to 500 milligrams of tryptophan to set up the brain for sleep. Above all, skip an all-carbohydrate snack, especially one high in junk sugars. With carbohydrate-only snacks, you miss out on the sleep-inducing effects of tryptophan found in high-protein foods, and you set off the roller-coaster effect, the ups and downs of blood sugar that release the rev-up stress hormones. Partner healthy carbohydrates with protein, and add some high-calcium foods like dairy products. Calcium helps the brain use the tryptophan to make melatonin.

Eat light and early. Eat a light dinner early, at least three hours before bedtime, especially if you suffer from reflux (heartburn) or other forms of indigestion. Observe the gut-friendly wisdom, "Don't dine after nine." If you have trouble sleeping, try making dinner your lightest meal of the day. But don't go to bed hungry, as hunger can keep you awake, stimulating stress (also known as waking) hormones. Balance is key.

Avoid junk food, especially in the evening. Eat junk food and expect junk sleep. Junk sugars (those that are not partnered with protein or fiber, such as sweetened beverages or doughnuts) trigger insulin. After the insulin effect wears off, the blood sugar levels crash, which triggers

MORE LEAN = MORE SLEEP

One of the most preventable causes of sleeplessness during prime time is excess weight. Not only does excess belly fat create a general hormonal imbalance that interferes with sleep, obesity can lead to one of the most severe causes of restlessness—obstructive sleep apnea (OSA). The accumulation of excess fat within the structures of the neck can obstruct breathing passages, causing air hunger during sleep. (During sleep, the muscles that keep the airway open relax a bit, causing the breathing passages to be narrower.) Because the brain is very sensitive to a drop in blood oxygen, it wakes the body up to tell it to breathe. Loss of sleep from OSA also weakens the immune system, just what we don't need during prime time. And studies show that obese people have decreased blood tryptophan levels, which can lower the quality of sleep. Even if you are lean, suspect OSA if you are a noisy, restless sleeper and are always tired.

the stress hormones adrenaline and cortisol to perk up the blood sugar. In people who are particularly sensitive to chemical cuisine, artificial food additives, such as MSG and aspartame, can cause poor-quality sleep. These chemical additives seem to interfere with normal melatonin production.

3. Forget the nightcap. Alcohol is not a sedative, as many people think. For most people, alcohol disrupts sleep rather than induces it. It may cause you to fall asleep faster, yet during the night it interferes with sleep cycles, resulting in lower-quality sleep and earlier awakening. Drinks before bedtime can also prompt you to get up to urinate frequently during the night and cause indigestion and heartburn. While one glass of wine or a bottle of beer is unlikely to disturb sleep, more than that probably will.

4. Cut down on caffeine. Some people are more caffeine-sensitive than others. Caffeine is a stimulant that promotes alertness and helps college students pull all-nighters. Yet, stimulation is not what you want during sleep. Caffeine increases cortisol and epinephrine, which trigger an increase in heart rate, blood pressure, breathing rate, production of stomach acids, urinary output, and brain activity. Since caffeine may take as long as twelve hours to clear your system (the half-life of caffeine is about six hours), get your java jolt in the morning, if you must.

5. Have an earlier bedtime. The saying "Early to bed, early to rise, makes a man healthy, wealthy, and wise" has a physiologic basis. Your rev-up hormone (cortisol) is highest at 6 a.m. and starts to dip in the evening. Physiologically speaking, turning in at 10 p.m. and waking around 6 a.m. would be most in tune with the body's natural hormonal cycles, although this may vary a bit from person to person. Once I got my own body into biochemical balance, that's what it told me to do. Most prime timers find that they naturally feel better on the ten-to-six regimen. As we age, our body tends to be reset to go to bed earlier and to wake up earlier.

6. Don't worry, be sleepy. Strive for a stressless evening. Keep your hormones (your on-off switches) balanced. As the production of cortisol (your body's "on" switch) increases around 6 a.m.

CAFFEINE CAUTION

Confessions of a coffee lover: This book was written under the influence of caffeine. I enjoy my cup of java on cold mornings and green tea on long writing days. Coffee and tea contain potent antioxidants such as flavenols. MRI scans of the brain show that caffeine increases activity in the areas of the brain associated with memory retention. Yet, as is true of any stimulant, balance is key.

FIVE REASONS TO BE CAREFUL WITH CAFFEINE

1. **Caffeine can act as a stimulant *and* as a depressant.** While caffeine in the appropriate doses can perk up the brain, high doses can leave you feeling depressed. (I use the word *dose* because caffeine is a drug.) The busy electrical activity in the brain has a sort of built-in brake that automatically slows down the thinking neurotransmitters from going too fast. Caffeine tells the brain to ignore the brake pedal and allows the neurotransmitters to speed. How much caffeine it takes to perk up the brain and how much depresses it varies considerably from person to person.

2. **The caffeine effect can be addictive.** As with any drug, the body habituates to caffeine, meaning

it takes higher and higher doses to achieve the desired effect. At first one cup of coffee perks you up, then it takes two cups, then three, and so on. The higher the dosage, the greater the side effects. This is why it's important to take "caffeine holidays" if you are a regular java jolter, so that you can gradually lower the number of cups you drink. Lowering your dosage too fast, however, can lead to withdrawal symptoms, such as extreme fatigue, depression, headaches, and jitteriness.

3. **Caffeine can be hard on the heart.** There is conflicting research as to whether caffeine is heart healthy or heart harmful. My advice is to follow the science of common sense: Caffeine increases the blood level of the stress hormone adrenaline, which speeds up not only brain activity but also heart rate and can raise blood pressure. Any drug that increases the circulating levels of stress hormones can't be good for the brain or the body. So go easy.

4. **Caffeine can bother the bones and upset the tummy.** For some people, excess caffeine can cause excessive excretion of calcium in the urine. Also, because caffeine can increase stomach acid

secretion, prime timers who already suffer from reflux or heartburn should limit caffeine or at least sip their coffee or tea *slowly* and not on an empty stomach.

The effect of caffeine consumed during the day causes the brain and body to act like they are in a state of "perpetual stress" in the evening. People who are already tense get what I call the "carryover effect" of caffeine, and it only makes them more tense, causing them to sleep poorly at night. This makes them more anxious the next day, and the cycle gets worse. Too much caffeine can actually zap rather than boost energy.

My advice on caffeine:
- If you don't already drink caffeine-containing beverages, don't start.
- Choose decaf coffee and tea. Coffee beans are decaffeinated in two ways: They can be

and decreases around 6 p.m., melatonin (your body's "off" switch) does the opposite, decreasing when it's light and increasing when it's dark.

A relaxing bedtime ritual that works for Martha and me is a bedtime prayer and Scripture reading. We take turns. Oftentimes the listener

soaked in water to leach out the caffeine or be processed chemically. Because I generally trust nature more than chemistry labs, I go for water-processed decaf. You can decaf your own tea: Pour a cup of hot water, dip the caffeinated tea bag into the hot water for 20 to 30 seconds, then discard the water. You've just removed most of the caffeine from the tea bag but retained the flavor and flavonoids.

- If you do have caffeine-containing drinks, limit your caffeine milligrams to no more than twice your body weight. So if you weigh 100 pounds, you should have no more than 200 milligrams of caffeine a day, which is about two cups of coffee or three cups of black tea.

(usually me) drifts off to sleep before the prayer/reader is finished. Prayer and meditation are the most time-tested methods to clear the brain of unsettling thoughts and set it up for sleep. (See meditation tips, page 415.) Prayer is also helpful for getting back to sleep.

High cortisol goes along with all the other "highs" of aging, such as high blood pressure, high cholesterol, and high blood sugar. If you continue your daytime stress into the evening, you're keeping your cortisol high at bedtime. High cortisol keeps you from enjoying enough of deep sleep, which is the most healing. Also, cortisol deprives the brain of the sleep-inducing amino acid tryptophan, which is found in the snooze foods we mentioned earlier.

Deep breathe your way to sleep. If you're revved up and can't wind down, enjoy the deep-breathing mood mellower described on page 210. Breathing slowly and deeply turns up the calming part of your central nervous system and turns down the excitement centers of the brain. If you awaken and start worrying, do the deep breathing again. Be aware of the insomnia-depression cycle: restless sleep lowers the happy hormone serotonin, which can cause depression and anxiety, which leads to more insomnia.

Your kids may be out of your house, but they're never out of your thoughts. Because we are a busy family with eight children, Martha and I agreed never to rehash family problems before going to bed. While before bed may be the only "free time" you have, it needs to be happy time. Martha and I agree to allow only happy talk and happy thoughts in the bedroom.

You should neither dwell on unfinished business nor anticipate the business of the next morning while trying to sleep. Go to bed enjoying solutions rather than focusing on problems. When getting into bed, I deliberately delete any worrisome thoughts from my in-box, knowing that I can access them again in the morning, if necessary. Then I replay my library of pleasant memories. My favorite is to imagine dozing off in a swinging hammock at a Caribbean beach resort.

7. Go to bed at the same time each night. People who go to bed at about the same time each night tend to enjoy more restful sleep.

8. Have a restful bedtime routine. We are creatures of habit. Even infants and toddlers are taught bedtime routines to set them up for sleep. In brain research, a bedtime routine is called a *setting event*. This means that the brain gets into the habit of expecting, after following a set routine (brush teeth, bath or shower, turn on music, turn down lights, get into bed, pick up a book), that sleep will naturally happen. A set bedtime routine might be considered like foreplay for sex: it sets up the mind and body for pleasure to follow.

9. Set up your bedroom for sleep. Try these sleep-inducing bedroom tips:

Make the bedroom boring. While some people find watching a movie before bed relaxing enough to help them go to sleep, ideally the bedroom should be reserved for sleep and sex and nothing else. Some people have an office in their bedroom, which is a reminder of daytime stressors, as are computers and TVs. In addition, the lights of computer screens rev up the brain.

Keep the bedroom dark. I'm like a rooster that wakes up with the very first ray of sunlight or moonlight, so we have blackout drapes on our bedroom windows. Light stimulates serotonin; darkness stimulates melatonin. This may be why some people sleep longer in the darker winter months than in summer. (This could also

PRIME TIMERS NEED SIESTAS

A recent study in the medical journal *Archives of Internal Medicine* showed that people who took a one-hour nap at least three times a week were 37 percent less likely to die from heart disease. In fact, sleep researchers found that as we age, our bodies naturally tell us to nap between 1 p.m. and 3 p.m. During these hours, the brain's natural sleep cycles are best programmed for rest. Listen to your brain. When it tells you to nap, nap.

be the basis for seasonal affect disorder, or SAD, during the winter months when people may produce less serotonin, the happy hormone.) Deep inside the brain is a peanut-size structure called the suprachiasmic nucleus (SCN), which acts like the brain's own alarm clock. This gland is light sensitive. It goes off when stimulated by light. Often even a small light, such as a computer light or a bright clock dial, can turn up the brain during a nightly trip to the bathroom. If you're having trouble falling asleep, avoid checking e-mail or watching TV. The bright lights of screen glare can tell the brain to stay awake instead of priming it for sleep. Try blackout curtains or blackout drape liners.

Keep the bedroom cool, airy, and allergen free. Fresh air is healthful; stuffiness is not. Remove potential allergens, such as all the fuzzy stuff, from your bedroom.

10. Get warm, then cool down. A warm bath or shower right before bed raises the body temperature. The natural cooling-down process that follows relaxes the body and induces sleep.

11. Clear a stuffy nose. A stuffy nose makes breathing more difficult and deprives the brain of sufficient oxygen to enjoy a restful sleep. (An oxygen-deprived brain tells the body to wake up and take a deep breath.) Open-mouthed breathing is not as restful. To keep your mouth closed and nose open during sleep, try Dr. Bill's dynamic duo, a nose hose and steam clean (see page 200). If you suffer from nasal stuffiness, before going to bed:

- Use a *facial steamer* to liquefy secretions that clog your nose and airways.
- To really flush your nose and sinuses of obstructive mucus, use a *Neti Pot*.
- If you have allergies, use a HEPA air filter in your bedroom.

12. Check for snoring or irregular breathing during sleep. One of the most commonly overlooked causes of restless sleep is obstructive sleep apnea. If you are a noisy sleeper and are tired the next day, ask your doctor to refer you to a sleep specialist. The specialist might recommend that you have a sleep study (monitoring your brain waves and blood oxygen levels overnight) to see if you suffer from sleep apnea. As a side note, sleep apnea is a common and treatable cause of high blood pressure.

13. Enjoy sounds to sleep by. If your mind is cluttered with worried thoughts, put on soothing sounds for sleep. Listen to music that you have learned by experience relaxes you. We enjoy flute, harp, and classical guitar as sounds to sleep by. Some people find white-noise machines (CDs of rainfall, babbling brooks, ocean waves, etc.) sleep inducing.

14. Sniff off to sleep. Each night Martha drifts off to sleep to the aroma of lavender oil drops on her pillow. Science supports Martha's sleepy sniffing. Japanese researchers at the

Meikai University School of Dentistry studied the saliva of people after they sniffed lavender oil for four to five minutes. Their fascinating results: the levels of the stress hormone cortisol in the saliva decreased, and the levels of anti-oxidants, called free-radical-scavenging activity (FRSA), increased. The essence of this research was that sniffing to sleep is both relaxing and healing. Aromatherapists recommend that you

---

WHAT ABOUT SLEEP MEDICATIONS?

The brain is naturally programmed to release neurochemicals at just the right time to promote quality sleep. Many mood-altering drugs, especially antidepressants and anti-anxiety medications, interfere with the brain's natural neurochemicals and may interfere with sleep. This is why sleeping medications are often prescribed along with these drugs. But then you get into the cycle of using one drug (which may have undesirable side effects) to counteract the side effects of other drugs. Sleeping pills are actually sedatives to relax the brain—they don't promote natural sleep cycles. If they are absolutely necessary, sleeping pills should only be used for a short time and ideally under the guidance of a sleep specialist.

---

use the lowest strength to get the effect. Smells that are too strong or unpleasant can actually disturb sleep.

15. Wake up to your body's own alarm. Think about what the word *alarm* means. You set off a series of alarms in your brain and body that increase heart rate and blood pressure. Being alarmed isn't an ideal way to begin the day. If possible, instead of setting an alarm, wake up when your body is ready. Your body's healthiest wake-up signal is the sunrise. Until you become tuned in to this inner wake-up call, set a musical wake-up call: music with gradually increasing volume will ease you into the day.

Rx FOR PRIME-TIME SLEEP

- ❏ Get lots of exercise during the day.
- ❏ Eat snooze foods.
- ❏ Don't dine after nine.
- ❏ Stay lean.
- ❏ Reduce caffeine and alcohol.
- ❏ Enjoy an earlier, consistent bedtime.
- ❏ Remove stressful thoughts before going to bed.
- ❏ Make the bedroom quiet, dark, cool, and airy.
- ❏ Clear a stuffy nose.
- ❏ Enjoy sleep-inducing music.
- ❏ Try lavender-oil aromatherapy.
- ❏ When possible, awaken to body's own natural "alarm."

CHAPTER 15

Subdue Stress

As we age, our bodies are less able to handle the wear and tear caused by stress. Let's call it *dis*-ease. Normally, the body, especially the brain, has built-in mechanisms to keep stress hormones at just the right level. But as we get older, these internal stress-hormone-reducing mechanisms gradually become less effective. The main primetime message? The older we get, the calmer we need to be.

TWO STRESS FACTS EVERY PRIME TIMER SHOULD KNOW

"Stressing out" is what happens to prime timers who don't handle stress in a healthy way. You stress your body out of hormonal balance, out of vitality, and out of longevity.

1. The body needs balance. Remember the three magic words for health and longevity? *Stable insulin levels.* Now add three more: *stable stress levels.* Healthy bodies need the right levels of circulating stress hormones — too little, and we get weak and slow; too much, and we get sick and fat. Your body's levels of stress hormones are regulated by the autonomic nervous system (ANS). Like a built-in computer, it keeps your body running automatically. You don't have to think about your heart rate going up during exercise or sweating when it gets hot. The ANS has two components that balance each other, the sympathetic nervous system (SNS) and the parasympathetic nervous system (PNS).

The SNS *turns up* your nervous system. It helps you handle what you perceive to be emergencies and is in charge of the flight-or-fight response. When you need to swerve to miss an oncoming car, your heart rate goes up, your pupils dilate, and you may sweat. All this good stuff occurs in your body to put you on red alert for survival.

Its counterpart, the PNS, *turns down* the nervous system and helps you to be calm. It promotes relaxation, rest, sleep, and drowsiness. Most stress management is aimed at turning up the PNS and turning down the SNS.

During a stress response, such as running from a tiger, your body is in strict survival mode. So it secretes cortisol to rev up your body; other hormones, such as endorphins, which blunt the perception of pain; and prolactin, which suppresses your desire and ability to reproduce. Glucagon, a hormone in the liver, releases sugar. This sends extra fuel throughout the body, especially to the muscles, that you will need to run from the approaching tiger. If your body is habitually revved up, that will take a toll, especially on your brain and blood vessels. Think of a car engine that's always running too fast and does not receive diligent maintenance or the right fuel. Obviously, it's going to break down sooner. The same thing happens in your body.

Stress management is a marvelous system. To better understand your body's stress mechanisms, I highly recommend Robert Sapolsky's *Why Zebras Don't Get Ulcers.* Informative and humorous, it explains what stress does to the body in a very easy-to-read way.

AVOID HIGH-C SYNDROME

People who spend most of their lives with high levels of cortisol are said to have what I call the high-C syndrome and must cope with these unhealthy physiologic actions of excess cortisol:

- premature aging
- decreased insulin sensitivity, causing diabetes
- growth of cancer cells
- decreased growth hormone
- increased appetite
- increased fat storage, especially abdominal fat ("toxic waist")
- increased reflux, heartburn
- weakened muscles
- slow wound healing
- poor quality sleep
- erectile dysfunction
- destruction of brain cells, especially memory function

Six ways to turn down high cortisol:

1. **Practice stress busters.** (See "Six Simple Stress Busters," page 404.)
2. **Cut down on caffeine.** Caffeine raises stress-hormone levels. The wear and tear on the body from the pick-me-up perks of caffeine, if over-used, aren't worth it.

3. **Reduce unnecessary noise.** Disturbing noises—like traffic sounds, train horns, and even loud music—can increase cortisol levels.

4. **Get enough rest.** When we spend less time in deep sleep, we produce less growth hormone, which throws the body out of endocrine balance. It's also important to relax in the late afternoon and evening. Normally, cortisol falls to its lowest level around 6 p.m., preparing the body for a relaxed state in order to fall asleep. Yet, afternoon and evening stress increases the level of cortisol, which can interfere with sleep. Spending the night with a high level of cortisol—and therefore having less restful sleep—also throws off the cortisol balance the next day.

5. **Enjoy a natural morning high.** The blood level of cortisol is naturally high in the morning (6 a.m.), which helps you start each day with a burst of energy. Take advantage of this morning high with exercise and productive work. (Most of this book was written in the morning.)

6. **Stay lean.** It may be news to you that fat cells produce excess cortisol. This causes overstressed and overfat people to get into an unhealthy cycle: excess stress produces fat (especially abdominal fat); these excess fat cells produce even more cortisol, and more cortisol produces more abdominal fat.

2. Prime timers need to control their cortisol. Once we are in prime time, we continue to produce just as much cortisol as we did when we were younger, yet we are unable to turn down its level as easily. As stress hormones get high, the brain puts on the brakes and tells the adrenal glands to stop pouring out so many stress hormones. As we age, this internal balance becomes less effective. "After every stressful situation, we become a little older," says stress researcher Dr. Hans Selye. I'll say it again: the older we get, the calmer we need to be.

HOW STRESS AGES EVERY BODY PART

As you read about how to care for your body from head to toe in part II, you may have noticed there was a section on stress management for nearly every part of the body. Here's a brief review:

Stress shrinks the brain. Chronic, unresolved stress can shrink the brain, a dementing process called *glucocorticoid neurotoxicity.*

Stress ages the heart. Uncontrolled stress gives you a bad case of the "highs": high blood pressure, high cholesterol, and high blood sugar. Chronic stress causes a chronically elevated heart rate, which eventually wears it out. Heart failure is particularly common following periods of sudden or prolonged stress, for example the death of a loved one or other personal losses.

Stress weakens the bones. Called stress-induced osteoporosis, high levels of stress hormones reduce calcium deposits in the bone bank, increase calcium loss by the kidneys, and interfere with calcium absorption through the intestines.

Stress makes you sick. People who suffer from chronic immune-system illnesses, such as asthma, rheumatoid arthritis, and even cancer, often notice a flare-up during a long period of unresolved stress.

Stress makes you fat. Stress can literally change the shape of your body, mainly by increasing belly fat. (See "Toxic Waist," page 92.)

Stress leads to diabetes. High levels of stress hormones raise blood sugar, which can lead to insulin resistance.

Stress is bad for the gut. Prolonged stress and anxiety can aggravate conditions such as reflux (heartburn), ulcers, and inflammatory bowel problems. People with irritable bowel syndrome often have flare-ups during times of stress.

Stress suppresses sleep. Stress hormones are designed to rev you up, not help you rest.

Stress suppresses sex. Stress hormones suppress testosterone and increase insulin, which can contribute to erectile dysfunction.

SIX SIMPLE STRESS BUSTERS

The expression "worried to death" has a biochemical basis. Chronic unresolved stress prematurely ages every vital organ. Optimists outlive pessimists. Anxious people are more likely to have a heart attack. Amped-up people who can't calm down are more likely than calmer people to get major illnesses. In fact, stress management is a key health secret of centenarians.

1. If you can't change it, don't worry about it. When a situation has passed or is beyond your control, come to terms with it. Recognize that you cannot change it, accept it, and move on. As I tell our eight children, "You can't always control situations, but you can control your *reactions* to them." How your mind reacts to a stressor is about the only thing that is totally under your control. Oftentimes, our reactions to stressful situations cause more problems than the situations themselves. Some people are overreactors, and this sets them up for the brain-damaging effects of chronic stress.

Try not to dwell on things that have gone wrong in your life in the past. The past is history. Don't feel guilty about something you can't change.

2. Focus on solutions, not problems. You can't fix a problem by getting yourself all worked up with "what-ifs" ("What if I..."), but you *can* look for solutions. After a problem occurs, immediately focus on finding a solution to regain a sense of control. The feeling of loss of control causes the stress to continue. By focusing on solutions, you divert your energy from the problem to how to fix it.

MUSIC MELLOWS THE MIND

We listen to lots of classical music in our home. Play music that helps you relax. Music opens up the endorphin-releasing pathways to the brain and mellows the same parts that control heart rate and blood pressure. To boost the brain's pleasure centers even more, *sing along.* Music reduces circulating inflammatory substances in the body. I have a "mood medley" playlist on my iPod. Some of my favorites include:

- "The Prayer," Andrea Bocelli
- "The Homecoming," Hagood Hardy
- theme from *Forrest Gump*
- *Heartstrings,* Jason and Nolan Livesay
- Moonlight Sonata, Beethoven
- "All I Ask of You," from *Phantom of the Opera*
- "Memory," from *Cats*
- "Elvira Madigan," Mozart
- The Swan, Saint-Saëns
- "Hawaiian Wedding Song"
- "What a Wonderful World," Louis Armstrong

Our family hobby is sailing, which affords us many life lessons. We often charter boats in the Caribbean for our family vacations. Part of the fun of boating is that something usually goes wrong and needs fixing. One day as we limped

Pleasant music can be very healing. The Mozart effect, touted for mellowing fussy babies, may have similar results in older minds. To soothe patients, hospitals are using music therapy during anxiety-provoking procedures such as cardiac catheterizations. Listening to pleasant music activates the part of the frontal lobe involved in moods and emotions. Can music muster up new brain cells? Possibly. PET scans show that some parts of the brain are larger in musicians than in nonmusicians. Music therapists suggest that melodies "warm up" the brain.

A certain song might remind you of a person or a pleasant scene, such as your wedding day or a memorable date. When I play Glenn Miller's classic "In the Mood," it mellows my mind as I replay the "happy feet" image of Martha and me swing dancing. When I hear "Thank Heaven for Little Girls," happy, cleansing tears come to my eyes as I relive my daughter's wedding day and the beautiful daddy-daughter dance we shared.

into a marina on a remote island hoping to find a mechanic to fix the boat's engine, I started worrying that the situation would ruin our whole vacation. As my stress rose, we were greeted by a friendly mechanic who said, "No problem, mon!"

That greeting de-stressed me. In fact, "No problem, mon!" became one of my stress-busting
refrains.

Focus on biggies, and downgrade smallies.
Ministresses don't deserve the mental effort you
give them. Smallies are life's little annoyances
that really don't hurt anyone. Because of a traffic
jam, you're late for a meeting. That's a relative
smallie compared to being delayed by a traffic
accident you cause while rushing to arrive on
time.

3. Redirect negative thoughts. Program
your mind so that when a stressor arrives, you
reflexively say, "Take five; don't go there." Instead,
in your mind, journey to a better time or place.
Draw from your most pleasant lifelong memories. This is known as *mental imagery.* As soon
as a negative thought or stressor arises, immediately click *instant replay.* Open your mental
library, and revisit pleasant scenes and thoughts
of happy relationships for a while *before* the
negative thoughts take over. These *serene scenes,*
such as your wedding day, or a favorite prayer,
are just what the stress doctor ordered. We

YOU *CAN* POSITIVELY CHANGE YOUR BRAIN

New research shows that you can actually change your brain by changing your thoughts. PET scans reveal that the "happy centers" of the brain light up during happy thoughts. These landmark neurochemistry studies suggest that filling the brain with happy thoughts (positive self-talk) builds more positive brain circuits and releases calming neurohormones, such as serotonin and dopamine. On the other hand, filling the mind with negative thoughts (negative self-talk) builds negative pathways. Grow as many positive connections as you can.

---

prime timers have a stress-busting advantage. Our library of instant replays is rich because we've had longer to stock it. Learn to quickly fill your mind with positive thoughts before negative ones get a foothold and run wild.

Trash "trash talk"! Suppose you receive a disturbing e-mail. Quickly delete it, ideally before you finish reading it and before it has a chance of infecting your thoughts. Immediately trash upsetting thoughts.

One day during a sailing vacation, I was walking along a beach, and I noticed that as the surf came in it washed my footprints away in the sand. Negative thoughts can be very much like footprints in the sand. Allow the surf of positive thoughts to come in and quickly wash them away.

4. Take a deep breath. As soon as a stressor enters your life, take a deep breath to activate your calming nerves. When you're stressed, your sympathetic nervous system, which is sort of a get-up-and-go mechanism that revs the body into high gear, overwhelms its partner, the parasympathetic nervous system, which normally relaxes bodily functions and lowers the level of circulating stress hormones. The SNS takes over and floods your body and brain with stress hormones, upsetting the balance.

Deep, relaxed breathing turns up the PNS and turns down the SNS. As a result, it allows more air into the lungs, relaxes the muscles, and gets more oxygen into your system. The next time you hear someone say, "Relax, and take a deep breath," don't hesitate. Do it. Something good and healthful happens to your body when you do.

At least ten times a day, I stop for a *breath break*, a moment to take a few deep, cleansing breaths during a meeting, while writing, or between patients. I feel the tension leaving my body as I exhale. Focusing on the breathing instead of the stressors enables me to relax and reload to continue working. (See page 210.)

5. Move to mellow your mind. You've heard the advice "Walk it off!" Exercise works like a prescription mood mellower but without the mood-flattening side effects. As an added perk, research shows that fit people are bothered less by stress biochemically than are more sedentary people.

ENJOY WALKING THERAPY

Moderate to vigorous exercise increases the blood flow to the brain, which secretes endorphins and other biochemicals that have a natural calming effect. It often requires more vigorous exercise to get this system going. Vigorous exercise also directly inhibits the stress response, causing a decrease in the alarm hormone (adrenocorticotropic hormone), as well as cortisol. I find walking and swimming the most relaxing. It also helps in decision making. Whenever I have an important choice to make, I think, *I'll swim on that.* If I get too tense, Martha will often say, "Go see your therapist—the pool."

ENJOY THE HELPER'S HIGH

When you help others, you usually get more than you give. The psychological term "helper's high" actually has a biochemical basis. When you give of yourself to help others, feel-good hormones, like dopamine, surge in your brain. Use your free time to help those in need. Prime timers who volunteer in hospitals, nursing homes, and with charitable organizations give a good feeling to everyone around them. Use knowledge gained from your own past challenges and struggles to assist those with similar problems. Honestly, this is one of the reasons we wrote this book. Knowing that somebody's life is better because of what we wrote is a priceless gift.

At my sixty-fifth birthday party, my children surprised me by dumping over my head a boxful of more than seven hundred letters from our readers around the world. They were written in response to a notice my daughter-in-law circulated that read, "If Dr. Bill has helped you...please write him." I treasure those "Thank you, Dr. Bill" letters and often reread them on a down day.

6. Surround yourself with upbeat, positive people. Emotions are contagious. Brain researchers use the term *mirroring* to describe how the brain reacts to people who reflect emotions, either positive or negative. Being around happy, uplifting people stimulates your brain to turn on happy emotions.

We travel a lot with friends. With flight delays and cancellations, travel can be stressful. It's a joy to travel with people who immediately click into "It's okay, we'll fix it" mode instead of infecting the whole group with "Oh, woe is me." Positive people improve the mood of everyone around them.

Compliment people who serve or help you, and you'll make others — and yourself — feel good: Great job! "Thanks, Joe!"

MEDITATE TO SELF-MEDICATE

Meditators live longer. At one time meditation was thought to be reserved for monks and hippies. Now, meditation is mainstream. Modern imaging techniques have enabled neurologists to delve inside the brain and discover that healthful things go on in the mind and body during meditation.

New studies show that meditation:

- lowers blood pressure
- boosts the immune system
- lowers heart rate
- reduces stress
- improves healing from heart disease and cancer
- slows the progression of cancer
- improves sleep
- relieves anxiety and depression
- accelerates weight loss
- lowers cortisol levels

How meditation mellows the mind. Fascinating PET scans show that during meditation, the blood flow to the areas of the brain that influence tranquility and emotions increases. PET scans and functional MRIs give a snapshot of the inner workings of the brain. During meditation, the left brain literally lights up. Simply put, meditation shifts the focus of thought from the right brain, where the stress centers are, to the left brain, which contains the peaceful centers. Meditation seems to protect the brain from disturbing environmental stimuli and thoughts. It turns down the SNS (the rev-up system) and turns up the PNS (the relaxing system).

While meditation is an ancient healing tool, it seems especially relevant in modern times. It can help us unplug from our iPods and Wiis and tune in to the wiring of our own minds. To get the most out of meditation, don't think you are wasting time or doing nothing. Just as you don't waste time going to the gym for physical fitness, neither do you waste time meditating for mental fitness.

Five Meditation Tips

1. Choose a place. Meditate anytime and anywhere that works for you. You may have a favorite meditation space in your home, with or without your favorite background music. Some prefer quietness without background music; others find that music mellows the mind to help them center. (*Centering* means tapping into the calm center of your mind, freeing you to focus on peaceful thoughts while blocking out disturbing ones.) Oftentimes, fifteen minutes before I'm scheduled to give a lecture, I retreat to the bathroom for a "men's room meditation." You can even meditate in a busy office building.

2. Choose a mantra. A *mantra* is a word or phrase that prevents your mind from getting sidetracked with anxious or disturbing negative thoughts. It's a centering device that helps quiet the clutter of competing self-talk. A mantra helps you switch to the happy center of your brain. Meditators describe it as being similar to purging your computer of junk mail, or as being silent so you can hear yourself speaking. Favorite mantras that are thought or said slowly include:

- Thank [inhalation] ...God [exhalation].
- Feel...good.
- Good...life.
- The Lord is...my Shepherd.

Anytime your mind wanders from your mantra, bring it back into focus. Above all, master meditators recommend suspending all judgments of whether you are doing it correctly and all expectations of what is supposed to happen.

3. Breathe with your mantra. Taking a deep breath while thinking your mantra turns down your excited nervous system and helps you relax. I find it helpful to use a two-word mantra — one on breathing in and the other on breathing out: "Thank" (breathe in), "God" (breathe out). Many meditators find it helpful to hum as they exhale. Choosing words that have an *o* in them helps you prolong your mantra as you breathe in and out: "Soo" (breathe in), "goood" (breathe out). This helps the mantra match the rhythm of breathing. (See "Take a deep breath," page 410, for the relaxing effects of deep breathing.)

4. Choose a posture. Sitting is usually better for meditation than is lying down, which is the position associated with sleep. Sit on the floor or use a chair. Relaxing most of the muscles in your body reduces tension traffic going to your brain. Meditation is a state of mind that is somewhere between being awake and being asleep.

5. Close your eyes. Your goal is to get in touch with what's inside your mind, not what's outside.

LAUGHTER IS THE BEST MEDICINE

Humor keeps you balanced.
A person without humor is like a
wagon without springs — jolted by
every pebble in the road.

—HENRY WARD BEECHER

Laughter is good for longevity. Dr. William Fry, a Stanford University psychiatrist, noted that children laugh more than four hundred times a day, whereas adults laugh only about a dozen times a day. As we round the corner into prime time, we need to get back to our childhood a bit. Norman Cousins, in his book *Anatomy of an Illness as Perceived by the Patient,* calls laughter "inner jogging" because a good-hearted belly laugh gives every system of the body a workout. During my cancer recovery, I was helped to heal by Cousins's book as he triumphed over a chronic disease through a strong belief in his own healing abilities and the empowering effects of humor. We added a joke-book section to our home library. I began each day reading jokes and read some more before going to bed.

Laughter is good for the brain. During the writing of this book, a friend of ours was suffering from reactive depression following the untimely death of her husband. When asked what helped her most, Susan joyfully replied, "I am momentarily distracted from my grief by the jokes my friends e-mail me." Depression is accompanied by suppression of the pleasure-enhancing neurochemicals in the brain. Persons suffering from chronic depression often admit, "Nothing is funny to me." Laughter reverses this process by triggering the release of feel-good neurohormones, such as endorphins and dopamine. Researchers believe that laughter activates the pleasure pathways in the brain.

Laughter is especially important in helping people get over chronic illness. It's often not the illness itself that overwhelms us and drags us down, but our fear and anxiety about the illness. This can set up a stressful cycle: pain, fear, and anxiety about the illness — illness worsens; pain, fear, and anxiety increases — illness worsens even more. Humor can break this cycle by triggering the release of endorphins, the body's natural painkillers. This is how physical exercise boosts a person's mood. It makes sense to make humor part of your daily exercise routine.

Laughter is good for the immune system. A fascinating new area of research, dubbed psychoneuroimmunology, finds that depression suppresses the immune system. Studies show that the stress hormones epinephrine and cortisol decrease during and following laughter. Researchers at Loma Linda University School of Medicine found that medical students who watched comedy videos had a significant increase in T-cells (cells that circulate through the body and gobble up germs) and lower levels of the stress hormone cortisol. Laughter boosts natural killer cells, which are suppressed during stressful experiences. Studies have shown that people with allergies experience fewer allergic reactions after watching humorous films. A study at Mount Sinai School of Medicine in New York showed that in widowers, the number of natural killer cells goes down for almost a year.

Laughter is good for the heart. Perk up your sense of humor. Laughter ("inner jogging," remember?) increases the heart rate and circulation, much like an aerobic workout. And, like exercise, after the laugh subsides, the heart rate drops below average, the improved circulation continues, and the body goes into a state of relaxation. Are you ever so angry at someone that you can feel your blood pressure rise? Let go of the anger (not so easy!), and read or tell a joke instead. Less-social and excessively serious people have higher rates of heart disease. Laugh for your health.

USE YOUR HUMOR LIBRARY

Having a down day or a sick day? Angry at someone? Feeling uptight? Visit your library—your humor library. Keep a folder of favorite jokes that your friends have told or e-mailed to you. Keep humorous articles and a rack of joke books. Stock your funniest home videos and DVDs on a shelf. Consider putting together your own home humor library as a "medicine cabinet" with no unpleasant side effects.

Laughter is good for the lungs. There is nothing more energizing than a good belly laugh. Laughter gives a good workout to the diaphragm

LOVE AND LONGEVITY

Many studies have proved what lovers have long known: love better, live better. Studies have shown that if you feel the love of another person, for example, when someone tells you, "I love you," it helps the immune system quiet down autoimmune diseases. Studies also show that happily married people are more likely to be in good health. The happier the relationship, the better the health. Strive for high-quality relationships. Studies have shown that people who are in the highest-quality relationships live the longest and stay the healthiest.

---

muscles. Also, laughter breaks up muscle tension in the face. The vibrating muscles of a hearty laugh give you an internal massage.

Laughter is good for you. Physiologically laughter is just the opposite of the stress response. Stress and tension elevate stress hormones, tighten muscles, constrict blood vessels, upset neurohormones, depress the immune system, and overload the heart. Laughter relieves tension, lowers stress hormones, improves neurochemistry, settles the heart, and boosts the immune system. So, the wisdom of "laugh it off" is healthy medicine.

EAT HAPPY FOODS

Enjoy foods for stress relief. While eating sweet and fatty foods may increase brain levels of feel-good neurochemicals, such as serotonin, uncontrolled emotional eating can make you fat and sick.

The best type of emotional eating is *grazing*. Grazers tend to have more stable blood sugar and therefore more stable moods. Here is a list of foods that we call "happy foods" — they contain a high level of the calming amino acid tryptophan and stimulate the happy and relaxing hormones dopamine and serotonin:

- whey protein
- seafood
- turkey
- whole grains
- beans
- rice
- hummus
- lentils
- nuts
- eggs
- sunflower seeds
- sesame seeds
- dairy products
- dark chocolate

Yes, chocolate! As a mood elevator, or "happy food," chocolate has some scientific merit. By a healthy biochemical quirk, while cocoa butter — the fat (stearic acid) that gives chocolate that appealing melt-in-the-mouth feel — is a saturated fat, it behaves metabolically like a healthy monounsaturated fat. Cocoa beans are loaded with flavonoids, the antioxidants found in fruits and vegetables. Proponents believe that some of the nutrients in chocolate stimulate feel-good hormones such as serotonin.

Here are our chocolate tips: the less sugar, the better. Dark, bittersweet chocolate seems to be the healthiest. The darker the chocolate, the higher it is likely to be in flavonoids. And, the nuttier, the healthier. Chocolate fondue (dipping chunks of fruit in warm, melted dark chocolate) is one of our "young food" delights. Look for dark chocolate that contains at least 70 to 80 percent cocoa solids; reputable brands list the percentage. The higher the percentage, the fewer junky fillers the chocolate has. Confession of a chocolate craver: several nights a week, I enjoy two small squares of dark chocolate after dinner.

As you get into the Prime-Time Health program and see its healthful effects on your mind and body, you will gain a sense of *control*. Being in control of your health and your life by the choices you make is itself a major stress buster.

Rx FOR PRIME-TIME STRESS BUSTING

❑ If you can't change it, don't worry about it.

❑ Focus less on problems and more on solutions.

❑ Click into "instant replay" of serene scenes.

❑ Enjoy mood-mellowing music.

❑ Deep breathe to de-stress.

❑ Have a helper's high.

❑ Enjoy mood-mellowing movements: dance, swim, walk.

❑ Love to live longer.

❑ Meditate several times a day.

❑ Laugh to live longer.

❑ Enjoy happy foods.

CHAPTER 16

Enjoy Better (and More) Sex

Getting older doesn't mean we have to get less sexy. By taking the same approach we know to take with the brain, the heart, and every other system in the body, we definitely can enjoy prime-time sex. While desire and ability may wane a bit, research shows that the more prime timers enjoy sex, the better their mental and physical health — *and* longevity. In this chapter, we focus on how to cope with the most common sexual changes that occur with age, starting with the ones that make the most headlines: menopause and erectile dysfunction (ED).

SEVEN WAYS TO MELLOW MENOPAUSE

It's important to realize that menopause is a natural stage in a woman's life. It simply means that menstrual periods pause and then stop. Most women go through menopause sometime between ages forty-five and fifty-five. This "pause" is caused by a gradually decreasing level of estrogen and progesterone. The body loves hormonal balance. As you may already know from having PMS and from being pregnant and then postpartum, when hormones change, your moods also change. How women experience menopause varies greatly, from minor discomforts to marked emotional and physical upsets. While there is no magic solution for every hot flash, as you learn to take charge of every other system in your body, so can you mellow your menopause.

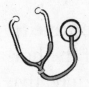

DR. SEARS SAYS...

Men, understand the changes that occur in women. Women, understand the changes that occur in men. Changes in one partner require a sensitive response from the other.

As women move into their forties, there is a natural decline in the sex hormones estrogen and progesterone. These changes can lessen libido and cause physiologic changes that can make intercourse uncomfortable, even painful. These hormonal changes may cause you to be less responsive. The following sexual-performance enhancers can help:

1. Have the talk. If your mate senses that you are less willing and less able to enjoy intercourse, he's likely to take it personally and blame himself, which can trigger in him the deflation cycle. Explain to him the normal changes that are occurring in your vagina and what he can do to be more sensitive. If you are shy or unaccustomed to talking this way, find a good book to help you become more familiar with what it is you want to say and the changes you want to consider in your need for better sex.

2. Help your vagina be more receptive to intercourse. Because there are less of the hormones that ready the vagina for entry, creative compensations are needed. The vaginal lining becomes less lubricated, thinner, and therefore less responsive. The vaginal tissues become less elastic. In some women, the size of the vaginal opening and canal actually decrease a bit. The same sexual arousal that used to turn on the "wetter" and "stretchier" vaginal responses don't turn on as easily. These changes make the vaginal tissue, if it becomes a bit traumatized, more sensitive and even prone to infection, which, in turn, makes the vaginal tissue, and therefore the whole woman, less ready and willing. But, while even the most sensual and sensitive partner cannot replace the hormones you are losing, your sex life doesn't have to go on pause.

Lubricate. The last thing you want is for your mate to rush into a dry, unprepared, and therefore unreceptive place. Liberally use a water-soluble lubricant, such as K-Y Jelly or Replens, to reduce any uncomfortable friction and to provide enjoyable foreplay.

Test out a new position. Try his and hers positions. Who says you don't need to experiment with different lovemaking positions as you age? When you're young, it's fun; when you're older, it's necessary. Because of increased sensitivity in a woman's vagina, a couple must learn which positions are most comfortable. Relax and have fun experimenting. This advice will benefit men who have difficulty maintaining an erection; they will also find certain positions are better. For example, the man-on-top position can allow gravity to maintain the pooling of blood in the penis and strengthen the erection. Yet, some men on top notice what is dubbed the "pelvic steal" syndrome, in which an erection softens because the activity of the leg and pelvic muscles steals blood from the penis. It seems that more blood flow to the muscles is needed for a man to be on top than on the bottom.

And for a woman, being on top means she can move more freely and with her own rhythm to achieve just the right amount of pressure and placement. She needs the same buildup of blood flow to her genitals to bring the engorgement that will resolve in the release of orgasm. Couples learn to take turns coming to climax — often the woman goes first (on top) then the man (also on top). Both may take longer to get there, but with loving patience it is worth the wait. Some things just cannot be rushed. If time is an issue, either make a "date" to make love when you have the time to dawdle or have a "quickie," and let both partners anticipate next time.

Realize that sex does not always have to mean orgasm. Because of the sexual changes that come with aging, many prime timers enjoy a healthy intimacy of emotional intercourse and physical touching (think back rub) that lead to mutual enjoyment and sweet time spent, especially when one or both bodies just aren't up for it (pun intended).

3. Cool it! You only wish! What we refer to here are the hormonal fluctuations that lead to hot flashes. Some women find that extremes of temperature (e.g., going from the cold into a heated building), hot coffee, excessive alcohol, and emotional upsets trigger hot flashes. Endocrinologists believe that hot flashes are like a withdrawal effect. The body was accustomed to a steady supply of hormones, and now it's getting less of these hormones and perhaps more stress hormones. Many women find that mood-mellowing practices like yoga and meditation can ease hot flashes.

Hot flashes and night sweats are so distressing for some women that they are the main reason women seek medical hormone replacement therapy (HRT). The subject of HRT is beyond the scope of this book. Speak with your physician for more information.

An alternative to HRT is support through supplements and natural forms of the hormones to keep levels optimal. If your doctor doesn't know about this, ask her to refer you to a doctor who specializes in integrative medicine.

4. Stay lean—but not skinny. Remember, fat tissue produces estrogen, which may explain why many women develop a "menopot" during menopause. So it's quite usual, and perhaps therapeutic, to be a bit more plump in your fifties than you were in your forties. Women who have more comfortably managed their menopause settle in to appreciate their slightly fuller bodies as a *menoplus.* Remember, *lean* means having the right amount of body fat for your particular body type, and that body may be better off with a bit more. Going up one skirt size may be just what your body needs. During menopause, many women gain about a pound a year, so ten pounds can sneak up on you. More than ten pounds may put you at higher risk for developing dis-ease in one or more of your systems, however, so this is the time to take our whole prime-time message about good nutrition and fitness seriously.

5. Don't smoke. Smoking further decreases hormonal output, just at the time when you need all the hormonal help you can get.

6. Kick in those Kegels. Remember those exercises you used to strengthen your pelvic muscles for childbirth? Replay them. Keeping the vaginal muscles strong can help to somewhat offset the tenderness that comes from having the thinner lining and smaller vaginal opening. Add Kegels to your anytime, anywhere exercises (see list on page 622). In case you've forgotten or never needed these exercises, here's a reminder: Squeeze your pelvic muscles like you're trying to stop urinating; hold for six seconds, then release. Repeat ten times.

7. Listen to the wisdom of your body. Whether to live with the effects of lowered hormones and gradually let your body adjust or to take prescription replacement hormones (estrogen, progesterone, testosterone) is an individual choice. If you start feeling worse or "not right" after trying hormonal replacement, your body may be telling you that it is not for you. Many women, instead of medical

HRT, first try diet and lifestyle changes. Work with your health-care provider to determine the right plan for you.

ANDROPAUSE

Even though the female "change" is the "-pause" that gets more press, between ages forty-five and fifty-five, men also go through a prime-time pause in their emotions and sexuality, called *andropause*. For men, it's more than a pause in hair growth. While many men think hormones are a female thing, we do experience a decline in andro-gens, which prompts changes in mind and body similar to what women experience: less desire and ability for sex, mood swings, sleep disturbances, and even a "menopot." These hormone changes occur more gradually in men than in women. But the diet, lifestyle, and stress-management strategies in the Prime-Time Health plan put the body in biochemical balance, which can help ease hormonal imbal-ances in men and women.

HOW TO PREVENT ERECTILE DYSFUNCTION

ED is an inability to either attain or maintain an erection sufficient for intercourse. It is estimated that about 30 million men in the United States have some degree of ED. Around 70 percent of men over seventy have varying degrees of ED.

How erections happen. Erections are a vascular marvel. When the mood hits the brain, it sends nerve signals to two tubelike spaces called cavernosa that run the length of the penis. Using the chemical messenger nitric oxide (NO), the nerves tell these tubes to dilate (or widen) and let more blood flow in. While these spongelike tubes are filling with blood and the penis is getting bigger, harder, and more erect, another signal tells the veins in the penis to constrict (or close) so the blood flowing into the expanding tubes stays trapped in there for a while — much like inflating a balloon and then holding the top so the air can't get out. Simply speaking, an erect penis is due to a lot of trapped blood.

NO is produced throughout the vascular system and is responsible for the cavernosa opening up and filling with blood. (As you learned in chapter 3, NO is a powerful vasodilator.) Both the duration and strength of the erection is proportional to the amount of NO released. The drugs Viagra, Cialis, and Levitra work by increasing NO's effect on the blood vessels. The erection is over when the veins open up and the cavernosa contract, allowing the trapped blood to quickly exit the penis and normal blood flow to resume.

In this mechanism, there are two main areas that can affect an erection: the nerves controlling it, and the lining of the blood vessels in the penis that produce NO.

EIGHT WAYS TO MAINTAIN A HEALTHY ERECTION

Despite what you read, ED should not be considered a normal complication of aging. It is usually due to lifestyle and medical problems that can be prevented or treated, including cardiovascular disease, high blood pressure, diabetes, depression, obesity, smoking, and excessive alcohol. It is also a side effect of some medications.

1. Have a healthy heart and a hard penis. Studies show that the healthier a man's cardiovascular system, the healthier his erections. This makes sense since erections are basically a vascular phenomenon. The connection between cardiovascular disease and ED is so strong that most doctors will evaluate a man's cardiovascular system if he is complaining of ED. Gentlemen, now that you know that hardening of the arteries leads to a softening of the penis, we hope you will be motivated to faithfully follow the heart-health suggestions in chapter 3.

THE CAD-ED CONNECTION

Research reveals that men with coronary artery disease (CAD) are *seven times* more likely to have ED.

---

2. Stay lean and stay hard. Studies show that obesity is associated with ED. Obesity increases inflammation, or wear and tear, in the lining of the blood vessels, shutting down the production of NO. In fact, obesity causes endothelial dysfunction as well as ED. The two go together.

In addition, excess body fat leads to decreased testosterone, which usually wanes a bit as men age. Leaner men tend to have higher testosterone levels as they get older. One reason for this is that the lower insulin levels associated with less belly fat allow more free testosterone to circulate in the bloodstream and do its job when needed. Excess fat also prompts the production of the female hormone estrogen, which accounts for one of the least favorite effects of male aging: increased breast tissue. This excess estrogen further decreases testosterone production.

3. Relax it up. Relaxing the mind can harden the penis. An erection begins in the brain, the

FOOD FOR SEX

The same foods that protect your heart and blood vessels protect your penis, namely the omega-3s in seafood and the antioxidants in fruits and vegetables. The amino acid L-arginine found in high-protein foods (such as seafood, lean beef and poultry, nuts, eggs, and beans) is one of the building blocks of NO, so the more of these you eat, the better your NO works. In fact, ED consultants often recommend that men take 3 grams of L-arginine as a supplement daily. We recommend that you get the L-arginine from food. A 6-ounce salmon fillet with wild rice and a salad containing high-protein foods such as beans and eggs will give you 3 grams.

body's largest "sex organ." It takes the right nerve impulses to get the blood vessels going. This is why men who are under the influence of alcohol, angry, anxious, or depressed often experience ED as a side effect. An increase in stress hormones can decrease testosterone and a man's readiness and ability to enjoy sex. That makes sense since stress hormones increase blood flow to the heart, brain, and muscles and divert it from the penis in men and the vagina in women. (No time for sex! Gotta run from the tiger!) Even men who are taking medications for ED often find that they work only if the brain is relaxed and they are mentally aroused in the first place. Simply taking a pill for the penis doesn't work until the brain sends the right signals.

Beware of performance anxiety. If a man is worried about how he is going to perform, it often becomes a self-fulfilling prophecy, a situation dubbed *performance anxiety.* Here's how this cycle happens: Because you've experienced varying degrees of ED in the past, your first thought when romance strikes is "Will it work?" Immediately, you've deflated your ego and your chances of getting an erection. The more the brain worries about the penis, the less the penis can perform. Eventually, if you're unable to get or sustain an erection, your brain shuts off its desire. Less libido leads to fewer erections, and the cycle worsens.

4. Move it up. Moving more blood around the body moves more blood to the penis. While you may imagine the opposite effect, a bout of strenuous exercise can often perk up the penis. A Harvard study of thirty thousand men ages fifty-three to ninety found that those who exercised vigorously were more likely to sustain an erection. Exercise increases NO and blood flow throughout the body. Remember the heart-healthy tip: *More NO, more blood flow.* (See page 54 to learn how movement stimulates the release of NO and why exercise can be called the "body's Viagra.")

The relationship between weight lifting and libido was popularized by Arnold Schwarzenegger. When he was a bodybuilder and before he became governor of California, he equated a good workout with a good orgasm. Apparently, fitness centers were deluged with applications after Schwarzenegger made this statement on national television.

5. Talk it up. Satisfying sex is such an important part of prime-time life that couples need to be both sensitive and frank about their needs and difficulties.

6. Think it up. The mental part of sexual arousal becomes even more important as we get older. It often takes more romance to get older organs interested. You'll have to perk up the setting for sex in order to better enjoy the physical part. Keep a mental list of your own personal perks — things in your day-to-day life that turn you on. For me, it can be as simple as looking at the "pinup wall" (a wall in our bedroom where we display favorite photos from romantic vacations). Sexual arousal begins in the brain, and in my case the eye. For Martha, it's having a lot of positive bonding time so that verbal intercourse leads naturally to sexual intercourse.

7. Don't drink it down. Even Shakespeare warned against alcohol. In *Macbeth,* he says it "provokes the desire, but it takes away the performance." Not only does the brain malfunction under the influence of alcohol, so does the penis.

This can be doubly frustrating since excess alcohol often relieves inhibitions and makes you want to enjoy sex but then prevents you from getting it up. Excessive alcohol disrupts sleep cycles, which also dampens the intricate neurovascular

PILLS FOR THE PENIS

For about the cost of a movie ticket, you can get the sluggish penis working again. ED medications have been available since 1998 and have both remarkable efficacy and safety records in millions of men. At this writing, the big three are Viagra (sildenafil), Levitra (vardenafil), and Cialis (tadalafil). An interesting feature of these pills is that they work locally within the penis, not in the sexual centers of the brain. Therefore, they do not work *unless* the mental part of sexual arousal is there, which further emphasizes the fact that sex begins in the eyes and brain. While all three of these medicines have similar biochemical actions, they differ in how they affect the timing of erections.

Precautions:
- Because as we age, our liver (the body's drug-disposal system) tends to work more slowly, the older you are, the more cautious you need to be about taking the proper medication and

mechanism that produces erections. This is why many men notice the absence of nocturnal erections after a night of bingeing. Just as you don't drink and drive, don't drink when you plan to enjoy sex.

---

dosage to avoid side effects. Be sure to discuss with your doctor which of these medications will work best for you.

- Read the package insert, the list of precautions that the pharmacist gives you with your medication. It will tell you which other drugs and which foods you must avoid when taking these pills, for example, grapefruit juice, which slows down the liver's ability to eliminate many medications.
- The most common side effects are headache, facial flushing, runny nose, heartburn, dizziness, and transient visual changes. Read the package insert carefully, so you know what to watch for and what to do in case side effects occur.
- Start with the lowest dose and, shall we say, work up.

---

8. Get a medical checkup. Before you dismiss your lessening libido and increasing limpness as male menopause, be smart and get a thorough medical evaluation. Oftentimes, changes in how the penis performs can signal underlying medical issues. Your doctor will first examine the area of your genitalia to see if there are any anatomical problems within the penis, prostate, or testes. He may also look for clues of underlying hormonal imbalances (e.g., androgenic and thyroid hormones), such as decreased genital hair and increased breast tissue. If the clues warrant, your doctor may measure testosterone levels, which normally decrease as men age anyway.

Nocturnal erections are most common in the early-morning hours just before waking when the state of light or REM sleep is most prominent. Your doctor will ask you about the frequency of nocturnal erections. The absence of early-morning erections may be a clue to an underlying hormonal or anatomical problem, yet it could also be normal. Your doctor will review your current medications to see if any of them might be causing ED. Medications that have been implicated in suppressing erections are antihypertensives (for blood pressure), diuretics, antidepressants, tranquilizers, chemotherapy agents, and cholesterol-lowering medicines.

One of the most satisfying perks of the whole Prime-Time Health program is a healthier sex life. Enjoy!

Rx FOR BETTER SEX

- ❏ Understand each other's "-pause."
- ❏ Be sensitive to each other's sexual needs.
- ❏ Experiment with novel positions and other strategies.
- ❏ Stay lean.
- ❏ Don't smoke.
- ❏ Seek professional help if hormone replacement is needed.
- ❏ Keep your cardiovascular system healthy to prevent ED.
- ❏ Move more.
- ❏ Remember that the primary sexual organ is the mind.
- ❏ Limit alcohol intake.

PART IV

Prime-Time Health Care

By now you have surely gotten the prime-time message that self-care is the answer to our health-care crisis. Our current health-care system is still in "fix it" mode instead of "prevent it" mode — it's a little like running a repair shop instead of a preventive maintenance program. We begin this section by shifting your focus from what you can *take* to what you can *do*. We call this the pills-and-skills model of health care. We realize that despite self-help efforts to prevent illnesses, most prime timers will eventually need some pills. We show you how to manage your medicines wisely and safely.

Next is a crash course in preventive medicine. We begin by showing you how not to be an iBod, a body full of inflammation. Imbalances in the immune system — runaway inflammation — are the root cause of most of the illnesses prime timers experience. We show you how to get your immune system back into balance to prevent all those "-itis" illnesses. To continue in proactive mode, we explain how to lower your risk of getting the four most preventable illnesses that account for the majority of doctor visits: high blood pressure, high blood sugar, high blood cholesterol, and cancer.

After you have read and practiced this section of the Prime-Time Health plan, you will feel like you are walking around with your own personal health toolbox. You will be able to access the right tool for the right ailment in the right "dosage" at the right time. You will feel more in control of your health care, so when someone asks, "Who is your primary health-care provider?" you can confidently reply, "I am!"

CHAPTER 17

Practice the Pills-and-Skills Model of Health Care

Doctors are desperately trying to find ways to reverse the costly and unhealthy trend they call "revolving-door medicine": prime timer enters doctor's office, gets pills but no self-help skills, goes back out the door, pops pills, returns next month for stronger pills (with more side effects), and the health-care system gets sicker. This medical model isn't working.

In preparing for prime time, most people rely on the marvels of modern prescription medicines and surgical procedures, yet neglect to stock their body's own medicine cabinet with knowledge and self-help skills. We often forget that longevity requires both pills and skills. Some people manage to live long and well without many pills, but no one lives long and well without self-help skills. At this writing, I'm happy to say that at age seventy, I take no regular prescription medicines. The pills-and-skills model means changing your mind-set from "Doctor, what can I *take*?" to "Doctor, what can I *do*?" The modern doctor welcomes this approach, for it motivates him to shift from "Here's what I *prescribe*" to "Here's what I *advise*"—certainly a healthier medical mind-set. After all, the word *doctor* originally meant "teacher."

WHY PILLS CAN BEHAVE BADLY IN PRIME-TIME BODIES

The ad says, "Ask your doctor if this pill is right for you." Some pills will not be right for you. A pill tested on younger people may not behave in the same way in the prime-time body. As we age, changes occur that cause medicines to be metabolized differently:

- The gut absorbs drugs differently.
- The esophagus is more prone to inflammation and is therefore more bothered by pills.
- The liver detoxifies drugs less effectively.
- The kidneys expel drug residues less efficiently.

Because of these quirks, the pills-and-skills model of self-care is even more important during prime time, in particular. Keep these points in mind:

1. Different folks require different dosages. While pills are designed and tested for the "average body"—whatever that is—they may not be appropriate for *your* body. There are different dosages for different folks. A 110-pound woman probably needs a lower dose than a 250-pound man, for example. In fact, women generally need lower doses, which is why women seem sensitive to some medicines. Certain female traits affect how drugs behave in their bodies: Women have more fat and less muscle, and some drugs are stored in body fat. A woman's garbage-disposal system, the liver, tends to work more slowly than a man's. And because the liver doesn't detoxify (eliminate) drugs as quickly in women, women taking the same dose as men tend to be affected more frequently by side effects.

2. Beware of the cocktail effect of pills. Pills are often partnered unsafely with other pills. As you will learn in the next chapter, the cause of most prime-time ills is inflammation, which leads to high blood pressure, high blood cholesterol, and high blood sugar. As a result, many prime timers are on two, three, or four pills to treat all these ills. The problem with this approach is that using drugs in combination is not the way they were tested and approved. Suppose the FDA approves a pill to lower high blood pressure. That drug was tested on people with high blood pressure and found to be safe and effective. It was not necessarily tested on people who were taking two or three other pills, which results in the "cocktail effect."

In real life, that same blood pressure pill is not only taken for a *longer* period than it was tested for, but it is also taken with other pills, such as blood thinners and anti-inflammatories. No one knows how this pharmaceutical soup behaves in the body because it was never tested. So, each prime-time patient on a cocktail of medications is herself an experiment. Do you want to participate in such a risky undertaking?

3. Is it the drug or the disease? The cocktail effect is an especially important consideration when prime timers are taking pills to lower the highs and to elevate "lows" such as depression. Here's a typical scenario, which I have seen many times in patients that I've tried to switch from pills-only to the pills-and-skills model. Susan is a fifty-two-year-old woman who was taking pills to lower her high blood pressure, high blood sugar, and high blood cholesterol. Initially, she seemed to do fine on these medications. Then she began getting depressed, and a fourth pill was prescribed. Because one of the side effects of the antidepressant was insomnia, a fifth pill was added to help her sleep. Her depression got worse, and she also began suffering from anxiety, so another pill was added to mellow her moods. She began experiencing heartburn, so antacids were prescribed. Then she developed arthritis, which required the frequent use of anti-inflammatories. Soon she was a walking polypharmacy, taking eight different pills daily.

Medically, I call this the "hole." When a person is on so many pills, it's nearly impossible for the doctor to sort out which of the patient's symptoms are due to the underlying illness and which are due to the side effects of the pills. The doctor is afraid to take the patient off the pills, and the patient is wisely afraid to stop taking the pills without the doctor's approval. Both the doctor and the patient remain in the hole. The only way to get out of the hole is by what is called the "washout method"— the patient gradually stops taking all or most of the medicines, then treatment begins again. Such a patient often suffers from withdrawal symptoms, especially from antidepressant medicines, and therefore may seem worse. This may prompt the doctor to put the patient back on the medicines and at a higher dose, which again leaves them in the hole.

Sometimes it's difficult for a doctor — and you — to tell whether a new symptom is a side effect of a drug, part of an existing disease, or just a new and unrelated symptom. Before you blame the drug, do some detective work to help your doctor. The drug has a high probability of being the culprit if:

- the reaction (muscle pain, insomnia, mood changes, etc.) appeared shortly after starting the drug;
- the symptoms were alleviated or went away after you stopped the drug or lowered the dose;
- according to your doctor, other patients have experienced similar side effects;

- your symptoms are on the list of possible side effects on the drug's package insert or website.

4. Pills help one body part but may harm another. No pill acts on only one organ. You may take a heart medicine that may bother the brain or a joint medicine that may bother the heart. "Anti-" pills (such as anti-inflammatories, antacids, anticoagulants, and antihypertensives) usually work as blockers or inhibitors of some enzyme's "on" switch. Yet, they also block the on switch in other parts of the body that need it. Antacids may lessen the production of stomach acids and thereby deprive the rest of the intestines of the healthful effects of these stomach acids. Anti-inflammatories may turn down the enzymes that cause inflammation so you don't have so much pain from arthritis when you walk, but they also upset the balance between the proinflammatories and the anti-inflammatories, so the blood vessels don't know whether to open up or close down. One such "anti-" was Vioxx, which was taken off the market because it threw the body out of inflammatory balance, causing blood clots and heart attacks.

The side effects of one "anti-," such as an anti-inflammatory, may be too much acid in the stomach, requiring you to take another "anti-," an antacid. Now you're in a vicious cycle: taking one pill to treat the side effects of the other. The good news is that the Prime-Time Health plan should replace many of the pills with self-help skills and put your body back into balance.

HOW PRIME TIMERS CAN TAKE PILLS WISELY AND SAFELY

Because pills behave differently in prime-time bodies, medications need to be prescribed and taken wisely. When a doctor prescribes a drug, ask, "What else can I try first?" The conditions that are most helped by self-help skills are high blood sugar, high blood pressure, and high blood cholesterol and depression. Whether your doctor perceives you as primarily a pills patient or a skills patient depends on how you present yourself. If you open the discussion with "Doctor, what can I *do*?" rather than "What can I *take*?" she gets the message that you want to take responsibility for your body. If after you practice the skills, your doctor also recommends pills, here are some guidelines:

Start low. Package inserts suggest lower dosages for most people over age fifty. In the liver and intestines, many enzymes break down a drug and discard its leftovers (called metabolites) in the urine or stools. Some people metabolize drugs more slowly than others. Because of their unique genetic programming, their drug-degrading enzymes aren't as fast. Slow metabolizers, therefore, need a lower dose of certain medications to prevent the drug from accumulating to toxic levels. Fast metabolizers, on the other hand, may need a higher dosage. You won't know which type of metabolizer you are unless you *start low and go slow.* While the package insert may specify an "average dose" of, say, 10 milligrams, ask your doctor if you can try a lower dose first to see how it works and how you react. Science is on your side. Studies show that most patients, especially prime timers, are helped by a lower-than-standard dose, especially of those medications for the highs and lows.

Go slow. Don't rush to double the dose if your cholesterol, blood pressure, or blood sugar isn't coming down. *Gradually* increase the pills. And double your skills.

HOW YOUR BODY MAKES
ITS OWN PILLS

If you're like most people, you assume that as you go through prime time, an increasing number of little amber bottles with white tops will occupy shelf space in your medicine cabinet. But that's not necessarily so. Here's an overview of the pills most prime timers take and what your body can do:

- Pills to lower *blood pressure.* The body can make its own (page 512).
- Pills to lower *cholesterol.* The body can be taught to make its own (page 517).
- Pills to lower *blood sugar.* The body can be taught to regulate its own blood sugar level (page 519).
- Pills to help the *heart beat stronger.* Your body can build a stronger heart that beats more efficiently (chapter 3).
- Pills to *steady your heartbeat.* You can eat foods that prevent your heartbeat from misfiring (page 78).
- Pills to *keep blood from overclotting,* to lessen heart attacks and strokes. The body makes its own blood thinners and certainly ones that are safer and more effective because they are tailor-made for you (page 60).
- Pills to *dilate blood vessels* to increase blood flow to organs. Here's where the body

really shines and makes its own vasodilators (page 59).

- Pills for the *"-itis" illnesses* (e.g., bronchitis, arthritis, colitis, and dermatitis). The body can make its own anti-inflammatories, which are better and safer than the ones you buy (page 470).
- Pills to *mellow your mood.* The brain can be primed to make its own "happy hormones" and natural antidepressants (pages 112, 128).
- Pills to perk up *cognitive* decline. Your body can make its own brain-saving medicines (pages 109, 127).
- Pills to heal a *hurting tummy*. You can get a handle on heartburn naturally (page 154).
- Pills to *kill germs*. Your body and nature's food *farm*acy make better antibiotics than you can buy (pages 470, 476).
- Pills to *cover up pain*. The Prime-Time Health plan helps your body make medicines that prevent the causes of pain.

Your body is a walking pharmacy, a storehouse of all you need to be happy and healthy. Learn how to unlock your body's medicines, which are tailor-made for you, by following the plan outlined in this book. Then you can say good-bye to disease, disabilities, and dysfunction.

Take only *one* pill if possible. Because prime timers tend to be slow metabolizers, try not to overwhelm your liver with too many pills. Two or more drugs may be metabolized by the same enzyme. These drug-degrading enzymes are part of the body's garbage-disposal system. If the enzyme is used up disposing of one drug, there may not be enough enzyme left over to eliminate the other drug, which can then accumulate to toxic levels.

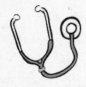

DR. SEARS SAYS…
The best way to lower your pill bill is to raise your self-help skills.

Consider the risk-benefit ratio. Every drug or treatment has one. Ask "What is the risk of damaging side effects versus benefits?" This risk-benefit ratio is particularly important with psychotropic drugs (antidepressants and antianxiety medications) and statins (cholesterol-lowering drugs). If you don't ask, you can't make an informed decision about what is right for you.

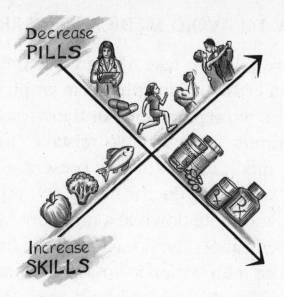

Add skills to your prescribed pills. Suppose your doctor prescribes a statin drug to lower your cholesterol. This class of drug is a prime example of why the pills-and-skills model is needed. Besides the pills, your doctor should prescribe increased exercise and diet changes, such as a more plant-based and less animal-based diet. He should also encourage you to eat more omega-3 oils and less omega-6 oils, a change that studies have shown helps statins work better.

HOW TO AVOID MEDICATION ERRORS

The more pills we take, the greater the chance of human error: patient, physician, or pharmacist. Taking the wrong medicine or the wrong dosage is a common yet avoidable mistake. To ensure that the medication a doctor prescribes is right for you, when the doctor hands you a prescription, ask and write down in a notebook the name of the medication, the dosage, and the frequency. Having this information in your own handwriting for your reference can be a help later. Then ask:

1. Why are you prescribing this?
2. Are there lifestyle changes I could try first?
3. Would you prescribe this drug to a family member?
4. Will it interact with my other medications?
5. Should I take it with food, or before or after eating?
6. What side effects can I expect? How can I avoid them?

Finally, be sure to tell your doctor if you are taking herbal or "natural" supplements — and which ones — as these may make the prescription drug less safe or effective.

Get to know your pharmacist. If possible, get all your prescriptions filled at the same pharmacy. This increases the likelihood that potential drug interactions will be detected, especially if different medications are prescribed by different doctors.

Ask the pharmacist for the package insert for the medication you're taking. When you pick up your prescription, be sure that you can read the directions. If the type is too small, the pharmacist can print them in larger type. Read the name of the medication, the dosage, and frequency while you're at the pharmacy and compare that information with your notes. This will ensure that you have the proper medication and that the pharmacist correctly interpreted the prescription. If you refill a prescription and the pills look different from the ones you had before, ask the pharmacist why. Read the complete package insert. It will inform you about the possible side effects, but it may also cause you to imagine that you're having one.

Develop a reliable method for remembering what to take when. Buy a medication organizer, or keep a log book and write down what you take when each day.

Keep a medical card in your wallet. Print the following information on a small card, attach it to your medical insurance card, and give a copy to your emergency contacts:

Name:
Major medical
    conditions:
Medications:
    [name, dosage,
    frequency]
Drug allergies:
	Emergency
	    contacts:
	    [names and
	    phone numbers]
	Doctor's name:
	Preferred hospital:
	Religion:

The American College of Emergency Physicians recommends that prime timers enter two emergency contacts into their cell phones and label them ICE: *in case of emergency.* Hospital emergency room staffs know this code.

DR. SEARS SAYS...

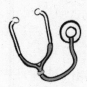

Show me the science. You may notice we mention only a handful of over-the-counter and natural remedies in this book. This is because the nutraceutical industry is undergoing more critical review. "Natural remedies" that were previously pronounced safe and effective are sometimes found to be either unsafe or ineffective. If a friend says, "Take XYZ — it really helped me!" respond with "Show me the science." Run the touted remedy by your doctor or try to find studies showing that a particular supplement works and is safe. For updates, see www.AskDrSears.com/Prime-TimeHealth.

Rx FOR PRIME-TIME PILL TAKING

❑ Practice the pills-and-skills mind-set.

❑ When it comes to drug dosage, start low and go slow.

❑ Write down your doctor's medication instructions.

❑ Keep a medical-summary card in your wallet.

❑ Only take supplements backed by solid science.

❑ What's the answer to the health-care crisis? *Self-care.*

CHAPTER 18

Free Your Body of Excess Inflammation

What "-itis" is in your body? Controlling inflammation ("-itis" illnesses) is the key to healthy aging. Evidence is mounting that inflammation contributes more to cardiovascular disease than does high cholesterol. And new research suggests that inflammation may be the number one cause of cardiovascular disease, cancer, and dementia, the big three challenges of prime time, as well as of many disabilities that plague us as we get older.

Inflammation, which literally means "on fire," is one of the main causes of premature aging. When excessive inflammation occurs, tissues that line certain parts of the body — such as the joints, the intestines, and especially the blood vessels — get "rough edges" and malfunction. It's that stiff and sticky stuff again. Most of the medical conditions afflicting prime timers — heart disease, arthritis, Alzheimer's disease, cancer, and diabetes — begin with excess inflammation or *cytokines*, the wear-and-tear chemicals produced by an immune system out of balance.

The right balance of inflammation protects and heals the body. Suppose you cut your finger. The injury signals the body to take action to cleanse and heal the cut. This is called the *inflammatory response*. Here's how it works: As soon as the skin of your finger is penetrated, the damage to the tissue and the potential entry of germs prompt local cells to send out chemical messengers (such as cytokines and histamines) to mobilize an infection-fighting army to the site. Then local cells, called macrophages ("big eaters"), act like miniature Pac-Men and engulf the germs at the wound site.

As you see your cut healing, marvel at the body at work. You'll notice *redness* from the extra blood flow to the injury site. Then you will see slight *swelling* from all those extra forces, like disaster workers, marshaled at the cut. All this commotion generates a lot of heat, or inflammation — it feels *hot*. This is why healing inflammation is dubbed "friendly fire."

ARE YOU AN IBOD?

As we age, not only do we have fewer of some immune-system soldiers (natural killer cells), but we occasionally produce too many cytokines, soldiers that overfight and trigger too much inflammation. For unknown reasons, the body occasionally overreacts by mustering up a bigger army than is needed to fight a little infection. Even worse, sometimes the body's inflammatory response gets confused and attacks its own tissues, causing buildup of battle debris (sticky stuff) in blood vessels (especially arteries of the heart and brain) and brain tissues (Alzheimer's disease), and leads to the ABCD "-itis" diseases (arthritis, bronchitis, colitis, dermatitis). I call people who have these illnesses *iBods,* inflammatory bodies.

For example, at the insistence of his loving wife, Mike, a forty-something restaurateur, came into my office for a "metabolic tune-up." He had sore joints, low energy, high blood pressure, and a big belly. "Mike," I said, "you're an iBod!" This caught Mike by surprise. He had no idea what an iBod was, but he didn't want to be one.

The key to a healthy immune response is

balance: just enough inflammatory response to fight infections and repair the normal wear and tear to tissues and slow aging — not too much to damage healthy tissues and accelerate aging. Premature aging, in a nutshell, is caused by the inflammatory response being out of balance. If the body is out of balance, it is said to be in a *proinflammatory state*.

NINE WAYS TO KEEP YOUR BODY'S INFLAMMATION BALANCED

Of course you could pop a pill each time you itch or ache. In case you haven't been following the news lately, "-itis" medicines such as Vioxx are not so safe. Here are nine ways to keep you from becoming an iBod:

1. Stay Lean

Staying lean is the number one way to keep from becoming an iBod. Americans are the most inflamed people in the world, and we are also the fattest. Any correlation? Excess belly fat promotes excess inflammation. While you may think that excess fat is just globs of extra tissue sitting there doing nothing but slowing you down, in fact these fat cells are chemical factories. Fat cells pump out proinflammatory wear-and-tear chemicals, like an overstaffed, restless army that goes around invading tissues and picking fights. The body, in its wisdom, regards excess fat cells as detrimental to its health, and therefore tries to fight them by producing more inflammatory chemicals. The fewer excess fat cells, the less excess inflammation. It's as simple as that. For young people who want to delay the infirmities of getting older and for older people who want to feel young, stay lean. It slows down the wear and tear on your tissues.

And remember to move. Studies show that exercise helps clean up that sticky stuff that accumulates in your brain, vessels, and joints. Reducing your excess waist size (or what I dub "waist management") is the best way to keep yourself from becoming an iBod. (See "Toxic Waist," page 92.)

2. Eat Fish

Omega-3 oils — especially those found in cold-water fish, such as wild salmon and tuna — are the most healthful anti-inflammatory foods you can eat. Omega-3s act like anti-inflammatories and anticoagulants. They prevent excess clotting and damage to the arterial walls, in effect keeping the surface of the road smooth and the traffic moving. Omega-3s act in much the same way that aspirin and some prescription drugs do but without the side effects. Studies show the higher a person's blood level of omega-3s, the less likely she is to be an iBod.

3. Change Your Oils

If you are inflamed like many prime timers, your body needs an oil change. Fish oils are anti-inflammatory; some factory-processed vegetable oils can be proinflammatory. To keep your body in balance, you need to have the right balance of omega-3 and omega-6 oils, as close as possible to a 1:1 ratio. (See a list of healthy and unhealthy oils, page 80.)

SPICE UP YOUR IMMUNE SYSTEM

By spicing up your diet, you can help reduce inflammation. Spices such as turmeric inhibit the D5D enzyme, which changes some of the oils in your diet to proinflammatory substances. (See "Spice Up Your Life," page 360.)

---

4. Don't Forget Your Phytos

Aging is rusting. Phytonutrients, or phytos (Greek for "plant") as I like to call them, are antirust nutrients found in plant-based foods. Rust (oxidation) is a natural by-product of cellular metabolism, like the exhaust from your car engine. Oxidation plus inflammation is a disastrous duo for premature aging. Healthy prime time requires developing an antirust program.

The antioxidants in foods often work better in the body than do antioxidants in vitamin pills because of the biochemical activity called *synergy*. The many different phytos in foods are like friends that work together to help each other be more powerful. See page 476 for a list of healing foods.

5. Change Your Carbs to Stabilize Your Insulin

The main hormone that determines whether your body is in anti-inflammatory and proinflammatory balance is insulin. A high level of insulin promotes a high inflammatory state — more wear and tear, less repair. Good carbs promote stable insulin levels. Bad carbs lead to a roller-coaster effect in both blood sugar and insulin. People with a steady diet of junk carbs,

JUICE UP YOUR DEFENSES

To keep inflammation down, drink a daily glass of pomegranate, grape, or carrot juice. Enjoy frequent sprinkles of lemon or lime juice in water or on salads. At this writing, I take only one nutritional supplement, an antioxidant-concentrated fruit and vegetable extract called Juice Plus. Even though I get the recommended nine daily servings of fruits and vegetables in my smoothie (see page 151) and my supersalad (see page 554), I believe I need extra antioxidant protection because of a biochemical quirk called *exercise-induced oxidative stress.* I exercise one to two hours a day. Just as a heavily driven car engine produces extra exhaust, a vigorously exercising body produces extra oxidation. A 2009 study in *Medicine and Science in Sports and Exercise,* the official journal of the American College of Sports Medicine, showed that taking this antioxidant concentrate lessened the oxidative damage of proteins (inflammation) after strenuous exercise.

---

especially those who are prediabetic or show a blood chemistry profile of insulin resistance, are more likely to be iBods. To tamp down inflammation, you need a diet high in good carbs and low in bad carbs.

Graze on good foods. Grazing minimizes swings in blood sugar and therefore keeps insulin stable by preventing the highs and lows.

Eat a high-fiber diet. Fiber slows the release of carbs into the bloodstream, stabilizing the blood sugar level, and therefore stabilizing insulin levels.

Eat a right-carb diet. Carbs partnered with protein and fiber are released slowly into the bloodstream and keep insulin from spiking. On the other hand, junk carbs have been shown to depress the immune system by decreasing the number of infection-fighting white blood cells.

Stay lean. Excess body fat churns out chemicals that make cells more resistant to insulin, and the pancreas has to produce more insulin to drive the sugar into the cells. Excess insulin promotes excess inflammation, and it also promotes excess hunger. It's a vicious cycle.

6. Move

People who exercise vigorously at least three times a week have lower blood levels of inflammatory chemicals than do people who sit too much.

HEALING FOODS VS. HURTING FOODS

Eat more healing, or anti-inflammatory, foods—a few nuts here, a sprinkle of spices there. It adds up. And those super-phyto foods work even while you're asleep, when the body clicks into *repair mode,* sort of like a self-cleaning oven, and rewards you for making good food choices throughout the day. Healing repair foods keep the linings of joints and blood vessels smooth. Think of them as "smooth" foods. In contrast, proinflammatory foods make linings rough.

Anti-inflammatory Foods	Proinflammatory Foods
Cold-water fish, especially salmon, tuna, sardines, anchovies	Animal fats, especially from feedlot animals
	Sunflower oil
Fish-oil supplements	Corn oil
Flax oil, flaxseeds (ground)	Safflower oil
	Soybean oil
Olive oil	Coconut oil
Nuts	Palm kernel oil

Exercise regulates the inflammatory response in several ways:

Exercise stabilizes insulin. Since strength-training exercises build muscle, the more muscle

Anti-inflammatory Foods	Proinflammatory Foods
Game meats	"Partially hydrogenated" oils
Fruits: blueberries, pomegranates, papaya, apricots, cherries, pink grapefruit, grapes	French fries
	Fried foods
	Most salad dressings
Vegetables: especially greens and high-fiber ones	Most fast-food meals
Lentils	Sweetened beverages
Onions	Most margarines
Sweet potatoes	Most shortenings
Spices, such as turmeric, curry, ginger, cinnamon	High-fructose corn syrup
Chili peppers	
Green tea	
Garlic	
Lemon and lime juices	

you have, the more carbs you burn, and the more stable your blood insulin level is likely to be. (If you exercise strenuously you need to eat more antioxidant-rich foods.)

Exercise burns fat. The leaner you are, the lower your levels of proinflammatories.

Exercise blocks the body's production of proinflammatory substances. Specifically, moderate exercise blocks the enzyme D5D that converts the omega-6 oils (proinflammatory vegetable oils, such as corn, safflower, and sunflower oils) into the inflammation chemical arachidonic acid. Even though very strenuous exercise produces oxidative stress, all levels of exercise help the body achieve inflammatory balance.

7. Breathe Clean Air

It's not only what you swallow that triggers inflammation, it's also what you breathe. Studies show that the blood level of inflammatory substances goes up after people breathe polluted air.

8. Stay Calm

Positive emotions such as joy and laughter can keep your immune system in balance. Excessive and unresolved stress causes the body to spew out excess stress hormones, mainly cortisol. A 2005 study from the Institute for Mind Body Medicine at Massachusetts General Hospital and

Harvard Medical School showed that people practicing relaxation techniques had higher blood levels of nitric oxide, that total-body health elixir (see page 54).

9. Take Care of Your Gums

One of the best ways to keep yourself from becoming an iBod is to have good dental health. Gingivitis is a common source of inflammation entering the body.

WHAT ABOUT
ANTI-INFLAMMATORY MEDICINES?

Americans spend over $20 billion a year on anti-inflammatory medicines. Imagine spending that much on lifestyle changes and nutrition for your body. The body churns out proinflammatory chemicals by using an enzyme called cyclooxygenase (COX). Most of the over-the-counter nonsteroidal anti-inflammatory drugs (NSAIDs), like aspirin and ibuprofen, and prescription medications, like Vioxx and Celebrex, inhibit the COX enzymes and therefore lessen inflammation. (These medications are known as COX inhibitors.) Anti-inflammatory drugs once thought to be the magic bullet for controlling inflammation-related pain, such as arthritis, have now been shown to have risks. Here's why:

They're hard on the heart. It would be nice if these medicines, and all prescription drugs, could be like smart bombs and target only specific enzymes. Yet, these drugs have been found to interfere with the part of the inflammatory response that has a beneficial effect, and in some cases to increase a person's risk of cardiovascular disease.

They're irritating to the gut. Excessive use of even over-the-counter anti-inflammatories, such as ibuprofen, can interfere with the way the lining of the stomach secretes protective sealants to keep from digesting itself. And, too much acetaminophen can damage your body's main garbage-disposal system, the liver. By suppressing prostaglandins, which regulate the balance of gastric acid and protective mucus, these COX inhibitors can *increase* gastric acid and *decrease* intestinal mucus — just the opposite of what you want.

I recently attended a seminar on the health benefits of omega-3s given by Dr. William Lands, an expert on fatty acids and author of *Fish, Omega-3, and Human Health.* Dr. Lands summed up the "-itis" and pill problem: "We take medicines such as COX inhibitors and NSAIDs to treat the inflammation caused by the dietary excesses of omega-6s and deficiencies of omega-3s." I agree. We take drugs to treat a dietary abuse. Why not just correct the abuse!

MEASURING YOUR INFLAMMATION

There isn't yet a routine lab test available that can measure your level of circulating proinflammatories. With the increasing awareness that inflammation is the root of most major diseases, it's only a matter of time before researchers come up with a reliable inflammation profile similar to the lipid profile used for assessing the risk of cardiovascular disease. For now, here are some general tests, called *markers,* that will give you a sense of whether your body's inflammatory response is in balance. These blood tests measure the average level of sticky stuff in your body:

AA/EPA ratio. Ask your doctor to order an essential-fatty-acid profile, which measures the relative amounts of AA (arachidonic acid) and EPA (eicosapentaenoic acid) in your blood. This is the ratio of the proinflammatory fatty acid AA and the anti-inflammatory fatty acid EPA. The more AA circulating in your blood relative to EPA, the more likely your body is to be leaning toward a proinflammatory state, and vice versa. Try to keep the AA/EPA ratio to less than 3:1.

Carbohydrate profile. Two tests give you a clue as to whether you have excess carbs floating around in your bloodstream: the fasting blood insulin level and fasting blood sugar level. Try to keep your fasting insulin level below 10 μU/mL and your fasting blood sugar level under 125 (ideally both of these measurements should be even lower for optimal biochemical health). If your carbohydrate profile is higher than these levels, you are at increased risk of developing insulin-resistance or type 2 diabetes, and biochemically your body is in the proinflammatory state.

Hemoglobin A1c. Called "glycated hemo-globin," this is a measure of the excess carbo-hydrates sticking to your red blood cells. If this level is high, it's a clue that your average blood sugar is too high. Ideally, HbA1c should be less than 6 percent.

Lipid profile. This measures fats in your bloodstream and predicts your risk of heart disease and gives a clue as to your risk of excess inflammation. These numbers include triglycerides (TGs), total cholesterol, LDL cho-lesterol, small-particle LDL, HDL cholesterol, and the TG/HDL ratio. The higher the TG/HDL ratio, the higher your risk of cardiovascular disease and heart attack, and the more likely your body is to lean toward an excessively proinflammatory state. Try to keep your TG/HDL ratio below 3.

C-reactive protein. C-reactive protein (CRP) is a substance produced by the liver as part of the body's inflammatory response. It normally goes up while the body fights an infec-tion. Yet, if the level of CRP — or the newer test called hs-CRP (high-sensitivity CRP) — stays high even when you don't have an acute infection, this is a crude indication that the body's inflammatory response is overactive. An hs-CRP *less than 3* mg/L (lower is even better) is considered okay. Higher levels are concerning and may indicate the body is in a chronic inflammatory state.

Waist size. This one measurement can give you a pretty accurate clue as to your level of risk for excess inflammation, since increased abdominal fat increases the risk of insulin resistance and skews the body toward a proinflammatory state. Generally, a waist circumference greater than 40 inches in men and 35 inches in women significantly increases this risk. (To learn how excess belly fat leads to inflammation, see "Toxic Waist," page 92.)

Rx FOR PRIME-TIME INFLAMMATION CONTROL

- ❑ Stay lean.
- ❑ Reduce your waist size.
- ❑ Eat more real food, less processed food.
- ❑ Graze on minimeals.
- ❑ Eat more fish than meat.
- ❑ Eat more fruits and vegetables.
- ❑ Drink water instead of sweetened beverages.
- ❑ Breathe clean air.
- ❑ Move more.
- ❑ Stay calm.
- ❑ Enjoy good dental hygiene.
- ❑ Have your blood inflammatory profile checked.

CHAPTER 19

Lower High Blood Pressure, High Blood Cholesterol, and High Blood Sugar

High blood pressure, cholesterol, and sugar are such a common triad for prime timers that there are rumors of pharmaceutical companies working to develop a polypill that contains medications to address all three. But while these "highs" are some of the most common ailments of aging, the good news is that they're also the easiest to control through diet and lifestyle. The recommendations for controlling high blood pressure, cholesterol, and sugar are very similar. That's because they are interrelated and often occur together. Four simple words are all you need to remember to lower these highs: *fish, pure, lean,* and *move.*

You may hear that diet and lifestyle changes alone won't lower the highs. Research has shown the opposite to be true. The fact is that many people are not willing to make the necessary changes for this approach to work. By lowering these highs, you can lengthen your life.

"But my blood tests are fine," rationalized one of my patients who was abusing his body. Don't wait for your body to hurt and your blood tests to show problems. By then, the damage has already been done. Better to *prevent* now than to linger in *repair* mode later.

KEEP YOUR BLOOD PRESSURE RIGHT FOR YOU

High blood pressure, or hypertension, ranks among the top causes of unhealthy aging and premature death in the United States. Consider these scary stats:

- About 25 percent of adults in the United States, more than 50 million people, have blood pressure that is too high. This alarming percentage increases with age: 50 percent of adults over age sixty and 80 percent of adults over age seventy have high blood pressure.
- After age sixty, women have a greater risk of high blood pressure than men.

- In the United States, high blood pressure is the most common reason that adults visit the doctor, and drugs to treat it are the most frequently prescribed. It often leads to heart failure, heart attack, and stroke.

Cardiologists estimate that 95 percent of people with high blood pressure could lower it with lifestyle changes. Healthy blood pressure is necessary to prevent target organ diseases such as stroke, kidney failure, and heart failure. For example, if the heart, a muscular organ, continually has to pump against high resistance, it will eventually fail.

Blood Pressure 101: What Every Prime Timer Must Know

Next time you water your garden, notice that you can regulate the water pressure in the hose by adjusting the opening of the nozzle. You can regulate your blood pressure in a similar way by opening (dilating) or closing (constricting) your arteries. The built-in sensors in the walls of your blood vessels do this automatically. But, if the vessel walls are stiff from an accumulation of too much sticky stuff, your blood pressure stays high. Again, it's back to our simple remedy for aging: keep the sticky stuff out of your body.

Know your numbers. The numbers that are considered normal for most adults are 120/80. The top number (120) is the systolic blood pressure, the maximum pressure reached in the arteries while the heart muscle contracts and pumps blood into them. It is the pressure when the heart beats. The bottom number (80), the diastolic pressure, is the pressure that occurs in the arteries when the heart relaxes between contractions, or the pressure between beats. The numbers 120 and 80 indicate the number of millimeters of pressure needed to push up a column of mercury. While you're wearing an old-fashioned blood-pressure cuff, you can watch the silver stuff climb up the column.

Low numbers are healthier. Of the two, the diastolic, or the bottom number, is the most meaningful. The heart relaxes for a longer period between beats than it contracts, so the diastolic pressure "presses" against the arteries for a longer time than does the systolic.

WHAT DO THE NUMBERS MEAN?

Blood-Pressure Classification	Systolic	Diastolic
Optimal (your heart is smiling)	Less than 120	Less than 80
Normal (your heart is still smiling)	Less than 130	Less than 85
Prehypertension* (heart "check engine" light is on)	130–139	85–89
Stage 1: Get serious about heart health	140–159	90–99
Stage 2: Get even more serious	160–179	100–109
Stage 3: Be sure your life insurance payments are current	Above 180	Above 109

*This new category of prehypertension is a signal that your cardiovascular system needs attention to keep you from progressing to the other stages.

If you develop high blood pressure, your chance of dying within a year is double that of a person who has normal blood pressure. If the doubling of death rate doesn't scare you into changing how you live, move, think, and eat, remember that the rate of disabilities also increases — kidney disease, stroke, heart attack, and a generally debilitated life.

What causes high blood pressure, and why it's harmful. Let's go back to the pressure in your garden hose. The following conditions would increase the water pressure within the hose: the faucet is turned up higher (your heart could pump harder); the thickness of the hose could be stiffer or less elastic (hardening of the arteries); or there might be a kink in the hose (a major artery is narrowed from either a congenital defect or plaque buildup). While fewer than 5 percent of people have high blood pressure because of kidney disease, hormone imbalance, or a congenital defect called a *coarctation* (narrowing of the aorta, a major blood vessel coming from the heart), 95 percent of people have high blood pressure because the blood vessels get too stiff, and that's the cause that's most preventable.

If you were to take your garden hose and deliberately put a kink in it, eventually there would be so much wear and tear from the high water pressure that the hose lining would weaken and pop. Or, the water might suddenly start to spurt out where the hose is attached to the faucet. This is what happens in a stroke caused by high blood pressure: a vessel in the brain pops, and the blood leaks out. In fact, *80 percent* of strokes are caused by high blood pressure. The best way to maintain a healthy blood pressure is to keep the blood vessels smooth and strong. This is exactly what the Prime-Time Health plan can help you do.

One of the ways a popular class of blood-pressure-lowering medications (called angiotensin-converting enzyme [ACE] inhibitors) works is by blocking the action of a potent vasoconstrictor called angiotensin, which the endothelium secretes to constrict, or narrow, the arteries. When endothelial function goes wrong, such as when too much angiotensin is secreted, high blood pressure results. Because angiotensin and nitric oxide have opposite effects, blood vessel health (tailoring the highway according to the amount of traffic) requires just the right balance between NO and angiotensin. The Prime-Time Health plan can help you to achieve this balance.

Many blood-pressure-lowering medications (called antihypertensives) have such unpleasant side effects that patients often stop taking them. The good news is that by taking care of your endothelium, you can help your body make its own antihypertensive medicines.

SMALL CHANGES LEAD TO BIG HEALTH BENEFITS

When it comes to reducing high blood pressure to a level that is right for you, small changes can make a big difference:

- A decrease of only 5 millimeters in diastolic blood pressure reduces the risk of heart failure by 52 percent and the risk of stroke by 40 percent.
- In the Trial of Nonpharmacologic Intervention in the Elderly (TONE), a small reduction in daily sodium intake decreased the need for hypertensive medications in 40 percent of people.
- A weight loss of ten pounds reduced the need for blood pressure medication by 36 percent.
- The combination of consuming less sodium and losing ten pounds reduced the need for blood-pressure-lowering medication by 53 percent.

CONTROL YOUR CHOLESTEROL

From the way the pharmaceutical companies pitch it, you might think that every prime timer should be on medication to lower their cholesterol. Food packaging hypes "no cholesterol" or "low cholesterol," and low-cholesterol diets are touted. Yet, cholesterol is not always as bad as it's portrayed to be.

Cholesterol 101: What Every Prime Timer Must Know

Your liver makes most of the cholesterol in your blood naturally. If cholesterol were really bad, your body wouldn't make it. It's an *excess* of cholesterol that can be harmful. To better control your cholesterol level, understand the following:

You need cholesterol. Biochemically, cholesterol is a sterol, a fatlike nutrient that helps build cell membranes. It can be considered the mortar that holds the bricks of the cell membrane together. The right amount of cholesterol does good things for you:

- Cholesterol is an especially important nutrient in the cell-membrane structures of the brain and the central nervous system. It is essential in myelin, the fatty tissue that insulates nerves and helps the electrical impulses of the central nervous system travel faster. Lowering cholesterol too much, and too fast, can rob the brain of this needed nutrient. This is why neurologists believe that some people suffer fuzzy thinking when taking cholesterol-lowering drugs.

- Cholesterol is a component of bile, which helps fat digestion.
- Cholesterol forms a vital part of sex hormones and adrenal hormones.
- Cholesterol helps the body manufacture vitamin D.

Cholesterol is an integral component of the cell membranes of nearly all animal tissue, but the cell membranes of plants are composed of fiber, not cholesterol. So when you see "no cholesterol" on labels for fruit, vegetables, vegetable oils, or grains, remember that there was no cholesterol in them in the first place.

The body makes all the cholesterol it needs. Your natural cholesterol — the

3,000 milligrams per day your body makes (ten times the maximum recommended daily amount of dietary cholesterol) — is more than enough for health. In fact, for most people, about 80 percent of the cholesterol in their blood is made by their own bodies. The rest comes from their diet.

Some people are more sensitive to dietary cholesterol than others. Normally, when a healthy person eats high-cholesterol foods, the liver reduces its cholesterol production to maintain blood cholesterol at a healthy level. Yet, in around 30 percent of people, this internal cholesterol-monitoring system doesn't operate efficiently; when such people eat high-cholesterol foods, their blood-cholesterol levels go up, so they need to closely watch what they eat. Only about 0.5 percent of all people have *familial hypercholesterolemia,* a genetic quirk that prevents the internal cholesterol-regulating system from being in balance, causing the liver to produce more cholesterol than the body requires. People with this condition most need the cholesterol-lowering statins. Sensitivity to cholesterol-containing foods varies greatly. In most people, a low-cholesterol diet and regular exercise are enough to reduce cholesterol levels, but others may also need medication.

There's good cholesterol and not-so-good cholesterol. The cholesterol in food travels to your liver, where it teams up with the cholesterol that the liver makes naturally. When your body needs cholesterol, it signals the liver to release some of the stored cholesterol. The cholesterol then enters the bloodstream, where it is transported by low-density lipoproteins (LDLs), forming LDL cholesterol, a nutritional ferry service that carries cholesterol from the liver to the cells. If a cell already has all the cholesterol it needs, it "refuses delivery" of the cholesterol cargo, and the cholesterol-laden LDL stays in the bloodstream, where it forms sticky stuff that can be deposited in the walls of arteries, causing atherosclerotic plaque. The more plaque that builds up, the stiffer and narrower the arteries become. While LDL is known as the "bad cholesterol," as you can see, in the right amount it does good things for the body. It is an *excess* of LDL that is bad. Lower amounts of LDL are better.

High-density lipoprotein (HDL), the "good cholesterol" (HDL should be *h*igher), travels through the bloodstream like a vacuum cleaner, sucking up excess cholesterol from fatty plaques in the arterial walls. The HDL carries excess cholesterol back to the liver, where it is eliminated in the intestines. How your liver handles cholesterol and how much stays in your bloodstream has to do with your family history (heredity) and what you eat. The genes you're stuck with, but the food you can control.

The *real* cholesterol/cardiovascular disease connection. The cholesterol/cardiovascular disease connection was first made several decades ago in the classic Framingham Heart Study, which showed that people who had higher blood cholesterol levels also had a higher incidence of cardiovascular disease. This was only a *statistical correlation,* not necessarily a cause and effect, yet it triggered worries about high cholesterol that birthed a whole industry of low-cholesterol diets and cholesterol-lowering drugs. And these diets and drugs worked. Many studies showed that lowering a person's high cholesterol also lowered the risk of heart disease. Cholesterol became an easy target. Doctors could measure it and prescribe medicines to treat it.

New studies have shown that the cholesterol/ cardiovascular disease connection is not so clear. Perhaps cholesterol is not the culprit. About half of people who have heart attacks have *normal* cholesterol levels. And despite the effectiveness of cholesterol-lowering drugs, the incidence of cardiovascular disease is rising. These observations have led many cardiologists to rethink the cholesterol connection. Could it be that people who eat high-cholesterol diets also have other more harmful habits that make them more prone to cardiovascular disease? In light of new research, many heart doctors now believe that inflammation causes more cardiovascular disease than high cholesterol, and that the anti-inflammatory, rather than the cholesterol-lowering, effects of statin drugs may be responsible for their cardiovascular benefits.

Know Your Cholesterol Numbers

Numbers are statistical guides, or red flags, that alert you to risks. They are also powerful motivators for change. When your doctor orders a lipid panel to measure the amount of various fats in your bloodstream, be sure you understand your numbers.

Here's what your doctor measures and the numbers that are healthy.

Lipid Panel	Heart-Healthy Numbers
Triglycerides	Less than 150 mg
Total cholesterol	Less than 190 mg
LDL	Less than 130 mg
HDL	More than 50 mg
Total cholesterol/ HDL ratio	Less than 4:1

While these numbers are nice to have, rather than using absolute numbers many cardiologists emphasize ratios. The number that seems to be most predictive of heart disease is the ratio of total cholesterol to HDL. For example, a total cholesterol of 200 and an HDL of 50 would give you a cholesterol/HDL ratio of 4:1. A total cholesterol/HDL ratio greater than 4.5:1 increases a person's risk of cardiovascular disease. Dropping the ratio by one full point, for example from 5:1 to 4:1, reduces the likelihood of heart attack by 50 percent.

A high HDL is one of the best numbers you can have. One study showed that the risk of heart disease was 38 percent higher in men whose HDL was under 35, even if they had normal to low total cholesterol. So shoot for a high HDL *and* a low total cholesterol.

Some studies suggest that the most predictive number for cardiovascular disease risk is the triglyceride/HDL ratio. A heart-healthy ratio is 2:1 or less. You can improve this ratio by exercising and taking omega-3 supplements.

As doctors learn more about the value of cholesterol testing for predicting heart health, more sophisticated tests are being developed. For instance, new insights into the cholesterol/cardiovascular disease connection reveal that it is the particle size of the cholesterol molecule that determines its plaque-producing qualities — larger particles (HDL) are better, since smaller cholesterol particles can worm their way into blood vessel walls. A new method to measure particle size is the small, dense LDL cholesterol test. The level should be less than 20 milligrams.

In July 2004, a federal panel of experts, including representatives from the American College of Cardiology, the National Institutes of Health, and the American Heart Association, lowered the

READING MY OWN NUMBERS

When I turned sixty-five, I wanted to upgrade my life insurance policy, and this required getting a lipid panel done. One day I received a call from a doctor at the insurance company who said that the computer rejected my application because of high cholesterol. As soon as I heard the words *high cholesterol*, I thought, *Oh, no! All my health theories on lifestyle and dietary changes to control cholesterol just went out the window!* The doctor went on, "Don't worry. It was a computer error. Your HDL, or good cholesterol, is so high [80] that it skewed the total cholesterol, and the computer flagged it. I personally wanted to call and ask you how a man of sixty-five has such a high HDL."

standard for LDL cholesterol levels. Yet, there is some flexibility in these numbers, as they depend on your particular cardiovascular risk factors. If you are very low risk, then an LDL of less than 160 is presumed okay. The higher your risk, the lower your LDL should be.

What cholesterol numbers are right for you? Because statistical studies correlated lower LDL cholesterol with lower risk of cardiovascular disease, "the lower, the better" became the cholesterol-treatment mantra. And because LDL cholesterol tends to creep up as we age, there is a movement to redefine the optimal level of LDL to less than 100 for prime timers, or even as low as 70 in people with severe cardiovascular disease.

So, should every prime timer be on a cholesterol-lowering pill? Absolutely not! Because the body needs cholesterol, dropping the level too low could be detrimental to your health.Also, increasing the drug dosage to decrease the cholesterol number may increase toxicity.

How to Make Your Blood Tests More Reliable

Each time you have your blood lipids measured, you may get different results, because various factors go into the numbers, such as the amount of fat in your diet during the days prior to the test. To get the most reliable results:

- Eat your typical diet for a few days before the test.
- Fast at least twelve hours before having your blood drawn.
- Take the average of three tests, done over a period of one week. I would not

WHAT YOU NEED TO KNOW ABOUT STATINS

Statins lower cholesterol by inhibiting the enzyme that helps the liver produce cholesterol. Use statins judiciously. Because statins can be heart saving and life saving for many prime timers, doctors understandably downplay their dangers. Yet, prime timers are particularly sensitive to statins and may suffer more side effects because their livers break down statins more slowly. Also, prime timers tend to take other medications, some of which can compromise how the liver discards leftover statin medicines. These drug-elimination quirks may cause statins to build up to harmful levels in the bloodstream.

- If your doctor agrees to this approach, first try to lower your cholesterol by using the lifestyle and nutrition skills on page 512. Eating more antioxidants (fruits, vegetables, and seafood) reduces the oxidation of LDL, making it less sticky to the lining of blood vessels.
- If you need cholesterol-lowering pills, use

them in addition to, never instead of,
skills.

- If you have familial hypercholesterolemia, you will probably need skills *and* pills.
- To take statins safely, *start low* and *go slow.* The standard dose recommended by drug manufacturers is often higher than needed for prime timers. Work with your doctor to start with a much lower statin dose (one-fourth to one-half the "average" dose), and slowly increase if necessary. The lower the dose, the fewer the side effects.
- If you take a statin drug to lower cholesterol, ask your doctor about pairing it with the over-the-counter supplement coenzyme Q10 (CoQ10) (100 mg/day). Research shows that statins reduce the normal level of the energy-producing enzyme CoQ10 in muscle tissue, which could be one reason why muscle weakness is a side effect of statins.

recommend taking cholesterol-lowering drugs based on only one measurement. While this may sound inconvenient, deciding whether you need cholesterol-lowering medications is a major decision.

Cholesterol readings during cold weather tend to be higher than during warmer months. Excessive change in weight or excessive drinking of alcohol can also change the cholesterol levels. If your numbers improve following lifestyle changes, this is a sign that your high cholesterol was due to your habits more than your genes. Good news!

LOWER YOUR HIGH BLOOD SUGAR

You may ask, "If blood sugar provides fuel for energy, doesn't *extra* blood sugar give me *extra* energy?" Not exactly! Just as the body needs optimal blood pressure and blood levels of cholesterol, so does it need optimal levels of blood sugar for health and vitality. Blood sugar that remains too high for too long ages your body. Before we explain how this happens, we want you to understand one of the most important concepts of healthy aging — hormonal harmony.

Hormonal Harmony Is the Key to Prime-Time Health

Let's review: The key to healthy aging is putting the body — and brain — in biochemical balance by promoting hormonal harmony. Hormones are like the body's Internet. Millions of times a day, organs send instant messages to one another to help the body function optimally. The Prime-Time Health plan keeps these hormones at the right levels — not too high, not too low.

Imagine that the body's chemistry is a symphony orchestra. Insulin is the master hormone and conductor, and every other hormone is an instrument in the orchestra. If one group of hormones is released at the wrong time or at a level that's too high, like the brass section coming in too soon or too strong, the body is out of sync. The conductor makes sure that the orchestra is in harmony and that beautiful music — or wellness — results.

High insulin and high blood sugar contribute to high blood pressure and high cholesterol. Insulin, the "wellness hormone," is secreted by a group of specialized cells in the pancreas. While insulin has many health-promoting functions throughout the body, its main job is to keep blood sugar at optimal levels for your individual, ever-changing energy needs. When insulin levels are too high, too low, or out of sync with the body's needs, the whole body is thrown out of biochemical balance.

Insulin balances blood sugar. Cells need carbohydrates. When carbs from food are absorbed from the intestines into the bloodstream, the blood sugar level rises, which triggers the release of insulin. Insulin then travels to the cells, where it opens the receptors, or "doors," on the cell membranes so the sugar can enter the cell as fuel. Cells are sensitive and let in just the right amount of energy. But if there are too many carbs, and too much insulin arrives in response, the cells *resist* as insulin attempts to open the doors. The carbs get the message and say, "We'll just go somewhere else in case you need us later." The insulin finds other storage sites in the body for the excess carbs, usually the belly and the liver, the body's storage bin for excess everything.

If excess carbs and excess insulin storm the doors of the cells repeatedly, eventually the receptors become even more resistant, and insulin resistance (also known as type 2 diabetes) develops. Then, normal amounts of insulin can't open the doors, and higher and higher insulin levels are needed. A chronically high insulin level can result, which over time can cause the insulin-producing areas in the pancreas to wear out, resulting in type 1 (insulin-dependent) diabetes.

High blood sugar makes you old. What happens to all that excess sugar that's floating around in your bloodstream? Like a lonely person, excess sugar looks for a partner to attach to. That partner is a protein that is also traveling around unattached. These sugar-protein pairs, biochemically known as AGEs (advanced glycation end products), are the sticky stuff and rust that lead to aging.

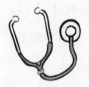

DR. SEARS SAYS...
Too much sweet stuff in your food causes too much sticky stuff in your blood.

High blood sugar makes you fat. Because your body doesn't want to waste food, if you eat more carbs than it can burn or store in the liver, insulin ushers the excess into the fat cells to be stored as extra fat. Consider insulin the body's energy-investment banker: insulin deposits the excess as fat around the middle, which is why people with big middles are often insulin resistant, or have type 2 diabetes.

Insulin stores fat by increasing the fat-storing enzyme lipoprotein lipase in the fat tissues, and it impairs the ability of muscles to burn fat — a double whammy. The good news is that when healthy blood sugar levels are maintained, excess belly fat is often the first to go.

Insulin regulates the satiety hormones. When blood sugar and blood insulin levels are just right, insulin alerts the brain to release satiety hormones that tell you you've eaten enough. When blood sugar levels are not optimal, the brain gets inaccurate signals that suggest you're hungry and should eat when in reality your body doesn't need to. Persistently high levels of blood sugar make you need more carbs to satisfy hunger.

High blood sugar makes you tired. When the levels of your blood sugar and blood insulin are stable, insulin acts efficiently, storing energy and releasing just the right amount when your body needs it. Insulin resistance leads to insulin *inefficiency;* sugar is not stored or released in amounts appropriate to your body's energy needs, so you get tired.

High blood sugar makes you sick. You've heard the phrase "sick and tired." That's exactly how persistently high blood sugar makes you feel. The incidence of just about every age-related illness goes up as your blood sugar rises: diabetes, cardiovascular disease, Alzheimer's, arthritis, and other "-itis" (inflammatory) illnesses. Insulin is also known as the retention hormone, because it keeps the body from excreting any excesses. For example, it can cause the kidneys to retain excess sodium, which can lead to high blood pressure. Excess insulin also stimulates the cholesterol-making enzyme in the liver. You can see how the three highs are interrelated.

Insulin is also one of your body's growth hormones. If you have cancer, have had cancer, or have a genetic tendency toward cancer, excess insulin can stimulate cancer cells to divide more rapidly.

Blood sugar imbalances can make you sad. Blood sugar levels are like the law of gravity: what goes up must come down. When blood sugar goes up too fast (from overeating junk food), it dives down too fast, causing the brain to be hungry. A hungry brain is an upset brain. Anxiety, depression, and quirky behaviors occur when the blood sugar level drops too low too fast. Erratic blood sugar and insulin levels can also trigger erratic stress hormone levels, which also contribute to mood swings.

High blood sugar makes you frail. High insulin levels lead to diminished levels of the muscle-building human growth hormone (HGH). Chronically high insulin can also lower blood levels of testosterone, the muscle-strengthening hormone. Last, excess insulin can interfere with calcium metabolism, which weakens bones.

FOUR WAYS TO LOWER THE THREE HIGHS

Now that you know that the causes of high blood pressure, high cholesterol, and high blood sugar are interrelated, it's easy to see why what's good for one is good for all three.

1. Lower Your Stress

Relax your mind, and relax your arteries. The nerves that surround the vessels are part of the sympathetic nervous system, and they regulate blood pressure. If the sympathetic nervous system is constantly and inappropriately stressed, on red alert, it causes the arteries to constrict and keeps blood pressure high. So, the mantra "relax" applies to both your mind and your arteries.

Unresolved stress can rapidly raise blood cholesterol levels by 10 to 50 percent. During stress, the liver and adrenal glands produce more cholesterol, which the body then uses to make more stress hormones.

Reducing stress can reduce blood sugar. Stress hormones, mainly cortisol, increase both blood sugar and insulin levels in addition to decreasing insulin sensitivity of the cells (see chapter 15).

Keep calm. Daily prayer or meditation can make a big difference. A simple exercise that helps me is to discipline my mind with the phrase "Don't go there." As soon as a toxic thought starts to enter, I flip the switch to "Don't go there," and I think of something else — a more positive thought or image. Keeping your stress level down is the best way to keep your arteries dilated and your blood pressure stable. Blood pressure often peaks in the morning when your stress hormones are naturally high. This is why morning meditation and exercise are so therapeutic. Studies show that daily yoga exercises can lower high blood pressure. Slower, deeper breathing turns down the sympathetic nervous system, which relaxes blood vessels and lowers blood pressure. (See "Six Simple Stress Busters," page 404.)

Marie's blood pressure had gone up to 196/100. She decided to take up yoga and to use yoga breathing to lower it. She said, "I would take my blood pressure before and after class. I was able to lower it twenty to thirty points each class. I could really feel my blood pressure coming down as I was feeling less anxious, more grounded, and more centered. Using breathing to relieve stress helps you take your yoga from the mat and apply it to everyday life." Her health changed for the better, and she's now a yoga instructor.

2. Stay Lean

Losing excess body fat lowers all the unhealthy highs. For every twenty pounds they lose, obese people can lower their blood pressure by ten points — this is called the 20/10 rule. The quickest way to lower your high blood sugar and high cholesterol is to get lean. (See chapter 21 for how to stay lean.)

3. Move

Movement is one of the best ways to help your body help itself.

Move blood pressure lower. When you pump your muscles, the blood, like rush-hour traffic, flows faster through your arteries. The faster-moving blood stimulates the glands in the endothelium, the lining of the arteries, to secrete natural biochemicals (called vasodilators) that relax artery walls and lower blood pressure. High blood pressure can lead to stroke. In the Women's Health Study, those who walked for at least *fifteen minutes a day* cut their risk of death from heart attack or stroke in half.

Move your blood sugar lower. Physical activity increases the sensitivity of the cells to insulin and stabilizes and lowers blood insulin levels, which lowers blood sugar.

DOGGONE HIGH BLOOD PRESSURE

In a classic pet study, cardiologists put one group of hypertensive patients on high blood pressure medicine and told another group to go out and get a dog. Blood pressure was lowered just as much in the pet group as in the pills group. This is proof-positive that the relaxation from having a dog, plus the exercise from walking it, lowers blood pressure.

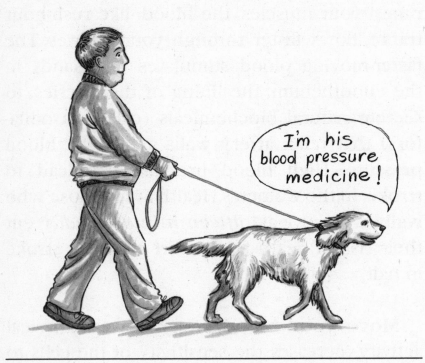

Move your cholesterol numbers. Exercise does double duty by increasing HDL and lowering LDL. Movement helps clear the heavy triglyceride fats from the bloodstream. Exercise often raises HDL cholesterol more than it lowers LDL cholesterol. In some people, exercise has little or no effect on the LDL; but by raising the HDL, exercise improves the total cholesterol/HDL ratio. The ability of movement to lower triglycerides might be even more significant. When you lower triglycerides, you automatically lower small-density LDL cholesterol, the most artery-clogging kind.

4. Change Your Diet

How did we humans, who are supposed to be so smart, get all these highs? Answer: We went from a real-food diet to a fake-food diet. Over the centuries, we've shifted from a diet rich in fresh fruits, vegetables, seafood, and wild (lean) animal protein to a diet of packaged foods, refined carbohydrates, canned vegetables, and caged (fat) animals. Here are the main dietary strategies that will lower the highs and improve your longevity.

Graze. Eat smaller minimeals throughout the day. (For more on grazing, see pages 86 and 144.)

Eat more plant-based foods and fewer animal-based foods. While animal fats raise cholesterol, most plant foods actually lower it. Especially avoid the factory-made hydrogenated or trans fats, which lower HDL and raise LDL.

Fruits and vegetables are naturally low in sodium and high in potassium, and they also are high in antioxidants, which slow inflammation and damage to blood vessels. We recommend, in addition to eating the real thing, a supplement called Juice Plus, a capsule with concentrated nutrients from fruits and vegetables. Because I operate on the "show me the science" principle, Juice Plus is the only supplement I presently take. Studies have shown that the immune system is boosted by Juice Plus, particularly in people with cardiovascular and blood vessel problems. Show your cardiologist the science. In the May 21, 2003, issue of the *Journal of the American College of Cardiology,* researchers at the University of Maryland found that taking Juice Plus daily (two capsules of fruits and two capsules of vegetables) improved blood vessel health. Specifically, this study found that Juice Plus improved after-meal vasodilation (opening of blood vessels). After you eat a large high-fat meal, the blood vessels can be in a state of vasoconstriction, which is risky for the heart. Remember, supplements are just that — use them *in addition to* not *instead of* a whole-food diet.

Avoid factory-made carbs. Factory-made food is often unhealthy because either chemicals are put into the food that raise the highs or healthy nutrients are taken out that keep the highs in check. Lower your cholesterol by lowering the amount of sugar you eat. Diets high in junk carbs increase the level of the small particles of LDL cholesterol in your blood, the type most likely to build up plaque in arterial walls. Junk carbs, also called high-glycemic carbs, are a triple threat: they increase triglycerides, decrease HDL cholesterol, and increase small-dense-particle LDL. In addition, insulin activates the critical enzyme responsible for making cholesterol in the liver; by reducing your insulin level, you reduce cholesterol. Just say no to white bread, white pasta, and sugary snacks and drinks.

Eat a right-carb diet. While you might think that the fewer carbs you eat, the lower your blood sugar will be, this is only partially true. Better for your overall health and stable insulin levels are right carbs, those that are naturally partnered with protein, fiber, or fat. Right carbs are absorbed more slowly into the

---

THREE NUTRIENTS THAT CAN LOWER HIGH BLOOD PRESSURE

Vitamin-C-containing foods. Studies show that vitamin C significantly reduces blood pressure in hypertensive people. The effective dosage in these studies was 500 milligrams a day, which is easy to get in vitamin- C-rich foods such as peppers, guava, papaya, strawberries, oranges, and kiwi. Vitamin C seems to stimulate the body's own vasodilating substances, such as nitric oxide (NO) and prostaglandins.

Coenzyme Q10. CoQ10 works by stimulating the body to produce vessel-relaxing biochemicals. Blood levels of CoQ10 decrease with age and tend to be lower in people with cardiovascular problems, such as high blood pressure, and in people who take statin drugs. Because statin drugs can deplete the body of its natural CoQ10 (muscle weakness

---

bloodstream, and this helps blood sugar and insulin levels remain stable.

Keep potassium up and sodium down. Eat foods that are high in potassium and low in sodium. To understand how an imbalance in biochemicals can cause your blood pressure

---

is a side effect of statins), it is now standard to recommend CoQ10 supplements if taking a statin. Studies showed that 100 to 200 milligrams of CoQ10 daily, taken with a meal, can significantly lower blood pressure without side effects. Peak blood pressure–lowering effects are usually noticed after four weeks.

L-arginine. Stimulating your body to produce optimal amounts of NO is one of the key blood pressure–regulating mechanisms. L-arginine, an amino acid, is the body's main building block (called a precursor) for NO. Studies show that eating a diet high in L-arginine (around 10 grams a day), either through supplements or food, can reduce elevated blood pressure. Top sources of arginine are seafood, lean meat and poultry, amaranth grain, nuts, pumpkin seeds, lentils, peas, tofu, wild rice, and soybeans.

---

to go out of balance, let's take a look at the average cell of the arterial muscles. On the membrane of the artery cell is a microscopic sodium-potassium pump. It is like a revolving door, pumping sodium out of the cell and letting potassium in. For optimal blood pressure, this pump needs to maintain the right balance of the biochemicals sodium and potassium. If the sodium is too high and the potassium too low, blood pressure regulation won't operate efficiently.

The sodium-potassium pump also drives the calcium pump, which causes muscle cells to contract and is most involved in maintaining optimal blood pressure. The calcium pump maintains the optimal balance of calcium inside and outside the cell. If the muscle needs to contract (raise the blood pressure), the revolving door lets calcium in; if it needs to relax (lower the blood pressure), it ushers calcium out. (Some of the newer blood pressure–lowering drugs are called calcium channel blockers; that is, they block excess calcium from entering the muscle cell so it doesn't contract as forcefully and elevate the blood pressure.)

If the sodium-potassium pump isn't working

correctly, too much calcium gets inside the muscle and nerve cells, causing them to contract and raise the blood pressure. Also, the increased calcium in the nerves stimulates hormones, such as epinephrine, that cause the smooth muscle

SEE SALT HIDING

Our bodies need only about 500 milligrams of sodium daily. Many prime timers consume five times that amount. It's best to limit your salt intake to less than 1,500 milligrams per day. As a general guide, the older you are, the less salt you should eat. To lower your dietary sodium:

- Instead of salt, use spices such as turmeric, coriander, and rosemary.
- Most canned foods are oversalted to make up for their bland taste. Remove much of the salt in canned vegetables, such as beans, by rinsing them first.
- Buy "low-salt" canned foods. (It's easy to exceed your daily limit of salt with one can of soup.)
- Even better, can most canned foods. Except for beans, we rarely open a can.

After a few months on a lower-salt diet, your taste buds will be retrained to prefer less salt.

of the arteries to contract even more. To add insult to injury, too much calcium in the arterial muscle cells increases scar tissue, which also contributes to hardening of the arteries. Finally, increased calcium in the cells can cause the cells to become resistant to insulin, causing insulin levels to rise, which further increases blood pressure. So you can see how an imbalance of these biochemicals can inevitably lead to high blood pressure.

The key to lowering the highs is to eat *real* foods. Foods that grow (fruits, vegetables, whole grains) are naturally high in potassium and low in sodium. Foods packaged in factories are the reverse. For example, fruits and vegetables contain several hundred times more potassium than sodium. The sodium content in most fresh fruits and vegetables is actually negligible. (It is just the opposite with canned goods. "Canned *bads*" would be a more nutritionally accurate description: they contain very little potassium and several hundred milligrams of sodium, depending on the serving size.) In one study, an increase of 400 milligrams of potassium a day (one banana) resulted in a 40 percent decrease in stroke-related deaths.

POWERFUL POTASSIUM FOODS

Try to consume an average of 3,500 to 4,500 milligrams of potassium daily.

Food	Potassium (in milligrams)
Salmon, 6 ounces	800
Potato, 1 medium, with skin	800
Figs, 5	650
Potato, 1 medium, without skin	600
Cantaloupe, 1 cup	500
Artichoke, ½ medium	500
Avocado, ½ medium	500
Yogurt, plain, nonfat, 1 cup	500
Banana, 1 medium	450
Raisins, ¼ cup	400
Papaya, ½ medium	400
Orange juice, 1 cup	400
Dried fruit: prunes, peaches, apricots	300–600
Squash, winter, ½ cup	300
Pepper, sweet, 1	300
Tomato, 1	275
Carrots, 1 medium	230
Beans, ½ cup	200–400
Orange, 1	200
Dates, dried, 4	200
Apricots, 3 medium	200
Nuts, 1 ounce	150

Magnify your magnesium. In addition to helping keep sodium, potassium, and calcium in balance, magnesium helps to strengthen cell membranes, preventing excessive leaks of other biochemicals into the cell membrane, which can upset the optimal balance of the cell and cause the artery muscle cell to contract more than relax. Studies show that increasing potassium and magnesium in the diet and lowering sodium can lower blood pressure. This biochemical fact is important to the DASH (Dietary Approaches to Stop Hypertension) diet recommended by the American Heart Association. Foods that are high in potassium also tend to be high in magnesium. Seafood, nuts, and greens (e.g., spinach and chard) are particularly rich in magnesium.

Change your oils. Incorporating more omega-3 oils in your diet and consuming less omega-6 is one of the best ways to lower the highs. Go fish! Eating a diet that is high in omega-3s (especially cold-water oily fish such as wild salmon and tuna) and monounsaturated fats (such as olive oil) and low in saturated fats and

MAJOR MAGNESIUM FOODS

Shoot for an average of at least 400 milligrams of magnesium a day.

Food	Magnesium (in milligrams)
Halibut, 6 ounces	180
Flaxseed, ground, 1 ounce (⅛ cup)	100
Tuna, 6 ounces	100
Quinoa, ¼ cup	90
Spinach, fresh or frozen, ½ cup	80
Nuts, almonds, 1 ounce	80
Yogurt, 8 ounces	43
Banana	33

omega-6 oils not only lowers LDL cholesterol, it raises the protective HDL cholesterol. A diet rich in omega-3s can also lower the artery-clogging triglyceride fats. "Go fish" is one of our top prime-time tips. Eating fish fats lowers blood fats. What a nutritional deal!

A recent article in the *Journal of the American Medical Association* found that eating one or two servings of oily fish per week reduces the risk of death from cardiovascular disease by

36 percent. The stability of the blood vessel's cell membrane helps regulate blood pressure. The stronger the cell membrane, the more likely is the cell to function optimally to relax and constrict the blood vessels to regulate blood pressure. Here's where omega-3s shine, since omega-3s are the structural component of the cell membrane.

You may have heard that taking 20 milligrams of niacin lowers LDL cholesterol and reduces the small, dense LDL particles that contribute most to plaque. This is true, yet some folks have uncomfortable facial flushing when taking niacin pills. A nicer niacin solution: 8 ounces of salmon or tuna, which contains 22 to 26 milligrams of niacin and does not cause flushing.

Omega-3s help regulate angiotensin, the vaso-constricting hormone that is medically inhibited by the blood pressure–lowering class of drugs called ACE inhibitors. In a nutshell, if you were to compare the mechanisms of how prescription drugs and omega-3s work to control blood pressure, you would be amazed by how similar they are, and omegas don't have any unpleasant side effects.

Eat a high-fiber diet. Fiber is filling without being fattening, and it steadies blood sugar levels. The steadier your blood sugar, the better your blood pressure. As an added bonus, fiber also lowers the bad cholesterol.

Avoid excessive alcohol. Excessive drinking raises blood pressure. It is thought that excessive alcohol can damage cell membranes throughout the body, and this can interfere with the sodium-potassium pump described earlier as well as disrupt the balance of the other blood pressure–controlling minerals calcium and magnesium. Also, heavy drinkers are more likely to be smokers and heavy eaters.

Cut cholesterol-containing foods. Here's how to trim excess cholesterol from your shopping cart:
- Eat more plant-based food and seafood and less meat.
- Trim the skin off poultry before cooking it.
- Choose white meat over dark.
- Choose turkey. Turkey meat is lower in fat than chicken.

- Buy lean meat. It's interesting that the priciest and tastiest cuts of meat are often the fattiest. "Select" is the leanest cut of meat; it is around 7 percent fat. "Prime" is the fattiest grade, and the one often served in restaurants. It can be as much as 35 to 40 percent fat. The leanest cut of beef is "round steak," sirloin and loin cuts are in the middle, and ribs are the highest in fat. If you're shopping for ground beef, ask the butcher to grind top round.
- Broil or bake instead of deep-frying or pan-frying.
- Opt for wild game meats. They are the lowest in total fat. Our favorite is wild venison.
- Eat real foods rather than packaged, fiberless carbs. In fact, new insights suggest that indulging in junk-food carbs may raise cholesterol more than cholesterol-containing foods.
- Rediscover eggs. Unless you have a hereditary trait that elevates cholesterol, an egg a day is fine. Recent studies have found the egg not guilty of contributing

to cardiovascular disease. Because whole eggs are very nutrient dense, most people should eat them. If you have familial hyper-cholesterolemia, egg whites or Egg Beaters is a better choice.

- Eat lots of foods containing soluble fiber, such as oats, barley, and beans, and most other fruits and vegetables. Soluble fiber acts like a cholesterol magnet and slows down the absorption of cholesterol in foods and escorts it out in waste.

Rx FOR LOWERING THE PRIME-TIME HIGHS

- ❑ Keep calm: use meditation, music, relaxation strategies.
- ❑ Stay lean.
- ❑ Move more.
- ❑ Care for a pet.
- ❑ Graze on frequent minimeals.
- ❑ Eat a *right*-fat diet: fewer animal fats and more seafood and plant-based fats.
- ❑ Eat more fresh fruit and vegetables.
- ❑ Be sure to get at least 500 milligrams of vitamin C (preferably in foods) daily.
- ❑ Eat a diet high in L-arginine.
- ❑ Eat more potassium and less sodium.
- ❑ Change your oils: more omega-3s and olive oil; less omega-6 vegetable oils (e.g., corn oil); no hydrogenated oils.
- ❑ Eat wild salmon three times a week, or take 3 grams of fish oil daily.
- ❑ Eat a high-fiber diet: at least 35 grams a day.
- ❑ Avoid drinking excess alcohol.
- ❑ Eat leaner meats.

CHAPTER 20

Cut Your Chances of Getting Cancer

In 1997, after surgery, chemotherapy, and radiation therapy for colon cancer, I decided to write this book to share what I'd learned — to help people prepare for prime time and prevent cancer. Like most cancers, mine was preventable. I consulted top cancer specialists around the country to find out what I could do to stay cancer free.

Because at least one-third of cancers are diet related, I started by asking for nutritional advice. One cancer specialist said, "Don't eat too many hamburgers." That was it. While the United States excels in the early detection and treatment of cancer, it gets failing grades when it comes to cancer prevention.

I realized I needed to do my own research and create my own anticancer program. No one is more motivated to put together a cancer-prevention program than a cancer survivor who wants to remain one. I only wish someone had shared this information with me when I was in my thirties or forties.

Do you want to avoid being among the one in three Americans shocked to hear the words "You've got cancer!"? Read on.

WHY CANCER OCCURS

We all have some precancer cells lurking in our bodies. But in most people, the body's defense department, the immune system, recognizes them as terrorist cells and destroys them before they have a chance to rapidly multiply and invade healthy tissues. You don't get cancer all of a sudden. It develops slowly, one errant cell at a time, until the cancer cells overwhelm the body's defenses.

Let's take a look at a healthy cell that is rapidly dividing and replacing itself in the lining of the colon. Inside each cell is a genetic code that tells the cell, "Increase and multiply, and when it is your time to die, make room so young, healthy cells can take your place." Apoptosis, or the replacement of old cells with young cells, occurs trillions of times a day throughout the body. But sometimes the genetic signal gets garbled and keeps turning on growth in a cell instead of turning it off. As a result, it becomes a cancer cell, multiplies out of control, and invades and damages surrounding tissues. Next, it creeps into the bloodstream and travels throughout the body — an often fatal turn of events called metastasis. Our prime-time anticancer program is aimed at keeping the genetic code in each cell healthy and, in case the code breaks down, strengthening the body's immune system to recognize the terrorist cells early enough to prevent cancer.

Some people have a family history of cancer. Both my father and Martha's mother died of colon cancer. So, we inherited so-called oncogenes, cells that are at high risk of going astray and becoming cancerous. You can lessen your risk of cancer through these mechanisms:

- Decrease your exposure to carcinogens — cancer-causing pollutants in your environment and in your diet that cause the genetic code to go haywire.

- Boost your immune system so it can eliminate the quirky cells that have mutated into cancer cells.
- Eat foods that talk to the genes and tell them to behave.
- Keep your body in hormonal balance. Cancer cells are hormonal hogs. An excess of the hormones insulin and estrogen can promote the growth of cancer cells.

WHO IS *LEAST* LIKELY TO GET CANCER?

Nonsmokers

Vegetable eaters

Seafood eaters

Grazers

Lean folks

Exercisers

Optimists

Sound familiar? These healthy lifestyle choices also prevent just about every other illness you don't want to get.

Despite the billions of dollars spent on cancer research, cancer prevention comes down to three simple steps:

1. Eat more fruits and vegetables.
2. Eat more seafood.
3. Go outside and play.

Your mother probably told you that!

HOW FOOD FEEDS AND FIGHTS CANCER

I pored through many scientific studies linking diet to cancer, and they all came to the same conclusion: what you eat can both cause and prevent cancer. My plan was simple: eat more cancer-preventing foods and fewer cancer-causing foods.

Research shows that diet can contribute to at least one-third of all cancers. Replacing an animal-based diet with a plant-based diet can lower the rate of the big bad four — lung, breast, colon, and prostate cancers — which account for more than 50 percent of all cancer deaths.

Diet promotes cancer-cell growth by generating free radicals that hit the genetic code of the cell with terrorist fire and cause it to misbehave. DNA codes are like switches that turn on cell growth, repair, and multiplication; other switches turn off the growth and division mechanism when it's not needed. Certain foods (fruits, vegetables, and seafood) feed the right switches and help them to function properly; others feed the wrong ones. For example, when oxidation of junk foods damages the cellular DNA, the signals can get out of control and turn on the "keep growing" switch instead of the "stop growing" switch.

There are two epidemics in America today: cancer and obesity. Is there any correlation? I believe there is. The main dietary disasters that have infected the standard American diet in the past three decades are a rise in fiberless, processed carbs (high glycemic) and a tendency to eat foods high in omega-6 oils and low in omega-3 oils. Both of these developments are carcinogenic and obesity producing.

To protect yourself, eat an anticancer diet. The anticancer diet is lower in animal fats and higher in plant-based foods. As a general guide, the more colorful the food and the more pungent its taste, the greater its anticancer properties.

This is because the very nutrients that give foods their color and zing also have medicinal anticancer effects. They help the cells to operate efficiently so they remember how to control their own growth — maintaining the proper size and number and dying on time. For example, the anthocyanins in blueberries act as a protective shield by reducing the ability of carcinogens to damage the genetic material inside the cells. The following superfoods have anticancer properties:

- colorful fruits and vegetables, especially beets, grapes, kale, and berries
- cruciferous vegetables: broccoli, cabbage, brussels sprouts, cauliflower
- garlic
- onions
- chili peppers
- leeks
- green tea
- seafood
- flaxseeds and flax meal
- nuts
- tomatoes
- soy foods
- turmeric
- curry
- yogurt
- shiitake mushrooms

THE STANDARD AMERICAN DIET CAUSES CANCER

The sad reality is that people who eat the standard American diet are three times more likely to develop cancer than are those who eat a more nutritious one. The standard American diet is a cancer-cell fertilizer.

Standard American Diet	Anticancer Diet
High in animal fat	Low in animal fat
High in fake fat	Low in fake fat
Low in plant-based foods	Higher in plant-based foods
Low in fiber	High in fiber
Low in omega-3 fats	High in omega-3 fats
High in omega-6 (processed) fat	Low in omega-6 (processed) fat

SIXTEEN WAYS TO PREVENT CANCER

These tips can help prevent all common cancers, especially cancers of the lung, breast, ovary, prostate, and colon.

1. Don't Smoke

The incidence of all cancers — and all other diseases — goes way up if you smoke. In fact, as the rate of smoking begins to drop in the United States, cancers related to smoking (nose, throat, and lung cancers) are also decreasing.

2. Graze

Researchers believe that grazing — eating less, more often — helps prevent cancer by lowering blood insulin levels. Insulin is a growth factor — a biochemical that, like a fertilizer, helps cells multiply faster, which is just what you *don't* want a precancer or cancer cell to do. For many prime timers, insulin levels rise with age. So, as we get older, we produce more grow-food for tumors. The solution: feed potential tumor cells less insulin. Fascinating studies revealed that experimental animals fed a junk-carb (high-glycemic) diet developed more cancers. Harvard researchers showed that women with the highest blood levels of IGF (insulin growth factor), a proinflammatory chemical that goes up when insulin is too high, were seven times more likely to develop breast cancer. Other studies have shown the same correlation with other hormonally driven cancers: colon, ovarian, and pancreatic cancers.

3. Blend

The sipping solution (see page 151 for smoothie recipe) is particularly helpful in preventing colon cancer. Making the food looser at the top end makes the waste softer and easier to pass through the lower end. Less constipation means less time for the waste products to irritate the lining of the gut and a lower chance that the cells lining the colon will become cancerous.

THE YOUNGER YOU START, THE BETTER

You don't all of a sudden "get cancer." A genetic quirk in an errant gene may lie dormant for decades and then suddenly become activated, resulting in cancer. This is particularly true of colon cancer. Even though 90 percent of colon cancer cases occur after age fifty, the damage was probably done in the thirties and forties. So don't delay. Improve your diet and lifestyle now.

---

4. Eat Lots of Fruits and Vegetables

When I surveyed the science of cancer prevention, the most outstanding statistic I found was that people who eat a plant-based diet have a much lower incidence of nearly all cancers. Here's how fruits and veggies work their anticancer magic:

They contain natural anticancer medicines. Plants contain phytonutrients, their own internal medicines, that evolved as natural defense mechanisms to help them to survive. These phytos are known as chemo protectors; they search out and destroy carcinogens, such as pollutants, before they reach the interior of the cell and cause damage. Savor the synergy of phyto foods. Eating lots of them together produces a greater anticancer effect than eating each one individually — chemotherapy without side effects. Think smoothies, soups, and salads.

They can crusade against cancer. The most anticancer vegetables are the crucifers: broccoli, cabbage, and brussels sprouts; and dark greens such as kale. Cruciferous vegetables contain protective biochemicals such as sulforaphane, which block carcinogens from getting into healthy cells, and indoles, which lower the risk of breast cancer. Researchers estimate that by eating lots of cruciferous vegetables, you can lower your risk of developing breast and colon cancer by 40 percent.

They can protect with phytoestrogens. Phytoestrogens, found especially in soy and cruciferous vegetables, can lower the risk of estrogen-dependent cancers, such as breast cancer. Estrogen is a cell-growth promoter. Phytoestrogens fill the estrogen receptor sites on cells, lessening the ability of the body's own estrogen to promote the growth of cells that have already become cancerous. This seems to be one of the reasons why people in cultures such as Asia who eat a lot of phytoestrogen-containing foods have a much lower risk of nearly all cancers.

They are high in fiber. People who eat more fruits and vegetables tend to eat less animal fat. Fruits and vegetables are fiber rich, and fiber is filling, fat free, and particularly important for colon health. The best fibers are found in beans, lentils, potatoes (with skins), and fruits. Also, fiber slows the release of carbs from the bloodstream, and this lowers blood insulin levels.

They are high in phytic acid and folate.
Think greens and beans. Legumes, such as beans
and lentils, have a high level of the cancer-
fighting compound phytic acid. Studies show
that people who eat four or more servings of
legumes weekly are 33 percent less likely to
develop colon polyps. Those who already have
polyps and eat more beans reduce their risk of
recurrence by 45 percent. And people who eat
the most high-folate greens get the least number
of cancers, probably because the folate in greens
interferes with the genetic mischief within the
cell that causes it to go cancerous. The lutein in
greens also contributes to cancer protection.

5. Savor Soy

Soy seems to protect against these cancers:
lung, breast, colon, rectal, stomach, and prostate.
In addition to the phytoestrogen anticancer effect
discussed above, soy contains isoflavones, which
seem to inhibit angiogenesis, the growth of new
blood vessels necessary for tumor survival (many
new chemotherapy drugs work by blocking
angiogenesis). The most potent isoflavone in soy
is *genistein*. Soy nuts are an excellent source of
genistein and a healthful snack food. Remember,

people in cultures with a lower incidence of cancer eat real soy, such as tofu and tempeh, not the processed stuff. Don't rely on highly processed soy foods, such as soy burgers, soy sauce, and soy beverages, which can contain much lower levels of the cancer-preventing isoflavones.

6. Eat Fewer Animal-Based Foods

People who eat little or no animal meat, especially red meat, have the lowest risk of developing cancer. This seems to be due to the carcinogenic stuff in meat. I was particularly motivated to change my carnivorous habits by the studies showing that when Asians —primarily plant eaters, with a very low rate of colon cancer— moved to America and started eating steak like Americans, they began to suffer colon cancer at similar rates as their meat-eating compatriots.

One of the largest and most influential diet and cancer studies, called the China Study, was a joint effort by universities in China, America, and Great Britain. This study concluded that the standard American diet contributed to the high incidence of cancer and cardiovascular disease. It also concluded that diet played more of a role in cancer development than did genetic tendencies. A study by my friend Dr. Dean Ornish at the Preventive Medicine Research Institute in Sausalito, California, found that the progression of prostate cancer could be slowed by switching to a more active lifestyle and a more plant-based diet. The famous Harvard Nurses' Health Study (of ninety thousand nurses) revealed that the women who ate the most meat got the most breast cancer. Other studies have found the same correlation in colon cancer.

What is it about meat that causes cancer? It's probably a combination of factors related to what we do to animals to make meat cheaper and tastier. Hormones, cheap animal feed, fatteners, and chemical preservatives are all carcinogenic. Cancer specialists believe that the increased fat in feedlot animals, namely LDL cholesterol, acts as a tumor fertilizer, fostering the growth of precancerous cells, such as polyps in the colon. Certainly, the nitrites added to cured foods, such as hot dogs, are not healthy. (I find the term *cured meat* ironic. What do they cure the meat of?) A high animal-fat diet increases the bile production needed to digest all that fatty marbling from the steak. Excess bile also feeds the growth of potentially cancerous cells. Besides, big meat-eaters tend to eat fewer anticancer fruits and vegetables.

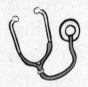

DR. SEARS SAYS...
Prime timers, eat less prime rib! If you are a meat lover, try wild game, such as venison. Its fat profile is much healthier, and it's free of chemical additives.

7. Go Fish

People who eat more seafood — especially cold-water fish like salmon and tuna — suffer fewer cancers. Here's what science says about the more seafood/less cancer connection:

- A 2006 Harvard study showed that men with the highest blood levels of omega-3s had a 66 percent reduced risk of developing colorectal cancer compared with those with the lowest blood levels of omega-3s.
- The twelve-year Health Professionals Follow-Up study of forty-seven thousand men showed that those who

ate the most fish had the lowest risk of prostate cancer.

- Studies show that people who consume more processed vegetable oils (omega-6s) and less fish oils (omegas-3s) get more cancers.
- A Swedish study showed that women who ate the most fatty fish had the least incidence of uterine cancer.
- People living in coastal villages who eat more fish have significantly less colon cancer than city dwellers who eat less fish. The European Prospective Investigation into Cancer (EPIC) is one of the largest more fish/less cancer studies. Researchers followed the dietary habits of thousands of people from ten European countries. Those who ate 10 to 20 ounces of fish per week were 30 percent less likely to get colon cancer.

Omega-3s are the ultimate health food for cellular genetic control mechanisms. If a cell gets quirky and starts dividing out of control, omega-3s help fix this genetic mistake before the mutated cells become cancerous. Omega-3s also help the body's garbage-disposal system — the immune system — to seek out and destroy mutated cells. As an extra nutritional perk, seafood is high in cancer-preventing vitamin D (see page 233).

8. Change Your Oils

People who eat more omega-6 oils (corn, cottonseed, soy, sunflower, and safflower) suffer more cancers than those who eat more omega-3 oils (fish and flax oils). Also, people who eat a Mediterranean diet, which is rich in omega-3s and other healthy oils, such as olive oil, have a lower rate of cancer. Greek women who consume lots of olive oil have a lower rate of breast cancer. One of the world's foremost omega-fat experts, Dr. William Lands, author of *Fish, Omega-3, and Human Health,* says that because of its high ratio of omega-6s to omega-3s, the standard American diet is basically carcinogenic. Fascinating research has shown that omega-6s not only promote the growth of cancer cells, they also decrease the immune system's ability to destroy these cells — a double fault of these processed oils.

9. Spice Up Your Diet

India enjoys low cancer rates, and researchers wondered why. Studies showed that curcumin, the hot stuff in curry and turmeric, suppressed the growth of cancer cells. Turmeric blocks the "turn on" switch for cancer cells and also has an anti-inflammatory effect (see page 361).

CANCER-SAVING SYNERGY

Most mornings I mix together a lot of colorful fruits, pomegranate juice, tofu, and flax into a smoothie (see page 151). Most evenings I enjoy a mixture of veggies in my supersalad (see page 554) and chase it with a green tea beverage. When you eat these foods together, you enjoy a powerful synergy of anticancer effects. Studies in mice with cancer showed that the greater the combination of anticancer foods they ate, the less their cancer progressed.

---

10. Get More Anticancer Nutrients

Here are some other nutrients that can lower your risk of cancer:

Calcium. Studies show that populations who eat more calcium-containing foods have a lower incidence of colorectal cancer. One study showed that people who ate an average of 1,200 milligrams of calcium a day enjoyed a 75 percent reduced risk of colorectal cancer. Calcium seems to prevent cancer in two ways: it keeps the surface cells lining the colon from multiplying out of control, and it binds bile acids and keeps them from irritating the lining of the colon. This is why I enjoy a daily cup of organic yogurt.

Nuts. The mineral selenium is a potent antioxidant. Studies show that people with high levels of selenium in their blood have a reduced incidence of various cancers. One study showed that men with the highest levels of selenium in their diets were found to have the lowest incidence of prostate cancer. Brazil nuts are a particularly good source of selenium. Shoot for 100 micrograms of selenium a day, the amount found in two Brazil nuts.

Vitamin C. Studies have shown that people with the highest intake of vitamin C have the lowest incidence of cancer. Vitamin C blocks the formation of carcinogens in the gut, such as those from nitrates and nitrites in processed meats. Vitamin C also boosts the immune system so that it can destroy cancer cells before they have a chance to spread.

Vitamin D. Vitamin D suppresses angiogenesis. People who live in climates with the most sunshine, and therefore the most vitamin D, enjoy lower rates of breast, colon, and prostate cancer. People with diets high in vitamin D enjoy a lower risk of breast and colon cancers. Because of its sources, vitamin D is called the seafood and sunshine vitamin.

Probiotics. Probiotics, those healthful bacteria found in yogurt, prevent cancer by promoting the growth of healthy bacteria in the colon. The more healthy bacteria in the colon, the more they crowd out carcinogens.

Flax. Flaxseed contains two anticancer compounds, omega-3s and lignans, which have been shown to reduce the risk of breast and colon cancers. Add two tablespoons of ground flaxseed to a smoothie or salad.

DR. BILL'S ANTICANCER SUPERSALAD

Serves 2

2 cups baby spinach,
  organic*
1 cup arugula
1 cup chopped tomatoes
½ cup kidney beans
2 teaspoons turmeric
½ teaspoon black pepper
¼ cup onion, chopped
¼ cup sunflower seeds
lemon or lime juice, sprinkle
2 tablespoons olive oil
1 tablespoon balsalmic
  vinegar

Special additions

4 to 6 ounces wild salmon fillet
Feta or goat cheese, sprinkle
2 tablespoons hummus (instead of
  olive oil)
¼ cup square tofu chunks
¼ cup raisins, organic
garlic, 1 clove, pressed
asparagus, slightly cooked
broccoli florets

beets   blueberries
pine nuts

Combine ingredients in a large bowl, toss, and enjoy!

*Use organic vegetables as much as possible

11. Reduce Your Waist

Lean is a top anticancer word. Remember, in order for cancer cells to grow out of control, they need to be fed. Excess junk food and the resulting excess body fat cause high blood sugar and high blood insulin levels, both cell-growth promoters. Increased body fat also leads to increased estrogen in women, which feeds cancer cells of the breast and colon especially. In fact, researchers at the University of North Carolina found that women who avoided putting on excess belly fat cut their risk of breast cancer by 48 percent. According to research in the *New England Journal of Medicine*, increased body fat from eating junk food increases the risk of cancers of the esophagus, colon, rectum, liver, gallbladder, lymph system, pancreas, kidney, prostate, and breast. And according to a recent study, for every four inches gained in belly fat, the risk of colon cancer increased 33 percent in men and 16 percent in women.

12. Move

Move is a top anticancer word because exercise helps muscles use excess insulin and lowers body fat. Movement increases the sensitivity of insulin receptors on the cell membrane, allowing insulin to work more efficiently. Lower blood insulin levels equal less food to feed the cancer. Dr. Lou Ignarro, whom you met on page 54, teaches that exercise releases the miracle molecule, nitric oxide (NO), a powerful antioxidant that prevents the growth of cancer cells.

In a study that tracked seventeen thousand Harvard alumni for twenty-five years, the group of men that burned at least 2,500 calories each week through exercise, the equivalent of forty-five minutes of exercise a day, had half the incidence of colon cancer when compared to their sedentary colleagues. Another study showed that men who had sedentary jobs had a higher risk of developing colon cancer than their more active peers. Movement boosts the immune system by increasing the circulating killer cells, those search-and-destroy soldiers that nip cancer cells before they get a chance to bud.

A study of thirteen thousand men and women followed for fifteen years by my friend and aerobics expert Dr. Kenneth Cooper at the Cooper Institute in Dallas found that the incidence of cancers closely correlated with a lack of physical fitness. These statistics show the truth of the saying "If you have no time for exercise, you'd better reserve more time for the hospital."

13. De-stress

While the body's immune system normally destroys quirky cells that can go astray and trigger cancer, stress can suppress the activity of the immune system and increase the risk of cancer. So don't sweat the small stuff. It's not worth it. (See a list of stress busters, page 404.) Eye-opening studies from a new field of mind-body medicine called psychoneuroimmunology reveal that the mind and the immune system are interrelated. Unmanaged stress turns on chemical cancer fertilizers and turns off the body's natural cancer-cell killers. Stress management strategies, such as meditation, do the reverse. Read *Molecules of Emotion* by neuroscientist Dr. Candace Pert for a fascinating discussion of this subject.

14. Sleep

Melatonin, the hormone that is naturally produced when you sleep, causes your immune system to produce anticancer proteins called cytokines, which inhibit tumor growth. A good night's sleep is good medicine.

15. Laugh

Laughter is one of the best anticancer medicines. A long-term study of women with breast cancer showed that those with a positive attitude were nearly three times more likely to survive than those with a fatalistic attitude. A study reported in the *Journal of the National Cancer Institute* showed that ten men who viewed an hour-long humorous video showed a significant increase in the immune-boosting and cancer-cell-fighting substance gamma-interferon, and this increase lasted into the next day. Long-term cancer studies show that people who convince themselves that they can beat this cancer do so more often than those with a fatalistic attitude. (For more on how humor boosts the immune system, see "Laughter Is the Best Medicine," page 418.)

16. Have Preventive Cancer Screenings

Along with not smoking, cancer screening is one of the top anticancer moves. The most preventable cancers through early detection are cancers of the colon, breast, prostate, and cervix.

Schedule your colonoscopy. Terminal colorectal cancer is a tragic consequence for those who put off regular colonoscopies. First, determine if you are at high risk for colon cancer. You are at high risk if you have:

- a personal history of inflammatory bowel disease
- a family history of colorectal cancer or colon polyps

If you have these risk factors, have your first colonoscopy at age thirty-five. (If I'd had regular checkups, I probably would have avoided getting colon cancer.) Also, beginning at age thirty-five, have a yearly fecal occult blood test (FOBT) as part of your annual physical exam. Colorectal cancer begins with polyps (fingerlike growths of precancerous cells) that grow slowly for five to fifteen years. Early detection of these precancerous polyps by colonoscopy can save you from getting colon cancer later on and spare you major surgery. Your doctor simply snips off the polyps during the colonoscopy. Because of early and aggressive cancer screening, the rate of colorectal cancer has been dropping slowly over the past decade.

Consider these recommendations from the American College of Gastroenterology (for updates, see www.acg.gi.org):

- If you're at low risk — that is, you have no family history of colon cancer or inflammatory bowel disease — have your first colonoscopy between ages forty-five and fifty.
- If a family member has had colon cancer, get a colonoscopy when you are ten years younger than that family member was at the age of diagnosis, or age forty, whichever is younger. For example, if your father was diagnosed with colon cancer at age forty-five, you should have a colonoscopy at age thirty-five.

- For people with severe inflammatory bowel disease, get screened eight to ten years after this diagnosis is made or by age thirty-five, whichever is younger.
- If your colonoscopy is normal but you're in the high-risk group, it is recommended that you have a colonoscopy at least every five years.

Make sure you get a mammogram. The American College of Obstetricians and Gynecologists recommends women get a mammogram:

- every 1 to 2 years between ages forty and forty-nine
- once a year at age fifty and older

If you have any of the following risk factors, your doctor may suggest you have the test at a younger age. These factors also may increase the risk of breast cancer in some women:

- personal history of cancer of the breast, endometrium, ovary, or colon
- postmenopausal obesity

- excessive alcohol intake
- recent hormone therapy
- recent use of birth control pills
- tall stature
- Jewish heritage

For updates, including how to perform a self-exam, see www.acog.org.

Get regular Pap smears. In a Pap smear, the doctor scrapes the lining of the cervix, and the cells are tested to detect early cervical cancer risk. The American College of Obstetricians and Gynecologists recommends:

- Pap smears beginning at age twenty-one or three years after the onset of sexual activity
- annual Pap screenings for women under age thirty
- Pap smears every two to three years when the Pap test is normal and negative for HPV (human papillomavirus) in women over thirty
- screening for HPV in conjunction with the Pap smear
- annual pelvic exam

Have a prostate screening. When prostate cancer is detected early, while it is still confined to the gland, the cure rates are extremely high. Once the cancer spreads beyond the prostate gland, the cure rates are very low. Because 98 percent of prostate cancer occurs in men over age fifty-five, it's important for men in their fifties to begin getting regular screening tests. As part of a general checkup, your doctor will do a digital rectal exam (DRE), feeling for a lumpy prostate. If your doctor suspects an abnormality on examination or if you are experiencing symptoms (a change in urinating pattern), he or she may recommend a prostate-specific antigen (PSA) test. A high PSA is only a clue and does not always mean that you have prostate cancer. According to a 2008 study, most men who have a prostate biopsy because of high PSA turn out not to have prostate cancer. Because of the uncertain reliability of the PSA test, your doctor will discuss what the test results mean in your individual case.

Rx FOR PRIME-TIME CANCER PREVENTION

- ❏ Don't smoke.
- ❏ Graze on frequent minimeals.
- ❏ Eat ten servings of colorful fruits and vegetables daily.
- ❏ Eat more real soy foods: tofu and tempeh.
- ❏ Eat less meat.
- ❏ Eat more seafood.
- ❏ Change your oils: eat more fish, nuts, flax, and olive oils; less processed vegetable oils.
- ❏ Spice up your cuisine: eat more turmeric and curry.
- ❏ Reduce your waist size.
- ❏ Move more.
- ❏ Stress less.
- ❏ Laugh more.
- ❏ Get screened.

PART V

Prime-Time Fitness

Fit is a powerful but tiny little word that economically describes how we should be in our prime time. In previous chapters, you learned how to be nutritionally fit, medically fit, and emotionally fit. Now, you will learn how to be physically fit.

We begin with a prime-time weight-management program that might be fittingly called "Waist Control." Because diet and exercise are the dynamic duo of prime time, we will also help you develop a personal workout plan that you can stick to.

You can be the fittest person in your neighborhood, but one careless slip, fall, and broken bone can set your whole program back for months. That's why learning how to design and maintain a safe living environment is an essential part of your overall health program.

Many of you may feel that the safety section is "too old" for you. While that may be true, you may have parents or friends whose environment requires a major safety overhaul, and you can learn how to help them do this.

What's the right diet and fitness program for you? One that you will consistently do.

CHAPTER 21

Stay Lean

Here's one of the most important health tips for prime timers: become leaner as you get older. As we age, we tend to accumulate extra body fat, especially around the middle. Called the *creep effect*, it's easy to put on at least a pound a year between the ages of forty and sixty. Yet the older we get, the more serious the health consequences of excess body fat become. The word that most accurately predicts longevity is *lean*. *Lean* does not mean skinny, which can imply not having enough body fat; it means having the right amount of body fat for your particular body type. A person who is thin is not necessarily fit, and becoming lean does not necessarily equate with weight loss. Muscle and bone weigh more than fat. You want to lose excess fat but not at the expense of losing calorie-burning muscle and strength-building bone, which will make you frail. Becoming lean in a healthy way actually makes you stronger because you are building stronger muscles and bones.

You will notice that we use the more descriptive and scientifically correct term *overfat* rather than *overweight* in this discussion. Excess fat is the real issue, especially for prime timers. Part of our program is to preserve and even gain muscle while losing excess fat, especially around the middle. Because muscle weighs a lot more than fat, the inches of fat loss that your measuring tape shows is a lot more meaningful than your weight in pounds. In fact, many people on the Prime-Time Health plan lose inches around their waist without a major loss of weight. If you practice all of the prime-time tips in this book, you're becoming leaner without even realizing it.

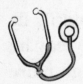

DR. SEARS SAYS...
Cut junk carbs! Besides exercising more, the most important nutritional change you can make to get and stay lean is to cut junk carbs. So-called high-glycemic carbs,

those fiberless, proteinless carbs listed on page 597, are the number one cause of being overfat. One of the biggest scientific break-throughs in weight management was the discovery that it's mainly dietary carbs, more than fats, that contribute to excess body fat.

Why lean? Lean and longevity go together. Excess body fat raises the risk of just about every disease you can get. An overfat prime timer is more prone to:

- Alzheimer's disease
- arthritis
- asthma
- breathing difficulties
- cancer
- cardiovascular disease
- diabetes
- gum disease
- heartburn
- high blood pressure
- skin sores
- stroke
- vision loss
- injuries

If that list is not enough motivation for you to remain lean, consider that illnesses related to overfatness are the number one cause of disability and a shorter lifespan.

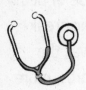

DR. SEARS SAYS...
"You're prediabetic!" In my medical practice, I no longer use the term *overweight*. Instead, I use a more medically accurate term when counseling patients with an excess waist size: *prediabetic*. That change of terminology gets their attention.

SIX SIMPLE DIET FACTS YOU MUST KNOW

Before we work out your personal weight-management program, there are a few basic principles about dieting you must know.

1. Most "Diets" Don't Work

Did you ever wonder why 90 percent of people who diet regain their lost weight within a year and often put on even more weight? More and more Americans are dieting than ever before, yet they're getting fatter, not leaner. Here's why most diets fail:

Most diets take the fun out of eating. The word *diet* comes from the Greek word *diaita*, which describes a person's lifestyle and eating style. In this book, we use the term *diet* to mean a healthier way of eating, not one full of restrictions. Humans are creatures of pleasure. Eating is supposed to be pleasurable, so it's only a matter of time until a dieter resents being on a typical diet, and resentment invariably leads to failure. Diets that take the joy out of eating don't succeed. Because the prime-time diet focuses on feeling good (with excess fat loss as a natural consequence), you won't resent it, you'll crave it. If someone asks, "What diet are you on?" reply, "The real-food diet!"

Most diets focus on fat and carbs. Americans went wild for *low-fat* diets, and they got fatter. Then they shifted to low-carb diets and got even fatter. A low-anything diet often doesn't taste good, doesn't work, doesn't last, and can be downright unhealthy. Consider the popular Atkins diet, which is scientifically incorrect and simply doesn't make sense. Eating a high-protein, high-fat, low-carb diet, as the Atkins diet recommends, causes the body to go into a biochemically abnormal state called ketosis, which kills the appetite and dehydrates the body. Any diet that makes you sick in order to get you lean won't work. Most fad diets fail because the body ultimately rejects what is not good for it. The prime-time plan for eating replaces *low* fat and carbs with *right* fat and carbs. For most prime timers, small, healthy daily changes — because they are good for us — are more likely to be accepted than rejected by the body.

2. Eat Right for Your Metabolic Type

Do you ever wonder why your lean friend can indulge in brownies, yet if you eat brownies you gain weight? That's because you each have different metabolic rates and burn calories differently. Some people are wired to be calorie burners, and others are calorie storers.

Genetically lean people — we dub them "bananas" — are natural calorie burners. More rounded people — we dub them "apples" (round waist) or "pears" (round hips) — tend to be calorie storers. And then there are the "yams" who are just big all over.

Why you start packing on fat after forty. Even though there are genetic differences in how we burn calories, don't rely completely on these tendencies after forty, when we all tend to become calorie storers rather than burners. It's common to marry a banana only to retire with an apple. It's often hard for bananas to stay lean. They've been so used to eating virtually anything they want that they start to put on extra middle fat when they hit middle age.

3. You Don't Have to Count Calories

Eating should be a pleasurable event, not a mathematical exercise. If you follow the prime-time diet, you'll automatically eat fewer calories without purposely trying to do so.

JUST EAT REAL FOODS!

These are the four magic words. Real foods (such as salads and seafood) are usually found on the perimeter of the supermarket, unlike fake foods (those packaged "bads"), which tend to be located in the center aisles. Perimeter foods are usually nutrient-dense foods—they naturally pack more nutrition in fewer calories—not calorie-dense foods, which pack more calories with less nutrition. Nutrient-dense foods tend to be more satisfying, so it takes less of these foods to fill you up. There are also what we like to call *free foods*—those you can eat as much of as you want (see page 594).

4. You Shouldn't Go Hungry

Many diets interfere with the basic principle of appetite control called the *fat point,* also known as the *set point,* the level of eating and fat your body has gotten used to. Because the body believes that this amount of eating and body fat is normal for you, it strives to maintain this level and resists any attempts to lose fat or to lower the fat point. When you start to eat drastically differently or start to lose fat, your body mistakenly concludes that it's famine time. Your metabolism slows (like that of a hibernating bear), and your appetite often increases. The goal is to *gradually* cut back on your calories so that your body doesn't think that you're making drastic changes. This approach is just the opposite of crash or starvation diets. When you replace quantity with quality foods, your body concludes, "Finally! You're feeding me right. Keep it up." You then begin craving those quality foods.

The key to getting and staying lean is resetting your fat point so you burn rather than store fat. With the prime-time diet, you first go through a stage of fooling your fat point. A stuck fat point is why some people on diets plateau. Your body decides that this is where it wants to stay for a while. It's a signal that you need to trick it again by stepping up the prime-time diet.

5. Change Your Cravings

The great thing about the prime-time diet is that it curbs your food cravings and actually changes them. You'll alter your gut-brain's perception about what's normal for you, and you'll begin to *crave* real food. This is known as *metabolic programming*. After a few months following the prime-time diet, I noticed that I craved the foods that were healthiest for me and shied away from foods that were unhealthy for me. In the first stage of this approach, you will have to eliminate or restrict junk foods and eat only healthy-aging foods. I guarantee that within three months or so, your gut will crave the very foods that are best for you. When that occurs, you'll know that the prime-time diet is working.

Rose's story. Rose was a 230-pound, five-foot-four-inch, forty-year-old mother of three who came into my office for a weight-loss consultation. Rose had heard about our prime-time diet and wanted to try it. Her initial laboratory values were alarming: triglycerides: 1,130 (seven times the healthy range); total cholesterol: 255; fasting blood sugar: 130; blood pressure: 160/92; waist circumference: 45. I called it like it was: "Rose, you are prediabetic." Within six months on the prime-time diet and exercise plan, she had dropped forty pounds, and her blood chemistry had improved. Rose was well on her way to being healthy.

Joe's story. Impressed with her success, Rose asked me to help her husband. Into my office came 330-pound, five-foot-six-inch Joe, the owner of a meat-packing plant, of all things. Joe's blood chemistries were even worse than Rose's. In addition to using the term *prediabetic,* I motivated Joe with his three daughters: "Joe, unless you make drastic changes in the way you live and eat, you won't live long enough to walk your daughters down the aisle." He got the point. Joe eventually shed pounds of fat off his body, inches off his waist, and added years to his life.

A few months into the program, Rose and Joe were ecstatic. They said, "You know, Dr. Bill, we just *can't* eat the way we used to." These leaner and happier folks had changed at the gut level. Their cravings had changed, and they didn't look back.

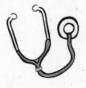

DR. SEARS SAYS...
Weight management should become *waist* management.

6. Reduce Your Waist

Many prime timers literally go to pot. Your waist size should be your most meaningful motivator. Using your personal waistometer — a belt, a skirt, or a pair of jeans — is more helpful than using a scale. The fat around your middle releases aging inflammatory chemicals into the bloodstream, which increase the risk of heart disease and diabetes. Men, especially in midlife, tend to store fat around the middle, while women tend to store excess fat on the buttocks, hips, and thighs. Yet, women going through menopause also tend to develop excess belly fat, a "menopot."

By eating too much and moving too little, you can easily put on abdominal fat, but the

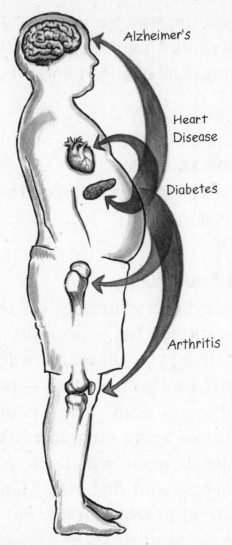

Alzheimer's

Heart
Disease

Diabetes

Arthritis

The Big Bad Four of Belly Fat

great news is that by eating better and moving more, you can easily take it off. (For a complete discussion of why abdominal fat is so unhealthy, see "Toxic Waist," page 92.)

THIRTEEN WAYS TO STAY LEAN

The prime-time diet is easy to learn and follow, contains no gimmicks, and is based on solid nutritional science. It is simply about eating what your body needs for a longer and healthier life. Loss of excess body fat will be a welcome perk. Let's get started!

1. Keep a Prime-Time Diary

Set your personal prime-time goals by creating a chart like the one below. In the first column, list the main goals you want to achieve (decrease in waist size, less aching joints, more energy, etc.). In the second column, list the current obstacles that are keeping you from meeting these goals (too busy, too lazy, putting it off, not a priority, etc.). In the third column, list ways you might overcome these obstacles. For example:

Your Goals	Your Obstacles	Solutions
Lose two inches off waist	Like big meals	Graze
More energy		
Pain-free walking		

2. Know Your Numbers

Consult your doctor about using the prime-time diet. Because it's not a crash or fad diet, we can think of no medical reason why you couldn't do it. *Every* body was designed to eat this way. Following are the medical tests and measurements you should record in your diary. Keep track of these before you start the program and for at least six months after you begin.

Before Prime-Time Diet	Three Months After Prime-Time Diet
Waist circumference (or size of skirt, pants, number of belt notches):	Waist circumference:
Height:	Height:
Weight:	Weight:
Blood pressure:	Blood pressure:
Fasting blood sugar:	Fasting blood sugar:
Complete lipid and cholesterol profile:	Complete lipid and cholesterol profile:
Fasting insulin level:	Fasting insulin level:

Before Prime-Time Diet	Three Months After Prime-Time Diet
Inflammatory marker profile:	Inflammatory marker profile:
Illness feelings: energy level, joint aches, heartburn, etc.	Wellness feelings: brain, eyes, gut, joints, etc.

Now that you've programmed your mind, let's get started on the body.

3. Graze

This can be the first major change you make. People who eat frequent minimeals throughout the day tend to consume fewer calories but are just as satisfied as those who eat larger meals less frequently.

Remember our rule of twos, the simplest way to start:

- Eat twice as often.
- Eat half as much.
- Chew twice as long.

The grazers vs. gorgers study. Obesity researchers studied two groups of overfat people.

Both groups ate the same foods and the same number of daily calories. Yet, the group that ate six mini-meals lost more body fat than those who ate three square meals a day. Grazing perks up your metabolism and turns you into more of a calorie burner than a calorie storer.

Try the sipping solution. We suggest that prime timers who need a major metabolic overhaul and must lose twenty to thirty pounds and three to four inches off their waist begin the prime-time diet by sipping on a smoothie for breakfast, snacks, and lunch for the first month. This is the simplest, most effective, and healthiest weight-control tip we can share with you. The sipping solution resets your gut-filling level so you are satisfied with less food, sort of like shrinking your stomach's "I'm full" gauge. Once you get used to the sipping solution, your gut will begin to protest if you try to eat huge helpings. Prime timers in our medical practice report that this is the top change that worked for them. (Read the background of the sipping solution and why it is so good for the gut, page 147; recipe, page 151.) Those who are trying to improve an already healthful diet may not need to make such a big change.

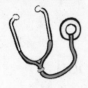

DR. SEARS SAYS...
Remember, your body tends to dislike drastic changes in eating. When using the sipping solution, start gradually, beginning with one day a week and progressing to four.

4. Eat Real Foods

The prime-time diet could also be called the real-food diet. Some foods keep you lean; others can make you fat. Lean foods are simply real foods that have gone from field and stream to your table without being messed with by some food chemist. To make our lean-food list, a food must meet all of the following criteria:

- be nutrient dense
- be fiber rich and filling
- contribute to steady blood sugar, and therefore, steady insulin levels
- promote fat burning rather than fat storing
- contribute to the physical health of the organs and tissues of the body
- contribute to the mental, emotional, and intellectual health of the brain

All fruits and vegetables belong on the

prime-time diet, but here is our list of top lean foods — true health foods:

- apples
- artichokes
- avocados
- beans
- blueberries
- broccoli
- cantaloupe
- carrot juice
- chickpeas (hummus)
- chili peppers
- cranberry juice
- eggs
- flax oil and ground flaxseeds
- garlic
- grapes
- lentils
- mango
- olive oil
- onions
- oranges
- papaya
- peanut butter
- pink grapefruit
- seafood (especially salmon and tuna)
- soy products (e.g., tofu)
- spinach
- sunflower seeds (raw)
- sweet potatoes
- tomatoes
- walnuts (raw)
- watermelon
- wild rice
- yogurt

Avoid or drastically cut down on "forbidden foods." These foods are harmful in one or more of the following ways. They:

- promote fat storage rather than fat burning
- promote erratic swings in blood sugar

- promote overeating because they lack fiber and are unsatisfying
- are calorie dense

To help you remember what to eat and what not to, consider real foods "young foods." The following items are "old foods." Avoid foods containing these additives:

- high-fructose corn syrup
- hydrogenated oils
- foods with dyes and numbers (e.g., red #40) on the ingredients list
- snack foods that are high in processed carbohydrates but low in fiber and protein

(For additional lists, see pages 306 and 476.)

SNACK SMART: THE RULE OF THREES

Be sure to include both fiber and protein with every meal and carbohydrate snack. Fiber fills you up for less (less calories, that is). Protein also has a high satiety factor, and it perks up metabolism and helps weight control. The body uses up more calories processing protein than it does digesting carbs. Be sure your snack contains at least 3 grams of fiber and/or 3 grams of protein.

Record your good-gut-feeling foods and bad-gut-feeling foods. Note which foods give you a good gut feeling and which make you feel uncomfortable. Eventually, your gut will tell you which foods belong on your personal prime-time list and which you need to cut down on or shun completely. (See related section, metabolic programming, page 15.)

Good-Gut-Feeling Foods	Bad-Gut-Feeling Foods

5. Eat Fill-up Foods

Fill-up foods are naturally high in protein and fiber. (Review the concept of satiety on page 158 and our list of fill-up foods on page 161.)

Fiber is filling without being fattening. Fiber curbs overeating. High-fiber foods require more chewing. Besides predigesting the food and burning more calories, prolonged chewing helps to satisfy the appetite so you eat less. Fiber-rich foods stay in the stomach longer, absorb water, swell, and help you feel full. Because of this feeling of fullness, when you eat a fiber-rich diet, you tend to eat more slowly and eat less. When you eat fiber with fat, you're likely to eat less of the fatty food. Martha makes pie crust with high-fiber whole-wheat or brown-rice flour (and uses hearty oats for cobbler topping), and I notice that I tend to eat a smaller piece and feel just as satisfied as I would with a regular pastry.

Studies show that people who eat an extra 5 grams of fiber a day (the equivalent of one serving of fiber-rich cereal) eat fewer calories that day. One study showed that people who ate a high-fiber breakfast cereal consumed an average of 150 fewer calories that day than those who ate a low-fiber cereal. (Eating 150 fewer

HOW MUCH FIBER?

The latest USDA guideline for prime-time health is to eat **14 grams of fiber per 1,000 calories per day.** This translates to 25 to 35 grams of fiber daily in a 2,000- to 2,500-calorie diet.

calories a day translates into more than a pound less fat per month.)

Protein is filling without being fattening. Protein has three perks, which makes it the darling of dieters:

- Protein has a higher satiety factor than fiberless carbs — it fills you up for less.
- Unlike carbs, protein does not trigger the roller-coaster effect of the insulin cycle. So eating a lot of protein does not give you the high-to-low feeling that you get after a rush of junk sugars.
- Unlike sugar and fat, excess protein in the diet is not stored as fat. Whatever protein your body doesn't need, it excretes as waste.

LEAN TIP: EAT FIBER AND PROTEIN FIRST

Fill up with fiber-rich and high-protein foods, such as salad and salmon, near the beginning of the meal. These filling foods help you feel satisfied early in the meal, and you will therefore crave fewer carbs.

---

6. Be Satisfied with Less

Eat *real* food. Real foods are more filling and satisfying. Fake foods are often less filling so you have to eat more to be satisfied.

Take time to dine. The faster you eat, the more likely you are to overeat. There is a mechanism in the hypothalamus of the brain dubbed the *appestat,* which controls your appetite. The appestat is designed to register when you have had your fill and cue you to stop eating. The problem is, there is a time delay of approximately twenty minutes between when you eat and when the appestat registers "enough!" Slowing down your eating allows time for the food to be registered by your appestat. Try these suggestions to slow down your eating:

- Start low, and go slow: start with a smaller portion; slowly refill as needed.
- Get up and go to the bathroom after twenty minutes into the meal.
- Put down your fork and stir up a conversation between bites. Focus on the people instead of your plate.
- Sip warm water or tea between bites.
- Take a few deep breaths between bites.

- Use your napkin between bites.
- Eat with the opposite hand.
- Keep the serving bowls on another table; it takes time to get up and serve yourself a second helping.

Chew your food longer. The longer food lingers in your mouth, the easier it is to digest and the less likely you are to overeat. Chewing breaks up the fiber that holds the food together and gives digestive enzymes easier access to the food. Chewing stimulates saliva, which has three digestive perks:

- It lubricates the upper digestive tract for smoother passage.
- It protects against the irritating effects of stomach acids.
- It is rich in enzymes that predigest the food, which means less work — and rumbling — in your stomach and intestines.

Saliva is your body's own health juice. Your mouth, stomach, and intestines are like food processors. The more work you do at the upper end, the less work the food processors have to do at the lower end.

Use smaller plates. Reduce your plate size to reduce your waist size. When you use smaller plates, you're likely to eat less. Reduce your prime-time plate by a couple of inches, and you're more likely to reduce your waist a couple of inches. When eating at buffets, I began using salad-size plates, even for the entrées. I noticed I was eating more slowly. And just getting up

---

CHOPSTICKS, ANYONE?

During a recent lecture tour of China and Japan, I noticed that using chopsticks made me take smaller bites and eat more slowly than I do with a fork. One evening during a traditional Japanese meal, I realized that it is not only what they eat (primarily vegetables and seafood with meat as an accent) but also *how* they eat (smaller bites, smaller plates, and taking more time to dine) that accounts for their longevity. I commented on these healthy-eating customs to our host, who summed it up very simply: "Be good to your body, and your body will be good to you!"

---

to refill the smaller plates prolonged the enjoyment of the meal.

Practice "out of sight, out of stomach." Obesity research proves that the more food you see, the more you are likely to eat. Until you reach your lean goal, avoid all-you-can-eat buffets. Serve yourself at the stove or kitchen counter rather than letting big serving bowls full of food on the dining table tempt you.

Practice "out of mind, out of mouth." Weight-control studies have also shown that the more we think about a particular food, the more intense our cravings get, and the more likely we are to give in and overindulge. You think about a hot-fudge sundae. The more you picture the indulgence in your mind, the more likely you are to give in and overeat. Instead, get up, take a walk, and feast your mind on some pleasant scene (fantasy or memory) completely off the subject of food. Simply changing mental pathways seems to trick the mind into forgetting about food. If after using this technique you still have a chocolate craving, give in to a minidose. We enjoy a guiltless square or two of dark chocolate after the evening meal.

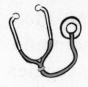

DR. SEARS SAYS...

Curb your carb cravings. Don't eat carbs you crave on an empty stomach or you're likely to overeat. Instead, save that square of dark chocolate for *after* your meal.

Enjoy happy meals. Relax while eating. The happier and more relaxed you are as you dine, the less likely you are to mindlessly overeat. Since stress diminishes saliva production, the more relaxed you are, the more saliva you produce. This gives you a head start on digestion and leads to a more comfortable gut feeling after eating. Keeping the conversation happy at mealtime gives you a better chance of eating less and enjoying it more. Put on some good music and dine by candlelight.

SPICE IT UP!

Hot spices, such as turmeric, curry, chili peppers, jalapeño peppers, and wasabi, increase metabolism and help the body burn calories. Spicing up your meals keeps the blandness out of your eating and helps you enjoy your lean cuisine.

7. Indulge in "Free Foods"

Value your veggies; savor your salads. All effective eating plans have one thing in common: lots of vegetables. Ounce for ounce, veggies contain fewer calories and more fiber than most other foods, so they tend to fill you up without putting on the fat. They're nutrient dense, meaning they pack more nutrition, including phytos, into fewer calories. In the prime-time diet, we call veggies "free foods" because you can eat all you want without counting calories. The lean little biochemical quirk in veggies that allows you this indulgence is the *thermogenic effect*. Your body uses almost as many calories to digest most vegetables as veggies contain in the first place. For example, you'll use up most of the 26 calories in a tomato just by chewing, swallowing, and digesting it.

Salads are perfect free foods. Here are some tips:

- Fill up on salad at the *beginning* of a meal, and you're likely to eat less of the main course and dessert.
- When eating out, choose a restaurant that has a nutritious salad bar, and begin

the meal with a hefty portion, sans the heavy dressing.

- Choose green greens. Generally, the darker the greens, the more nutritious the salad. The best greens are spinach, arugula, beet greens, watercress, endive, and romaine.
- Steam your salads. Lightly steamed greens, such as spinach, swiss chard, and beet greens, are a nutrient-dense, filling, and low-calorie side dish.
- As a salad dressing, choose 1 tablespoon of olive oil and add balsamic vinegar. A nutritious and tasty alternative to commercial dressings is a tablespoon of hummus.

(See supersalad recipe, page 554.)

8. Eat a Right-Carb Diet

For most prime timers, eating too many of the wrong carbs can make you fat. Think more in terms of a *right*-carb diet, not a low-carb or a bad-carb diet.

Don't insult your insulin. Insulin is your body's investment banker. It stores excess

FOLLOW THE FRENCH

The French paradox puzzles many nutritionists. How do the French, who drink wine with meals and eat saucy foods like beef bourguignonne, stay leaner and enjoy a much lower incidence of cardiovascular disease and other ailments than Americans do? The French eat *real food,* usually from a neighborhood market or a farmer's produce stand—which they often walk or bike to. Home cooking is prized; fast-food restaurants are shunned. For the French, eating is a social affair. They take time to dine and digest their food rather than wolfing it down. Finally, they are satisfied with smaller portions. So, it's not really a paradox after all.

food as fat, which is your energy bank. Not only does the body not function well with too much insulin, it also doesn't function well with too little. Grazing on good carbs steadies insulin levels. With the Prime-Time Health plan, insulin doesn't get high enough to store excess fat or low enough to trigger hunger pangs.

You've probably heard the term *glycemic index* and the advice "eat foods with a low

Lean Carbs	Fat Carbs
Fruits	Sweetened beverages
Vegetables	White breads
Oatmeal	Sugar-loaded icings
Flaxseed meal	Cereals and snack foods
Soy foods	that are highly
Yogurt	sweetened, low in fiber,
Whole grains	and low in protein

glycemic index." This just means you should eat *real foods.* Foods with a low glycemic index are slowly absorbed into the bloodstream and don't trigger an erratic insulin cycle as do foods with a high glycemic index that rush quickly into the bloodstream.

For many of us, taking a number like the glycemic index into consideration detracts from the joy of eating. Instead, stick with the simple designations *good carb* and *bad carb*. Good carbs have a lower glycemic index because they're partnered with protein, fiber, or fat. Also, it's the glycemic index of the *whole* meal or snack that counts, not just a particular food. This is why a carb-only meal or snack, such as guzzling a sweetened beverage (very high glycemic index and very bad carb), is the worst thing you can do for your blood sugar and your weight. If you must indulge in a sweetened beverage, sip it *slowly* with an otherwise healthy meal. (See page 118 for a simple way to tell a "lean carb" from a "fat carb," and page 158 for "bad words" to watch out for on food labels.)

SODA: SAD FOR PRIME TIMERS

On the checkout counter of our family medical office, we display a large bottle of soda around which is a printed label that reads, "Diabetes in a bottle." Our patients get the message. Here's why soda is so sad for prime timers:

Soda makes you fat. Remember to always partner carbs with fiber, protein, or healthy fats; sodas contain just sweeteners. It's these unpartnered sweeteners, such as sugar and high-fructose corn syrup, that can be stored as extra fat and rev up the roller coaster of sugar highs and lows. Sweetened beverages don't contribute to *satiety*. Interesting research disclosed an unfortunate quirk about sodas: the calories from sodas don't register on the body's daily calorie counter, your built-in signal that says, "You've eaten enough today!"

Try sweet substitutes. While we never completely outgrow our sweet tooth, we can reshape
our tastes a bit as we age. Instead of sugar or
high-fructose corn syrup, try these healthier
sweeteners:

- cinnamon (see health benefits of,
  page 363)
- agave nectar

Soda makes you frail. Soda weakens your bones. Because
prime timers are already prone to osteoporosis, the last thing
we should do is eat or drink foods that age our bones. When
I was a child, we used to call sodas phosphates because the
phosphoric acid is what makes sodas fizzy. Phosphates get
in the bloodstream and leach calcium from the bones.

Soda weakens your teeth. The same acids in soda that
weaken the bones can weaken dental enamel.

Don't do diet drinks. You may think that diet sodas are
okay because they are low calorie, but the artificial sweeteners, such as sucralose and aspartame, are, in my personal
opinion, not safe for prime timers. And, diet drinks are
likely to increase your cravings for sweet drinks, making it
hard for you to break the soda habit.

- fruit toppings, such as blueberries, instead of sugar on oatmeal
- *xylitol.* It occurs naturally in many fruits and vegetables. While it is just as sweet as table sugar, xylitol has some biochemical traits that could make it a healthier choice for baking. Xylitol has 40 percent fewer calories than table sugar, and unlike table sugar, it is absorbed more slowly and completely through the small intestine into the bloodstream, and it doesn't trigger the roller coaster of blood sugar and insulin levels. However, eat xylitol-containing foods slowly and don't overindulge; eating too much xylitol too fast can cause it to accumulate in the gut, ferment, and cause uncomfortable gas and diarrhea.

9. Eat a Right-Fat Diet

A good fat comes from a food that *swims* in the sea, *runs* in the forests, or *grows* in fields. A bad fat comes from a source that sits and eats junk food all day (e.g., penned-up livestock) or one that may have started as a good fat but after going

CAN ALCOHOL MAKE YOU FAT?

Yes. Alcohol is basically strong sugar water. Alcohol averages 100 calories per standard drink, which is 12 ounces of beer, 5 ounces of wine, and 1.5 ounces of hard liquor. Because alcohol is a sugar and gets into the bloodstream fast, excess sugar from alcohol is often deposited as fat, especially around the middle. And the gut brain doesn't count the calories in alcohol toward your daily needs. In addition, excess alcohol can override your inhibitions, prompting you to make less healthful food choices and overeat during a meal.

---

through the food-processing plant becomes a bad fat. The worst factory-made fat is hydrogenated, or trans fats.

Here's why right-fat eating rather than a low-fat diet is the better option as we age:

Fat makes food taste better. Fat gives food a pleasant mouth feel and brings out the flavors. And, some fat can make foods work better in the body. For example, olive oil increases the intestinal absorption of the nutrients in salad.

Fat is filling. While it's true that fat contains twice as many calories as carbs or protein, fat in a meal or snack is digested more slowly so you feel full longer. Fat has a higher satiety factor than carbs do. Fat added to carbs (e.g., peanut butter with jelly) slows the rush of carbs into your bloodstream. If done wisely, you really can eat fat to lose fat.

Fat keeps the brain smart. See page 107 for how the right fat protects the aging brain.

Right fat is good for the body. Good fat helps build healthy skin and facilitates the absorption of vitamins A, D, E, and K from foods. Healthy fat also helps the body make important hormones. Finally, fat provides energy when your carb stores run out.

HOW MUCH FAT DO YOU NEED?

While this may vary somewhat based on your own tastes and medical and dietary needs, I have found a healthy daily ratio of food nutrients to be around 50 percent healthy carbs, 25 percent protein, and 25 percent healthy fat.

10. Make Little Changes for a Lot of Fat Loss

Most likely you have passed the stage of life when you might be tempted to go on a crash diet to quickly shed 20 pounds to fit into a smaller wedding or prom dress. Remember to start low and go slow. Dropping 1 to 2 pounds a month is the most doable diet. If you're 10 pounds overweight, aim to drop 100 calories a day; if 20 pounds overweight, shed 200 calories a day (for example, 100 calories less of junk food and burning an extra 100 calories through 15 to 20 minutes of exercise). This small-change diet will do it.

Recent research has proved that shedding 5 to 10 pounds of excess fat can reap huge health benefits in terms of lowering your risk for certain diseases or slowing their progression, especially diabetes. Making small changes in your eating habits can result in big changes in your waistline — and your health. For example, ten fatty potato chips a day is an extra 100 calories, which translates into 10 pounds of extra fat a year. Lose the chips, and you'll lose the pounds. Cutting out just one slice of bread a day is a pound of fat lost a month, 12 pounds a year, 24 pounds in two years.

Instead of...	Try...
Whole milk	Low-fat or nonfat milk
Whole-milk yogurt	Low-fat or nonfat yogurt (see yogurt tips, page 335)
High-fat cheeses	Low-fat cheeses
Fatty beef	Lean beef with fat trimmed
Farmed fish	Wild fish
French fries	Sweet potato fries (these are really baked)
Dark-meat poultry	White-meat poultry
Beef (select round is leaner than choice cuts; prime is the fattiest)	Wild game meats, lean meats
Beef stir-fry	Tofu stir-fry
Beef burger	Veggie burger
Chicken	Turkey white meat
Sour cream	Greek yogurt
Salad dressing	Hummus, olive oil, and vinegar
Deep-frying	Stir-frying
Frying	Poaching or baking

Instead of...	Try...
Frying in oil	Sautéing with chicken broth
Butter on bread	Dip bread lightly in olive oil and balsamic vinegar
Butter on popcorn	Air-popped popcorn
Canned fruits in syrup	Canned fruits packed in water
Tuna packed in oil	Tuna packed in water

11. Eat Breakfast

Your mother was right, breakfast *is* the most important meal of the day. Here are three benefits of a healthy breakfast:

Breakfast gets the gut going for the day. Studies show that people who begin the day with a balanced breakfast — protein, carbs, and fiber — tend to eat less junk food during the day. This makes sense since a healthy breakfast sort of talks to the body and tells it how to eat for the rest of the day. A person eating a veggie omelet and whole-grain toast instead of coffee and a doughnut will actually send a healthy message to the brain and gut about the food to expect for the rest of the day.

Breakfast jump-starts your brain. Breaking your fast revs up your metabolism, which perks up your body and brain, preparing them for the day. Start your day smart. Feed those neurotransmitters, the neurochemical messengers that rev up your brain and steady your moods. Eat a healthy, balanced breakfast, and you'll feel energized and relaxed.

Breakfast keeps you lean. You may think that skipping breakfast will help you lose weight. Wrong! It's just the opposite. Studies show that breakfast eaters tend to be leaner than breakfast skippers, because by "front-loading" they prepare their bodies for the rest of the day. In a study comparing breakfast skippers to breakfast

---

"LIGHT" IS NOT ALWAYS RIGHT

Be suspicious of foods that display "light" or "lite" on the labels. More often than not, these diet foods are lean on nutrition and heavy on artificial sweeteners. To save a few calories, don't harm your health with junk food.

---

eaters, the skippers ate more food during the day, gained more weight, and generally had a higher incidence of heart disease, various "-itis" illnesses, and diabetes.

12. Shed Stress

Shedding stress sheds belly fat. Randy, a fifty-two-year-old stockbroker, came in for consultation. He said, "Dr. Bill, I exercise for an hour four days a week, my wife cooks nothing but wholesome meals, and my weight is stable, but I'm putting on a bigger spare tire each year. What's going on?" Randy didn't have the usual causes of toxic waist: eating too much (of the wrong foods) and moving too little. He was a healthy eater and a vigorous mover, yet Randy had a lot of stress in his life. Randy was trapped in a job that didn't suit him. He was a New York stockbroker swimming with the sharks. His unresolved stress levels were so high that his otherwise healthy exercise and eating habits couldn't compensate.

Long-term unresolved stress causes your body to have high levels of the circulating stress hormone cortisol. Cortisol is the good news/bad news hormone. Just the right amount is good for the body, but too much for too long is bad for the body. Excess

THE RECIPE FOR A PRIME-TIME BREAKFAST

- Eat protein-rich foods. Protein perks up the brain. And, because the body takes longer to digest protein than carbs, it helps you stay comfortably full for a longer period. You'll be less likely to overeat, and you'll be spared that midmorning carbo-craving crash.
- A high-fiber breakfast of slow-release carbs prevents midmorning crashes and sugar cravings.
- A calcium-rich breakfast jump-starts brain biochemistry.

Try these healthy combos:
- nonfat or low-fat plain, organic yogurt topped with blueberries, honey, and a sprinkle

---

cortisol stimulates the accumulation of abdominal fat. Randy's large belly was due to the unresolved stress in his life. Once he started shedding the stress, his belt size dropped down a few notches.

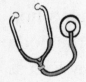 **DR. SEARS SAYS...**
Those who move more move longer.

of slivered almonds or chopped walnuts

- scrambled eggs, whole-wheat toast, and calcium-fortified orange juice
- a high-fiber, high-protein cereal with low-fat milk and fresh fruit
- a veggie omelet with whole-wheat toast and a side of guacamole
- whole-grain pancakes or waffles topped with berries and yogurt, and a glass of calcium-fortified orange juice
- two soft-boiled eggs, stewed tomatoes, and whole-wheat toast
- peanut butter and banana slices on a whole-wheat English muffin with low-fat milk
- crockpot oatmeal
- breakfast smoothie (see page 151)

13. Move

Diet and exercise are codependent health factors. The older we are, the more we need to move, for two reasons: prime timers tend to put on excess body fat, especially around the middle; and muscle mass diminishes as we age.

Muscle is your main calorie-burning source. If you lose muscle, your metabolism weakens, and you become a calorie storer instead of a calorie burner. Also, when you eat less without moving more to lose weight, the strategy can backfire. Eating less sends a signal to your body to burn fewer calories, mainly by decreasing your resting metabolic rate. This signals your body to click into calorie-storage mode. To make matters worse, if you eat less than your body actually needs, the body turns to its reserve tank, the muscles, and, in effect, cannibalizes the muscles for fuel.

SCALE DOWN!

Promise yourself you won't get on the scale more than once a month. Weigh yourself at the beginning of each month at the same time of day (preferably before breakfast) and in the same clothing (preferably none). Because body weight normally fluctuates during the day and from day to day, it is meaningless and often self-defeating to weigh yourself often. A change in a tape measure, belt notches, or clothing size will be more accurate than the scale and is the best indication of fat loss.

Store more muscle, and store less fat. Active prime timers do not experience the usual age-related decline in resting metabolic rate. This means they don't regress from being calorie burners to calorie storers. One of the best ways to stay lean is to increase muscle mass, because muscle burns more calories than fat.

Movement burns excess body fat. Obesity researchers have found that movement is the *best way* to decrease belly fat. Fat tissue, especially belly fat, contains a fat-storage enzyme called lipoprotein lipase (LPL). Exercise slows down LPL enzyme activity in the tissue, making it harder to store fat. When we stop exercising and start sitting for long periods of time, the LPL in fat tissue increases, so keep moving.

WALK AWAY FROM OVEREATING

The key is to make movement a natural part of your life. When you feel the urge to indulge, simply walk off the urge. Walk past the pantry door and out the front door. Food cravings usually last less than ten minutes, so take a ten-minute walk to distract yourself from your craving. Research shows that a brisk walk reduces the urge to snack.

Movement slows the appetite. Exercise can deaden appetite the way appetite-suppressing medicines do. Movement activates the norepinephrine and dopamine systems in the brain. Exercise seems to turn on the body's adrenal hormones for action, and as a perk these hormones turn off appetite. While it's true that vigorous exercise can sometimes make you hungrier, it can also stave off an indulgence if you're hungry but really don't need the food. Because exercise lessens the likelihood of overeating, weight-control experts recommend a vigorous workout before a tempting large meal. (Want another motivator? See how being lean affects erectile dysfunction, page 437.)

Rx FOR STAYING LEAN DURING PRIME TIME

- ❏ Cut out junk carbs.
- ❏ Eat real foods; shop the perimeter of the supermarket.
- ❏ Don't go hungry.
- ❏ Follow the rule of twos: eat *twice* as often, eat *half* as much, and chew twice as long.
- ❏ Try the sipping solution.
- ❏ Follow the rule of threes: be sure snacks contain at least *3 grams* of protein and *3 grams* of fiber.
- ❏ Eat more fiber and protein at the beginning of a meal.
- ❏ Spice up your meals with turmeric, chili peppers, wasabi.
- ❏ Shun sweetened beverages.
- ❏ Dis diet drinks.
- ❏ Make small daily changes.
- ❏ Enjoy breakfast.
- ❏ Shed stress to shed belly fat.
- ❏ Move more.
- ❏ Do muscle-building exercises.

CHAPTER 22

Stay Fit

This whole book is really about fitness — keeping your brain, heart, and all your other parts fit, as well as keeping your muscles and bones strong, your joints flexible, and your balance stable. Movement helps with all of it. You may already have a fitness plan that works for you. If not, here's how to start.

TOP TEN FITNESS STARTERS

Before you get started with exercises and with designing your personal fitness program, consult your physician. Here are some general guidelines to get fit safely and comfortably:

1. No excuses, please. One of my tips to our kids is never say you don't have time for xyz. That excuse really means that it isn't important to you. Even ten minutes a day will help. For those pressed for time, I recommend *The 10-Minute Total Body Breakthrough* by my trainer, Sean Foy.

Excuse	Rethink
But I don't have time.	Then you better reserve more time for the hospital.
But it's too expensive.	If you think wellness is expensive, try illness.
But I don't like exercise.	So, you like to take medicine?
I enjoy sitting.	Do you also enjoy hurting?
But I have a desk job.	The desk can't move, but you can.

2. Make fitness your priority. You spend time keeping your financial plan up to date, you make sure your health insurance is current, and you take your medicines as prescribed, don't you? Make movement your medicine too.

3. Use your brain before your muscles. One day our son Stephen, then nineteen, challenged me to wrestle. Impulsively, I got into a match, or mismatch, with this hunk of a teen. It took six months for my torn shoulder muscle to heal. I should have thought, *I haven't used these muscles this way for years; don't do it!*

4. Don't worry, and be happy. In the beginning, you may think of exercise as a chore, but with health and fitness programs your attitude matters. Think of movement as the best medicine you'll ever take and one that has only pleasant side effects. I consider my workout as my prime-time playtime. Initially, you may have to go through a month or two of forcing yourself to move more. Eventually, your body will become habituated (a nicer term than addicted) to the emotional and physical well-being movement provides. I guarantee that you will evolve from a need-to-do-it person to a want-to-do-it person. If you're experiencing low days of depression, strenuous exercise is by far the best perk-up pill.

5. Start low, and go slow. Ironically, I was on vacation while writing this chapter, and the resort had a fantastic fitness center with some state-of-the-art strength-training equipment I'd never used before. I was fascinated by the hip-muscle weight machine; I just had to try it. But I started with weights that were too heavy, and I went too fast. I limped for two days. A safer approach would have been to start with a lower weight, do fewer reps, and do slower movements for a shorter time. I could have come back in two days and bumped up the workout. I had used (or abused) my hip muscles in ways I never had before and paid the painful price. If you are just beginning a strength-building program, the key words are *thoughtful, slow,* and *gradual.* Older muscles are more easily injured if you do too much too fast. If you lift improperly and tear or injure a tendon or muscle, it could take at least six weeks to heal, which is quite a setback. It's not worth the risk of injury to overdo it.

6. Keep it safe, and make it fun. While your life on the job may be full of multitasking, during exercise keep your focus on your muscles. Workout accidents (falls, muscle strains, cuts, etc.) happen when you let your mind wander off the routine or weights. And try to get

SHALL WE DANCE?

While a variety of movements and exercises are good for longevity, if I had to pick just one, I'd choose dancing. At Martha's urging, I took up ballroom dancing at age fifty-five. I went from a klutz to a very accomplished dancer. Even when I was sixty-five, we beat a bunch of young couples in a swing-dance contest—three times. Dance is appropriately called "romance for the whole body." Rhythmic workouts have an extra perk in muscle maintenance: The tiny nerves that feed muscles often diminish with aging. Fewer nerves lead to weaker muscles. Dancing preserves these nerves as well as our ability to make sudden movements and adjust our posture. Dancing:

- strengthens bones, muscles, and joints;
- improves posture, balance, and coordination;
- maintains memory (you have to learn and remember the dance steps and sequences);
- reduces tension/stress (dance your worries away);
- builds social skills and networks; and
- helps healthy aging. One study showed that people who danced regularly cut their risk of developing Alzheimer's disease in half.

Our favorite dance doctors are the Glenn Miller orchestra and Fred Astaire. We once told our grandchildren, "We not only want to be there for your weddings; we want to dance at them."

into a fitness program that you enjoy and look forward to every day. Martha uses her walks to do some praying. I look forward to walking on a golf course.

7. Always warm up first. Cold, tight muscles are more prone to injury. Do lighter versions of the muscle exercises for a few minutes before starting your regular, vigorous workout. The increased blood flow to the warmed-up muscles makes them less prone to injury.

8. Make it accessible. Who says playrooms are just for kids? For those of you who don't like the sights and sounds of commercial gyms, put together your own home gym. Used and reconditioned home-gym equipment is available at a reduced cost. If you add up all the unnecessary — and often unhealthy — stuff you spend money on, in a year you could more than pay for a home gym. Remember, illness is more expensive than wellness. My playroom, which occupies only a ten-foot-by-ten-foot area, contains:

- a Precor all-in-one strength-training system
- an elliptical exerciser (my favorite "medicine")
- a fit ball
- exercise bands
- a TV (to enjoy while I move)

9. Personalize your program. In addition to the activities of daily living, I try to fit in at least 60 minutes of exercise a day. When you are putting together your personal fitness program, try to incorporate all three types of exercise at least twice a week:

- strength-building exercises for strong muscle and bone
- endurance exercises (also called aerobics or "cardio"; e.g., walking, jogging, swimming) to improve stamina
- stretching to improve flexibility (e.g., yoga)

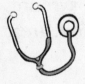

DR. SEARS SAYS...
The best exercise for *you* is the one you will *do*.

My own weekly program varies somewhat, but it generally runs like this:

- Strength training for 20 minutes, six days a week — three days upper body and three days lower body, alternating days. One day a week of complete rest from strength-training exercises.
- Walking (either just plain walking or golf) for at least 30 minutes, three days a week.
- Fit ball or stretching, 10 minutes, three to four days a week (see "Have a Ball," page 642).
- Swimming six days a week for at least 10 minutes each day.
- Exercise bands a few minutes three to four days a week while watching TV, for example (see "Strike Up the Bands," page 648).
- Yoga, when time permits.
- Taking stairs instead of escalators when possible, and parking a greater distance away so I have to walk farther to the store (see "Anytime, Anywhere Exercises," page 622).
- Isometrics (see page 654) and anytime, anywhere exercises when time and circumstances permit.

ANYTIME, ANYWHERE EXERCISES

Here are my favorite exercises for killing time usefully:

- **Walk while you wait.**
- **Flex while you stand or sit.** While waiting around, do squats, and go up and down on your toes and flex your knees. While sitting, arch your feet up and down, which flexes the muscles in the front and back of your legs. This exercise reduces the likelihood of blood clots in your legs, a prime-time health hazard during long air travel.
- **Squeeze while you sit.** While sitting and reading, squeeze a firm rubber ball. (See ball and finger flex exercises, page 648.)
- **Weight-train while you wait.** If you are really bored, use your bag or briefcase as a

10. Build muscle to burn fat during idle time. Little moves add up. Suppose you simply move your muscles an extra ten minutes a day. Those minimoves could translate into losing *five pounds* of excess fat each year, especially around the middle. Did you ever think about

dumbbell. While sitting, place it over your ankle and extend your legs.

- **Enjoy "band-aids."** Strategically place stretch bands around your home/hotel room and "flex a few" as you pass by.
  (See stretch-band exercises, page 648.)
- **Enjoy stair-stepping.** Make a few extra trips up and down the stairs. Before getting on an airplane or bus, walk around the waiting area for a while.
- **Practice isometrics** (see page 654).

Little movements throughout the day can help you stay fit. Imagine, 10 minutes a day of stretching, gripping, and flexing could translate into 5 pounds less of fat gain per year and be the difference between flabby and fit muscles.

how much time you waste standing in line? You could get in some movement medicine during this time. Say you're standing in line at the supermarket or checking in at the airport. Stretch and move during this otherwise wasted time. Flex your feet and legs up and down to strengthen your thigh and leg muscles. Shrug your shoulders or stretch your neck muscles. One day I was standing in a long line for an international flight. I began my muscle-flexing regimen — shrugging shoulders, flexing up and down on my toes, and even walking around in minicircles. One of the airport attendants, watching my ritual, kindly offered, "Sir, if you're afraid of flying, we have counselors who can help you." (Maybe I overdid it with the walking in circles.) After reassuring her that I did not have airplane anxiety but was just exercising my muscles before sitting for a long time, we both laughed and continued our respective tasks.

NINE SIMPLE STEPS TO WONDERFUL WALKING

Brisk walking is easy exercise. To get the most from it:

1. Cushion your heels. Buy a good running shoe — a half size larger than you normally take to allow for swelling — with a cushiony heel to lessen impact and prevent injuries to the knee and ankle joints. Avoid heel pounding.

2. Choose speed before distance. If your goal is to get fit and burn calories, walking *fast* is more efficient than walking *longer*. If you can carry on a normal conversation or sing while walking, you're probably not walking fast enough. Imagine you are walking to an important appointment, and you don't want to be late. Your breathing should be heavy enough to make it difficult to carry on a conversation. If you're walking for relaxation, walk at a leisurely pace that you enjoy.

Walking seems to have a dose-related effect. The faster and the longer you walk, the greater the heart benefit you get. During my visit to the Cooper Institute in Dallas, Texas, my friend and aerobics guru Dr. Ken Cooper presented studies showing that simply moving 30 minutes a day can cut the risk of heart disease in half. You don't have to run a marathon. Even no-sweat activities can yield tremendous health benefits.

3. Perk yourself up. Walking and swimming are the perfect movements for *mood*. Walking relaxes the mind when it's tense, perks it up when it's down, and boosts the body's energy when needed. Try an "unwind walk" when you

RUN SAFELY

Here's a healthy prime-time statistic from *USA Running:* four hundred thousand Americans finished at least one marathon in 2007, and 46 percent of these finishers were over forty years old. So much for slowing down as we age! Running, if you enjoy it, can be a good prime-time activity. My friend Terry Howell, age fifty-four, who has run competitively for more than forty years without any joint-related injuries, has these tips:

- Wear the proper shoes for your foot shape, foot plant (how your foot meets the ground), and body weight. Consider whether you pronate or supinate when choosing a running shoe. That's the first line of defense against

get home after a tense and draining day at work. Don't exercise just to burn calories. Exercise to feel good and stay healthy. Focus on how much better the exercise makes you *feel* rather than how many calories you *burn*.

4. Try spring walking. Flexing up on your toes during each step strengthens more muscles and burns more fat. You'll feel all the muscles of your legs and buttocks working.

running injuries. Most cities have running stores, staffed by runners who can make sure you get the right shoe.

- Do most of your training running on soft surfaces, such as grass, dirt, and yes, even treadmills. This helps to lessen the impact.
- After a 5-minute warm-up, stretch for 5 minutes before running.
- Keep yourself well hydrated.
- Pay attention to your diet, aiming for foods high in nutrients that help refuel and repair your body after every run, such as nuts, fruits, vegetables, lean meat, and seafood.

5. Step it up. If you like motivators or little gadgets to get you walking more, put on a pedometer. Try to increase your total number of steps by 500 per week. A good walking goal is 10,000 steps a day.

6. Walk while you work. Suppose you're saddled with a long cell-phone conversation. Find a quiet area, and walk while you talk. Walk up and down the stairs when you can. During a

MOVEMENT TIP: ENJOY
A BRISK MORNING WALK

Vigorous exercise in the morning before breakfast is likely to burn fat rather than sugar. The overnight fast uses up much of your body's sugar, allowing you to burn the excess fat around your middle. In addition, the mood-elevating perks of movement click your brain into happy mode and get it ready for work after a night's rest.

meeting break, walk the hallways or stairs. Walking fosters clarity and creativity in planning and decision making. Whenever I drew a blank while writing this book, I got up from my desk and thought while walking. (Martha calls it pacing.) During one of my infamous pacings around our living room, which is adjacent to my writing room, a houseguest asked, "What's Bill doing?" Martha explained, "He's planning a lecture."

7. **Buddy walk.** You may find it more motivating and enjoyable to walk with a partner, although sometimes walking with a friend can slow you down physically or possibly exhaust you mentally.

PUT ON A PEDOMETER

A pedometer is a matchbox-size battery-operated device that attaches to your belt or waistband and records how many steps you take each day. It is the perfect incentive for goal-oriented people who want to keep track of how much they're walking. A sedentary person may take only 5,000 steps a day. Try to increase this to a goal that averages 10,000 steps per day. This is roughly equivalent to five miles of walking. Walking uphill would naturally count for more. If you're a goal-oriented person, paste a pedometer chart on your refrigerator and enjoy watching the graph go up as you increase your walking and record your steps.

---

8. Stay lean. Walking may not be the best exercise for overfat people, since too much pounding on the ankles, knees, and back can cause joint injury. But there is one fat-burning perk: the more overfat a person is, the more energy he or she burns during exercise. A 200-pound person will burn more calories walking at the same speed for thirty minutes than will a 150-pound person. If you are overweight and can't walk fast for thirty minutes, walk slower for an hour. (See related section on how being lean is good for the knees, page 251.)

9. Swing your arms. Back injury specialist Dr. Stuart McGill teaches that walking faster while swinging your arms forward and back is healthier for the spine. It results in less strain on low-back structures than does strolling or walking slowly with your arms quiet.

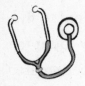

DR. SEARS SAYS...
Mind your walking posture: chin up, eyes down.

SIX HEALTH BENEFITS OF BUILDING BETTER MUSCLES

When I was putting together my own Prime-Time Health program and studying scientific research on what works and what lasts, one of the refrains that kept cropping up was the best way to lose excess belly fat is to gain more muscle.

What's one of the dreaded downfalls of prime time? It goes by the terrible-sounding name *sarcopenia.* It literally means "flesh wasting," or becoming frail. Once upon a time, it was believed that older folks lost muscle as a natural part of aging. Not necessarily so! Studies from the Tufts University Human Nutrition Research Center on Aging found that older people can maintain muscle with the same amount of strength training as younger folks. Other studies show that with the same amount of strength training, people over sixty-five can build just as much muscle as younger folks. Muscles are meant to move — the "use it or lose it" principle again. The more muscle you retain, or even gain, the healthier your prime time will be. Which exercise is better to burn fat, strength building or cardio (e.g., running)? you may wonder. Both! Yet to prevent the usual prime-time pot and to preserve those precious muscles that can waste away during prime time, remember, strength training is king; cardio is queen.

1. Build more muscle, store less fat. The main reason people go to pot during their prime time is because they lose muscle. Many prime timers suffer the disastrous duo of less muscle and more belly fat. Muscle tissue is your body's main calorie burner. Because muscles metabolize calories at a higher rate, a pound of muscle burns three times more calories than a pound of fat. Here's why: Inside muscle cells are fat-burning microfurnaces called mitochondria. The more muscle you build, the more mitochondria you make, and the more calories you burn. When you build muscle, you burn calories even while you sleep.

Try this muscle math: an increase of three pounds of muscle throughout your body will burn around 100 extra calories a day, which can translate into a loss of ten pounds a year of excess

POWER UP WITH PROTEIN

To maintain your muscle, you need to maintain enough protein in your diet. As a general guide, eat *at least three-quarters* of your body weight in grams of protein daily. For example, if you weigh 120 pounds, eat *at least* 90 grams of daily protein, more if you strength-train vigorously. With nutrient-dense food choices, this is easily achievable: 6 ounces of salmon (40 grams of protein); 8 ounces of Greek yogurt (20 grams); a bowl of whole-grain cereal with milk (15 grams); salad with beans and cheese (10 grams); 2 tablespoons of peanut butter (9 grams); 2 eggs (12 grams), 1 ounce of nuts (7 grams), and so on. (See "Power Up with Protein," page 345.)

fat. Sitters in particular need more muscle building. If you have a desk job or any type of employment that prohibits a lot of moving throughout the day, you need a diligent muscle-building routine. That extra muscle that you build up before and after your work hours helps you burn extra calories even while you're sitting.

2. Build more muscle and have stronger bones. Prime timers also tend to lose bone mass — osteoporosis. Because bones and muscles are codependent, building more muscle requires stronger bones for support.

3. Build more muscle and beat diabetes. It's a scary but preventable fact that most prime timers will become diabetic at some point in their lives. The main way to prevent this is to maintain, or even increase, your muscle mass. More muscle equals less belly fat, and less belly fat means more stable blood insulin levels.

4. Build more muscle and lower the highs. The three highs are the diseases that affect most people during prime time: high blood sugar, high blood cholesterol, and high blood pressure. If you're not yet pumped up to pump iron, consider this fact: studies have shown that people who maintain or gain muscle strength lower their blood sugar, blood lipids, and blood pressure.

5. Build more muscle and fall less. Our risk of falling increases as we age because of a loss of balance and coordination. Studies show that increasing muscle strength decreases the risk of falling.

6. Build more muscles and build a smarter brain. When you fatigue a muscle, you exhaust the mitochondria, those millions of microscopic energy furnaces within the muscle cells. These exhausted mitochondria send a chemical messenger to the brain (called trophic factor or growth messenger) and tell it to secrete human growth hormone (HGH), yes, the same HGH you see touted in all those feel-younger/look-younger ads. HGH builds muscle and also sends a growth messenger (brain-derived neurotrophic factor, or BDNF) that stimulates the brain to grow more brain tissue. So when you exercise to exhaustion, you not only build muscle cells, you build brain cells.

STAIR-STEPPING

One of my favorite anytime, anywhere exercises to strengthen the glutes, thigh, and leg muscles is stair-stepping. Place one foot onto a step or any stable surface that is elevated 15 to 18 inches from the ground. Step up with only a slight flex in your knee, bearing all your weight on that leg (if necessary, touch the floor with the opposite toe for balance). Hold for a couple of seconds, then ease back down to touch the floor with the opposite leg. Repeat 8 to 10 times with one leg. Then change legs and repeat. Put your arms out to the side or out in front of you to help with balance.

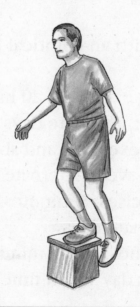

SIX STRENGTH-BUILDING TIPS
BEFORE YOU START LIFTING

My trainer reminded me that half of us will have to temporarily quit our strength-building programs within two weeks of starting because of injuries. Safety first!

1. Develop a set routine and try to stick with it as much as possible. Consider your workout routine your most important prime-time medicine. Try to devote at least 30 minutes a day to your strength-building routine, but alternate muscle groups. Take a day off between each group.

- warm-up with an elliptical trainer: 5 minutes
- upper-body exercises: 20 minutes, three days a week, alternate days
- lower-body exercises and abs: 20 minutes, three days a week, alternate days
- fit-ball exercises: 5 minutes, three days a week, alternate days
- exercise bands: 3 to 5 minutes, at least every other day when time and mood permit

2. Start low, and go slow. The older you are, the lighter the weights should be when you begin, and the more careful you need to be. Three variables to consider are:

- amount of the weight (called "load")
- repetitions: how many times you repeat the moves (called "reps")
- sets: how many times you do each rep

I suggest this safe progression: First, increase the number of sets. Next, increase the number of reps.

- Begin an exercise with a weight with which you can comfortably do one set of 8 to 12 repetitions. Stick with that for a week.
- Then increase to two sets for a week or so.
- Next increase to three sets.
- Once you can comfortably do three sets of 8 to 12 reps, increase the weight by 2½ to 5 pounds. Then repeat the above steps to increase the number of sets. To build more muscle, increase the weight rather than increasing the number of reps or sets.

If your goal is to increase your muscle strength, you need to gradually increase the weight and the sets to the point of fatigue; that is, you really have to work at completing the final few reps of each set. In fact, if you can easily do the twelfth rep, that is a sign that you need to increase the weight. While the dictum "no pain, no gain" is no longer acceptable advice in strength training, when it comes to building muscle you do need to feel the growth. A bit of muscle soreness the day after a workout is a signal that you have worked your muscles to their maximum intensity and they are undergoing repair and growth to meet that level of intensity.

3. Train strong and long. To build muscle faster, using a gradual progression of heavier weights and taking longer to do fewer reps will build more muscle than exercising with lighter weights and doing more fast reps. You will build more muscle if you do each rep slowly. Healthy muscle building is like healthy eating. Just as you get the most bang for your nutritional buck by eating nutrient-dense foods, so do you gain more muscle in less time by lifting the right weights in the right way. I call a good muscle workout dense and intense. For more muscle, think *time under tension*.

Many fitness trainers encourage high-intensity interval training (HIIT). Alternate intervals of moderate cardio workouts with short bursts of near maximum effort. HIIT expends more calories by keeping your metabolism revved up longer.

4. Don't jerk the joints. Don't bounce as you lift weights. Avoid locking your joints when you straighten them. Always keep a slight bend, especially in your elbow and knee joints.

5. Be extrasafe with shoulder exercises. The shoulder joint is the most complicated and easily injured joint in the body. It is also composed of muscles and tendons that are slow to heal once they are injured. Go particularly easy on overhead shoulder presses and any exercises that require lifting your arm above the level of your shoulder. Because the shoulder joint is so vulnerable to injury, many prime timers wisely stick to swimming (we're not talking marathon overarm strokes here!) rather

THE BEST MUSCLE-BUILDING TIP I'VE EVER HEARD

One day I was pumping iron when I heard a familiar voice say, "Bill, slow down! Let me show you a better way." To my rescue came my friend and former Olympic weight lifter Dr. Vince Fortanasce. I needed to listen to this guy. He said, "Instead of quickly going through a bunch of reps, especially with the major muscles of the arms and legs, try *the rule of fours.*"

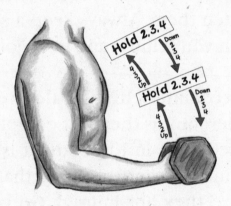

Lift weight up halfway while counting to four; pause and hold while counting to four; finish lift while counting to four; pause and hold while counting to four. Repeat the same sequence when lowering the weight.

DR. BILL'S SUGGESTED TWENTY-MINUTE WORKOUT

If the most time you have is 20 minutes, concentrate your workout:

- 10 minutes on an elliptical trainer, gradually increasing the resistance
- 10 minutes of muscle-building flexion/ extension exercises. One day do the upper body; the next day do the lower body.

Throughout the day, try to fit in many of the anytime, anywhere exercises listed on page 622 and a few stretching movements listed on page 656.

---

than free weights when it comes to exercising the shoulder muscle.

6. Use machines rather than free weights. As a prime timer, I'm getting less and less enthusiastic about free weights, such as dumbbells and barbells, and more enthusiastic about using resistance bands and weight machines to strengthen my muscles. Machine weight lifting is more steady, easier to control, and less likely to bounce and jerk the joints. Machines also allow you more flexibility in adjusting the progression of weights and tailoring the exercises to your own abilities and needs. Unless used under professional guidance, free weights can actually injure muscles and tendons and cause inflammation of the joints. Also, strength-building systems allow you to sit and support your back during exercises. Still, a few dumbbells strategically placed around the house will remind you to grab and flex as time allows.

HAVE A BALL

Several exercise balls occupy center stage of my home gym. They not only add fun and variety to my routine, they also help stretch stiff muscles and tendons and improve balance.

I particularly like to use a ball when doing abdominal crunches and back exercises. Instructions for other ways to "play ball" will be included with your exercise ball, and you can find others online. Here are a few of my favorites:

Play back ball (also called "airplane" or "Superman"). Lie across the ball on your chest. Spread your legs for stability. Then "fly." (See page 280 for illustration.)

EXERCISE-BALL TIPS

- Before buying a ball, go to a gym to try out different sizes, then choose the one that is most comfortable for you. A 55-centimeter ball works well for most people; a 45-centimeter ball is a good choice for smaller folks.
- Consider getting three balls: a standard 45- to 55-centimeter ball; a medicine ball, or several balls of various sizes and weights; and a dynamic-stability ball that is weighted to prevent easy rolling.

Play belly ball. Sit stably on the ball, lean back with your arms at your side or overhead; then sit up slowly as you contract your

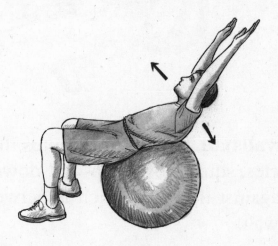

abdominal muscles. Keep your hands away from your head to avoid the temptation of pulling your neck forward. (See the 1-2-3-4 technique, page 640.)

Play side ball. This exercise strengthens the oblique abdominal muscles beneath your "love handles." Stabilize one or both feet against the wall, and brace your hips against the ball. Lift your shoulders toward the ceiling. Keep your hands away from your head.

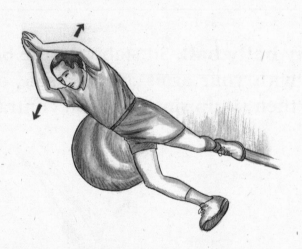

Play wall ball. To work your glutes, thigh, and leg muscles, squat slowly up and down while leaning against the ball, which is between you and the wall.

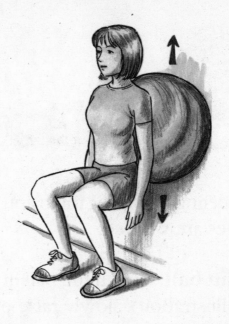

Play leg ball. Lie on your back. With the ball between your legs, slowly lift as you feel your abdominal and thigh muscles being worked. Hold for 10 seconds, then slowly return feet to floor. Turn over onto each side and do the same

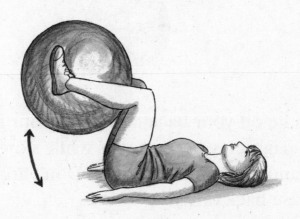

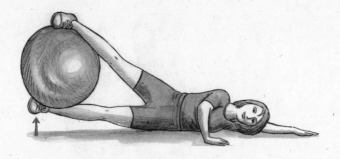

exercise, feeling how your thigh and side abdominal muscles are worked.

Play butt ball. Get on the ball in bridge position (see illustration). Slowly raise one leg. Hold for 10 seconds, then lower. Repeat with other leg. Then do both.

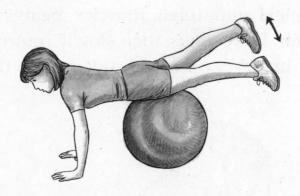

Then lie on your back and place your feet on the ball. Tighten your buttocks while slowly raising up, and hold for 10 seconds. Don't arch your back! Ease back down.

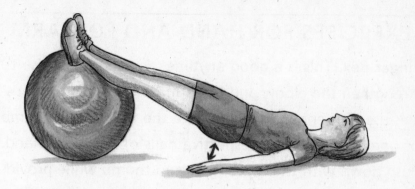

Next, lie on the ball on your side, raise one leg, keeping the knee and hip in line, and hold for 10 seconds, then lower. Repeat with other leg.

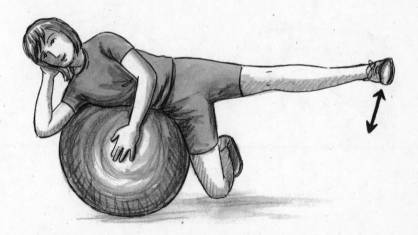

As you get more comfortable with ball exercises, gradually increase the number of repetitions and how long you hold each position. (For a complete workout of all muscle groups, using ball, band, and stretching exercises, see AskDrSears.com.)

EXERCISES FOR HAND AND FOREARM

Finger flex. This is a good anytime, anywhere exercise to strengthen the elbow and forearm tendons and the muscles used in tennis and golf. Place the fingers and thumb of one hand over the respective nails of the other hand. Push down with the top fingers and thumb while providing resistance from the bottom hand (A). Push until all fingers come together. Then reverse the process by opening the bottom fingers and thumb against the resistance of the top fingers (B). Do at least ten reps with each hand

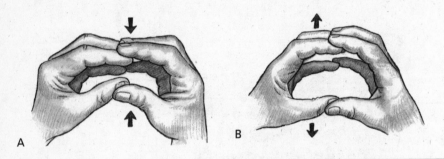

STRIKE UP THE BANDS

Band exercises, with resistance bands or tubing, are the safest way to begin strengthening your muscles. The risk of injury to muscles and joints is much lower with bands than it is with free weights or machine weights, and the bands allow for more gradual resistance, so there is less danger

several times a day. This strengthens the muscles important to the hands, fingers, elbows, and forearms.

Squeeze-ball finger flex. Hold a rubber ball and squeeze it with both hands until tired, rest briefly, then repeat (C). Alternatively, squeeze the ball with one hand, then the other (D). I squeeze a ball while reading. Notice how the muscles of your entire forearm, all the way back to the elbow, are exercised by this gripping motion.

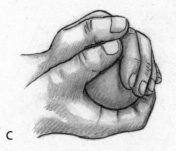

C

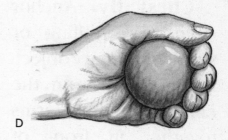

D

of jerking the joints. I leave resistance bands hanging around the house, especially in the TV room, so I can grab one and do a couple minutes of muscle-strengthening stretches while I'm standing around. When traveling, I pack my resistance band. I've even enjoyed an occasional five-minute workout in the airport men's room while waiting for a flight. All these little moves add up to a big gain in muscle strength — and longevity.

For many resistance-band exercises, you'll begin with feet hip- or shoulder-width apart, band taut; you can increase resistance by shortening the band. (Depending on the exercise, you can also add resistance by increasing the distance between your feet.) Try these basic exercises and customize as desired:

Chest fly. Anchor band to a railing or strong stationary object. Facing away from the railing, fly both arms together in front of your chest. For another exercise, punch with alternate arms as if you are boxing.

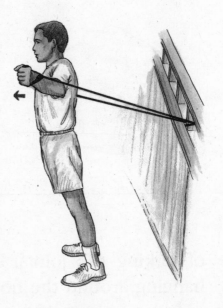

Back fly. With band still secured, face the railing, and fly both arms back, keeping elbows bent slightly. For another exercise, punch with alternate arms as if you are boxing.

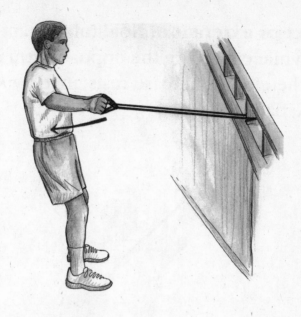

Biceps curls. Keeping your elbows close to your body and at the same level, curl your arms up, then down, in a controlled motion.

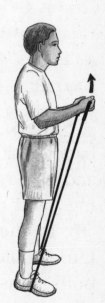

Triceps extension. Hold tubing taut behind back while extending the opposite arm forward from the elbow. Increase resistance by shortening the band.

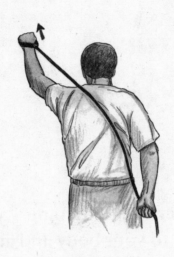

Squats. While gripping band, tuck elbows near sides and squat down while keeping band taut (A), then stand (B). In the same position, go into shoulder press by raising both arms above head until elbows are only slightly bent (not locked; C).

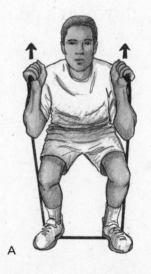

A

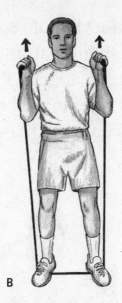

B

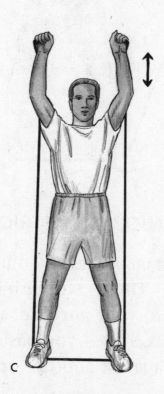

C

Rows. Stand on band, and bend forward 45 degrees at hips. Pull bands up while squeezing shoulder blades together. Raise band up toward shoulders keeping elbows bent slightly. Widen your stance to increase resistance (see illustration).

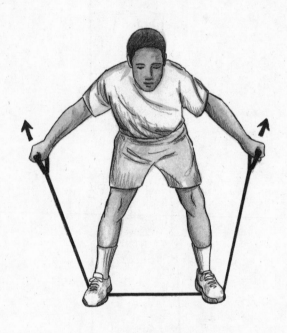

ENJOY ISOMETRICS

Isometrics means tensing muscles without moving them. These strength-building exercises can fit into your anytime, anywhere portfolio. In these exercises, you basically press one muscle group against another or against a wall or other surface and hold the compression for 10 seconds. Standing on your toes and tensing your muscles is a good lower-body isometric. Even professional weight lifters use isometrics as a way to build a bit more muscle during idle time. Here are my favorites:

Chest and arm press. Place hands and arms as shown and tighten arm and chest muscles as you press your palms together. Hold for 10 seconds. Repeat three times.

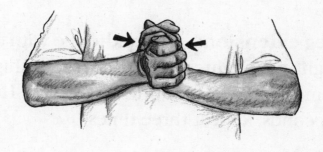

Biceps and triceps curls. Position hands and arms as shown. Flex or extend one hand against the other. Hold for 10 seconds. Repeat three times. Or if you're just standing around, make a fist, flex your biceps, and hold for 10 seconds.

Do this in private, or someone might think you're anxious or angry.

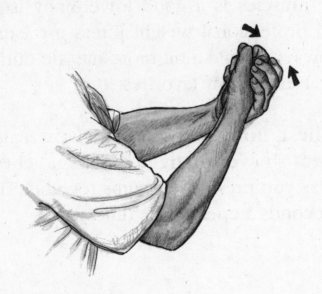

Leg extensions. Sit, stand, or lie with one leg straight out. Tighten the front of the thigh and calf muscles while you flex your foot. Hold for 10 seconds. Repeat three times.

STRETCH THOSE TIGHT MUSCLES

We are a generation that sits too much. As a result, by the time we reach prime time, muscles not only become weaker, they become tighter and shorter. Many of us are slumped, humped, and stiff. In fact, there is a medical term that describes people with aging muscles and joints — "stiff man syndrome." Fashion is also a factor in muscle shortening. It has been shown that women who spend a lot of their day in high heels actually have shorter Achilles tendons and more difficulty flexing their feet. This is why we need to stretch as well as strengthen our muscles.

Orthopedists have observed that in cultures in which people walk or bike to work and in which squatting and sitting cross-legged (Indian style) are part of the daily lifestyle, there is a lower incidence of arthritis and a much lower incidence of hip replacements. Many back, hip, and knee problems can be prevented by properly moving and stretching the muscles. Strong bones need support from strong and flexible muscles and tendons.

DR. SEARS'S STRETCHING PROGRAM

To view an illustrated total-body stretching program, see AskDrSears.com/Prime-TimeHealth.

Rx FOR PRIME-TIME PHYSICAL FITNESS

- ❏ Commit to at least 20 minutes a day of strenuous movement.
- ❏ Dance.
- ❏ Throughout the day, squeeze in anytime, anywhere exercises: stretching, flexing, and isometrics.
- ❏ Do endurance exercises: brisk walking, elliptical training, or swimming at least 10 minutes a day, six days a week.
- ❏ Do strength-building exercises at least 10 minutes a day (3 days a week, upper body; 3 days a week, lower body, back, and abdominals).
- ❏ Try high-intensity interval training.
- ❏ Use the 1-2-3-4 strategy to build more muscle in less time.
- ❏ Do stretch-band movements 5 minutes a day while watching TV or to pass the time.

CHAPTER 23

Stay Safe

The more absentminded (and older) I get, the more I deserve to be called Doctor Band-Aid by my favorite nurse, Martha Sears, RN. Although I dislike the statistics showing that the risk of just about everything goes up as we age, it is true that the risk of a serious injury from home accidents goes up more than five times between the ages of fifty and seventy-five. The leading causes of serious accidents at home, especially in people over age sixty-five, are falls, fires and burns, poisoning, and choking. Accident prevention is best put in place before the forgetfulness sets in. So, as you learned to accidentproof your home when you read our parenting books, now it's time to accidentproof yourself.

WHY PRIME TIMERS ARE MORE ACCIDENT-PRONE

Let's take a quick head-to-toe look at why we are more accident-prone as we age and what to do about it.

Brain and balance will be a bit off. The eye-muscle-brain communication pathway slows as we age — we have diminished *proprioception,* meaning the ability to adjust our posture to compensate for changing surfaces underfoot. Say you're about to trip over your grandchild's toy. Your legs send a message to your brain that quickly notifies your muscles, joints, and bones to catch yourself before you fall. This nerve-muscle-transmission signal slows as we age. Our adaptive reflexes also get slower and our ability to regain balance diminishes. In addition, the structures within the middle ear that help us maintain our balance — the vestibular system — also weaken with age. The best way to keep your proprioception and sense of balance intact is to keep your muscles and nerves strong through reactive games, such as tennis and Ping-Pong. Also, high blood sugar resulting in diabetes can lead to a condition called *peripheral neuropathy*, which simply means that the nerves to the muscles are slower to react, thus increasing your risk of falling. Keeping your blood insulin and blood sugar stable also helps to maintain your sense of balance and proprioception.

You may not hear an accident about to happen. Just as those tiny hairlike filaments, called cilia, that line our respiratory passages stiffen with age, so do the cilia in the ears. Normally, these cilia vibrate in response to sound and then send a message to the auditory nerve. As we age, the weakened cilia can result in diminished hearing.

Martha noticed a drop in her hearing seemingly overnight, at around age fifty-two or fifty-three. It's not bad enough to need a hearing gadget. She relies on seeing a speaker's face to hear better.

Your nose may not smell an accident coming. Our ability to smell unusual odors helps us prevent accidents — you smell gas coming from the leaky stove, or even the smoke of a fire starting. As we age, our sense of smell diminishes, increasing the risk of these types of accidents.

Your eyes may not see an accident about to happen. Between the ages of forty and fifty, some people develop presbyopia (aka old eyes), which slows the eyes from accommodating to sudden changes in focus distance and changes of scenery. Add to this other vision problems such as cataracts and age-related macular degeneration, and your eyes will be less able to protect you from falls and other accidents. (See chapter 6 for more about aging eyes.)

You may develop an accident-prone heart. Many prime-time falls occur when people quickly change position, such as from sitting to standing or hopping out of bed. Normally, a sudden change in position, from down to up, gives a signal to the heart to pump more blood to the brain. Yet, as we age, this signaling system weakens, causing *orthostatic hypotension,* also known as postural hypotension. (Many younger people have this too.) When you change position, the blood pressure suddenly drops, blood flow to the brain is insufficient, and you get lightheaded, or even faint and fall. Postural hypotension is worsened by plaque buildup in arteries, atherosclerosis, and diabetes. Some medications to treat blood pressure, called vasodilators, have postural hypotension as a side effect.

PRIME-TIME TIP: MOVE SLOW AS YOU GET UP AND GO

Always change positions *slowly* to give your heart advance warning that your brain needs adjustment of blood flow. This is especially true for men with impulsivity issues, like me, Martha points out. Once ADHD, always ADHD.

If you drink up, you're more likely to fall down. As we age, our body's ability to detoxify alcohol diminishes. Some prime timers find that they get off balance and woozy after having one or two drinks, whereas previously the same amount never bothered them. The reason that prime timers often need to lower the amount of alcohol they drink at any one sitting is that their liver's ability to get rid of the excess blood alcohol weakens with time. A higher level of blood alcohol can slow your reaction time, preventing you from recovering your balance if you should trip, for example. It goes without saying that we should be even *more* conscientious when contemplating driving after having just one drink.

Bones will weaken. Most people reach their peak bone mass by age thirty, and thereafter bones begin to soften and weaken, leading to the risk of fractures from a fall. The combination of sitting too much, eating too little calcium and vitamin D, smoking and drinking too much, and even taking certain medications can weaken the bones.

You need to urinate more often. Being half asleep when getting up during the night also raises the risk of falling.

NINE WAYS TO PROTECT YOURSELF FROM FALLS

Take fall prevention seriously. I have several friends who were very healthy until they had a preventable slip-and-fall hip fracture; they never completely regained their health.

1. Reduce your risk. Most accidents begin in the head. Think about where you're going. If the road is full of potholes or the steps are loose, avoid them if you can. It's easy to let your guard down when rushing to an appointment or trying to catch a plane. Before you rush and fall, click into a vigilant mind-set. Tell yourself, "I'm entering risky territory. Be careful."

MEDICINES THAT INCREASE THE RISK OF FALLING

Many of the most common medicines prescribed for prime timers can increase the risk of falling, either by causing postural hypotension or interfering with a sense of balance. If you are taking any of the following medicines and find that you are getting dizzy, light-headed, or that your walking and balance are affected, consult your doctor about lowering the dose or changing medications.

- antidepressants (SSRIs and tricyclics)
- antipsychotics
- blood pressure–lowering medicines
- sleep medications

2. Watch your step. Focus on the moment. Mental multitasking while walking up or down stairs or along challenging terrain is a recipe for falling. Think about *where you are* rather than where you're going. Even talking on a cell phone while going downstairs can be risky.

3. Move more slowly. As we get older, our body and brain can't compensate for sudden movements as quickly as when we were young. *Always* change positions slowly. Ease out of bed instead of jumping out of bed, particularly in the middle of the night. Sit on the edge of the bed for a few seconds, flex your calf muscles, and move your feet before you get up. (This is always done in yoga class, even for young people.) When the doorbell or the phone rings, instead of jumping off the sofa, be more deliberate. Take your time after getting up from the toilet. As you age, when getting up after sitting or lying down, it's a good idea to hold on to something.

If you become less active than usual for more than a few days — for example, if you are recuperating from an injury or flu — you'll be even more prone to falls and injuries because your muscles haven't moved for a while. Be even more mindful as you resume your regular activities, or you might wind up back in bed.

4. Keep fit. The stronger your muscles and bones are and the more muscle-coordination activities you do to improve your balance (such as yoga, Pilates, and dancing), the lower is your risk of falling and of being injured if you do fall. Fit folks suffer fewer fractures.

5. Light your way. Keep a nightlight on for those middle-of-the-night trips to the bathroom. Avoid walking around the room in the dark. Better yet, make sure the path to the bathroom is clear before you hit the sack. If regular nightlights keep you awake, get one with a motion sensor so it will come on only when you need it.

6. Think before walking on slippery surfaces. When walking around pool decks or slippery surfaces, use a *plop-plop* step instead of the usual rhythmic heel-toe gait. Plop one foot down at a time or even shuffle a bit so that you don't raise your feet off the ground as much. Whatever gait can plant the whole foot at once and keep both feet on the ground longer during your walk is the safest for slippery surfaces. Walking on icy sidewalks must simply be avoided, but it will take discipline to talk yourself out of chancing it. The stakes are too high to risk that kind of skull-splitting, hip-snapping, sacrum-crushing, wrist- or knee-breaking fall. Older and wiser comes in here. But if you have no choice but to go out when the weather is icy, look into Yaktrax or a similar traction device for your shoes or boots.

7. Install railings on porch steps. Many falls occur on steps without railings. While you used to hold your head up high while going down steps, for safety's sake now look at your feet.

8. See where you're going. Be sure your glasses match your activity. Bifocals, for example, may help while you're reading but can blur your path while walking.

9. Wear fallproof shoes. Be particularly careful when wearing high-heeled dress shoes with smooth leather soles. Flats are more fashionable with younger women anyway (I'm thinking of our teenager). You can be sensible and sexy at the same time, even elegant. My favorite shoe for safety and comfort is a casual style called "Loaf Off Road," available at www.simpleshoes.com.

FALL-PROOFING YOUR HOME

Let's walk through a typical home or apartment to try to make it supersafe.

- Put nonskid backings on rugs so they don't slide.
- Keep rooms and entrances well lit, especially around stairs.
- Keep floors clear of toys and other clutter.
- Cover any temporary extension cords you are using with rugs or duct tape and keep other cords and tripping hazards tucked carefully out of the way.

Bathroom safety. Many accidents and injuries occur in the bathroom. To make yours comfortably safe:

- Install nonslip adhesive strips on the floor of the shower and bathtub or use an adhesive nonslip mat.
- Install grab bars on the inside wall of the shower or near your tub to help you pull yourself up.

- Use nonslip rugs on the bathroom floor.
- If necessary, put grab bars near the toilet seat to make it easier to get up and down. Or, try an elevated toilet seat. If you find it more comfortable to elevate the toilet seat to the point that your feet dangle, put a footstool in front of the toilet to rest your feet on. Dangling feet tighten rectal muscles and make it more difficult to defecate.

Stair safety

- Make sure the handrail runs the full length of the stairway.
- Light the stairway well so that you can see each step. Be sure there is a light switch at both the top and bottom of the stairway.
- Consider luminescent tape or nonskid strips on outdoor stair edges so you can see where you are stepping.

Bedroom safety

- Have your bed at the right height — not so high that your feet can't touch the floor when you sit on the edge or so

low that it is awkward to get in and out.
Ideally, your feet should be flat on the
floor when you are sitting on the side of
the bed.

- Be sure your nighttime path is clear.
Your bedroom can be a particularly
high risk after you've packed for travel
the next day. You get up for your
nightly bladder-emptying, trip over
the suitcase that was in your path, and
the injuries from the fall ruin your
vacation. This precaution also applies
to hotel rooms.
- Avoid placing pillows, shoes, and other
clutter at the side of your bed where you
could trip over them when getting up.
- Make sure the switch for your bedside
lamp is easy to reach. You can injure
your back by suddenly twisting to turn
your lamp on or off.

SAFE-ALCOHOL-DRINKING TIPS

It's time to rethink your drinking. If you don't
already drink alcohol, don't start for medicinal
purposes — poor excuse. Enjoy a handful of

grapes instead. The effects of alcohol, especially in excess, outweigh its alleged health benefits.

Alcohol behaves differently in the body as you age. Alcohol is actually the by-product produced by the fermentation of yeast. As you recall, our simple definition of aging is a weakened garbage-disposal system. So it stands to reason that you should put less garbage in your system as you get older. Also, there are gender and genetic differences in how alcohol affects us. Since women under age fifty have less of a liver enzyme called alcohol dehydrogenase that detoxifies alcohol, younger women tend to be more sensitive to the effects of alcohol than younger men. Over the age of fifty, men are more sensitive to alcohol than women because the activity of alcohol dehydrogenase decreases with age and after fifty drops below the level of that of women. People in some cultures, such as Asians, have lower levels of enzymes that detoxify alcohol. Try these safe-drinking tips:

Drink for taste, not effect. If you enjoy a glass of wine because it goes well with your meal, fine. Drinking for effect is like taking a dangerous and addictive drug.

Different shots for different folks. Because there is such a wide variation in how quickly the gut breaks down alcohol and how quickly it gets into the bloodstream, know your tolerance. If one drink bothers you, your body is telling you to drink smaller amounts more slowly.

Sip rather than guzzle. Just as the sipping solution is good for your gut, it's also good for your body when drinking alcohol. Sip slowly to enjoy the aroma and to slow down the absorption of alcohol into the bloodstream. Also, drinking too much too fast overwhelms the mucous protective lining of the stomach and the detoxifying enzymes in the intestines and liver, which can cause indigestion.

Drink while you eat. Never drink alcohol on an empty stomach at any age, especially when you're older. The presence of food in the stomach slows the absorption.

Avoid the "holiday heart syndrome." Avoid binge drinking during festivities; doing so is often associated with life-threatening irregularities of the heartbeat.

Drink less if overweight. If you are already overweight, it's best to avoid the extra carbs from alcohol.

Put a lid on it. Watch out for the *creep effect,* where you get used to one glass of wine or one drink a day, then two, and then find yourself wanting or needing more and more. If you can go four or five days or even a week without craving alcohol, okay. If you can't, suspect the creep effect. That's a red flag. Periodically take wine breaks. At one point I realized I could not eat fish without having a glass of wine. Now I occasionally enjoy a fish dinner without the wine just to decouple my tastes.

Drinking and drugs don't mix. Prime timers should be particularly careful about drinking alcohol while taking medicines, especially since we tend to take more medications as we get older. Certain medications disable the alcohol-detoxifying enzymes in the intestines. Common medicines, such as aspirin and antacids, can raise the blood alcohol level if alcohol is taken within an hour of taking the medicine.

Get the gas out. Carbonated beverages can increase alcohol absorption, presumably because carbon dioxide increases gastric-emptying time, causing alcohol to reach the small intestine more rapidly and be absorbed more quickly.

How much is too much? I suggest no more than an average of one drink a day. A drink translates to 5 ounces of wine, 12 ounces of beer, or 1.5 ounces of 80-proof spirits.

Rx FOR PRIME-TIME ACCIDENT PREVENTION

- ❑ Think before you move.
- ❑ Beware of medications that lessen coordination.
- ❑ Watch where you walk.
- ❑ Change positions slowly.
- ❑ Keep fit to maintain balance.
- ❑ Wear safe shoes.
- ❑ Fallproof your home and workplace.
- ❑ Limit alcohol to one drink a day.

PART VI

The Prime-Time Plan

Throughout this book you've learned hundreds of health tips. Together, these timely tips will help you live healthier, happier, and longer. Now let's put the whole Prime-Time Health plan into an eight-week course. What to do in which week is a matter of personal preference and medical needs. The week-by-week suggestions are the same ones we use in our medical office; they work for most people most of the time. Still, you can customize your own plan. Remember, the Prime-Time Health plan for you is the one you will do.

CHAPTER 24

Put Together Your Personal Eight-Week Prime-Time Plan

After you've read about all of the scientific studies and personal stories that support this important work, I hope you're beginning to see why the Prime-Time Health plan is your personal individual retirement account for health. It's your protection plan against disease and disability. Doctors have known for decades that eating the right foods, exercising regularly, getting good sleep, managing stress, and self-managing medical problems all work together to improve health, boost mood, increase energy, and even extend longevity.

Now we organize all of the major Prime-Time Health tips in this book into a doable program. Check off each step as you complete it. We ask you to make an eight-week commitment to your prime-time health. By the end of eight short weeks, you will feel so much healthier that you will just have to continue.

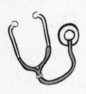

DR. SEARS SAYS…

Remember, the program that is for you is one that you will do. It's okay to pick and choose. For example, you can be a 90/10 eater (90 percent pure, 10 percent less pure) if that works for you, and you'll keep it up. Do as many of these steps as you can. Make it fit *you.*

WEEK 1: TAKE A HEALTH BREAK — MAKE HEALTH YOUR HOBBY

Once you've decided to prepare for prime time, plan to take a few days to a week off. Take a vacation for your own health. Learning how to make health your hobby is the main goal of your time away, whether you go somewhere or stay home. Your goals during your health break are:

❑ 1. Read this book from cover to cover. Highlight the points that are most meaningful to you — those "wow" points that make you say, "That's *me!* I've got to make that change."

❑ 2. With Post-it notes, flag and reread the sections that relate most to your own health concerns, whether joint stiffness, heart problems, or gut aches.

❑ 3. Really think about the importance of making health your hobby. Imagine how you want to spend your prime-time years. Visualize all the activities you want to do. During this time, immerse yourself in thoughts of wellness scenes: jogging, dancing, playing sports — all the great things you enjoy doing now and are looking forward to having more time for in the coming years. While you want to keep your mind filled with mostly positive thoughts, as a further motivator occasionally think about your friends who have not prepared for prime time and are spending it coping with illness and disabilities. Again, how do *you* want to spend your prime time?

❑ 4. List the most important changes you need and want to make. For example:
• Eat less junk carbs.

- Don't worry so much.
- _____
- _____
- _____
- _____

❑ 5. List the obstacles that are keeping you from following this Prime-Time Health plan, and counter them with specific solutions. For example:

Obstacle	How I'll Fix It
Pressed for time; financial commitments; lack of energy, motivation; spouse won't do program with me	Realize that illness wastes more time and is more expensive than wellness. Make wellness my priority. Just do it! Once my spouse and I feel and see the benefits, we will both be motivated to continue.

Obstacle	How I'll Fix It
But I don't have time to cook.	Taking time to cook is better than wasting time being sick.

❑ 6. Begin writing your own story. Don't let your experience and wisdom go unrecorded. Keep a prime-time journal, and track your daily journey. Topics might include what got you motivated to make a change, the obstacles you've had to overcome, how you bounced back from setbacks, what personal health strategies you've learned along the way. This is a journal you'll start during your health break, but one that you'll continue past then. Trust me, you'll be surprised how far you've come and how much better you feel as you record the changes that occur over just a few weeks. Chart your progress weekly. Do you have more stamina, happier feelings, clearer vision, and less joint stiffness, for example? Share your diary with your spouse, children, and friends. Let your loved ones share in and learn from your accomplishments. (I guarantee that once you feel the effects of the Prime-Time Health plan, you won't be able to keep the good news to yourself.)

❑ 7. Do the Prime-Time Health plan with your spouse, a friend, or a colleague at work. During your health-care break, spend as much time as possible discussing your personal prime-time plans. The best results will occur when both you and your partner use *Prime-Time Health* as a workbook. Agree to keep each other motivated. Perhaps even engage in a friendly competition, for example, to see who can lose the first inch of "toxic waist." Exercise together: walk and enjoy the beautiful sunset, go dancing, or play tennis.

❑ 8. Schedule a health checkup. Use the chart below to record your test results before beginning the Prime-Time Health plan, and then update them a month or two into the plan.

Baseline Measurements (Before Prime-Time Health Plan)	Eight Weeks into the Program
Waist circumference (or size of skirt, pants, number of belt notches):	Waist circumference:
Height:	Height:
Weight:	Weight:
Blood pressure:	Blood pressure:
Fasting blood sugar:	Fasting blood sugar:
Complete lipid and cholesterol profile:	Complete lipid and cholesterol profile:
Fasting insulin level:	Fasting insulin level:
Inflammatory marker profile:	Inflammatory marker profile:
Illness feelings: energy level, joint aches, heartburn, etc.	Wellness feelings: brain, eyes, gut, joints, etc.

❏ 9. Assemble a prime-time library. Now that you've made health your hobby, read more about it. Here are some of our favorites:

Newsletters

Vital Choices (an informative newsletter about the health
benefits of seafood; subscribe at vital-choice.com)

Wellness Letter, University of California, Berkeley

Bottom Line/Health

The Blaylock Wellness Report

Johns Hopkins Medical Letter: Health after Fifty

Environmental Nutrition

Books

- *The Spectrum,* Dean Ornish, MD
- *Love and Survival,* Dean Ornish, MD
- *The Anti-Alzheimer's Prescription,* Vincent Fortanasce, MD
- *NO More Heart Disease,* Louis Ignarro, PhD
- *The Jungle Effect,* Daphne Miller, MD
- *The 10-Minute Total Body Breakthrough,* Sean Foy
- *In Defense of Food,* Michael Pollan
- *The Source,* Woodson Merrell, MD

- *You* series, Mehmet Oz, MD, and Michael Roizen, MD
- *Ultraprevention,* Mark Hyman, MD, and Mark Liponis, MD
- *Save Your Hearing Now,* Michael Seidman, MD, and Marie Moneysmith
- *The Second Brain,* Michael Gershon, MD
- *In Bad Taste: The MSG Symptom Complex,* George Schwartz, MD
- *Buzz: The Science and Lore of Alcohol and Caffeine,* Stephen Braun
- *Genetic Nutritioneering,* Jeffrey S. Bland, PhD
- *The Sinatra Solution: New Hope for Preventing and Treating Heart Disease,* Stephen T. Sinatra, MD
- *Younger Next Year: A Guide to Living Like 50 Until You're 80 and Beyond,* Chris Crowley and Henry S. Lodge, MD

Magazines

Prevention

Life Extension

Women's Health

Men's Health

Websites

AskDrSears.com   AARP.org

WebMD.com   MayoClinic.com

AmericanHeart.com   MEG-3.com

Jump ahead to Week 3 by sneaking in some exercise; if you don't get exercise yet, park your car farther away in order to walk a bit.

PRIME WORDS FOR PRIME TIMERS

Paste this list of happy and healthy words on your wall. Read them several times a day. Enjoy them and live them:

love	sing
walk	dance
graze	pure
lean	create
fish	help
swim	sleep
laugh	pray

WEEK 2: EAT PURE

Once you are committed to making health your hobby — and your top priority — it's time to change your eating habits. While changes in long-term eating habits are often the most challenging to make, they are the changes that yield the quickest results. You can change gradually or go totally pure right now. The more changes you make, the sooner you're going to notice their positive health effects.

❑ 1. **Avoid "bad words" on food labels.** Remove from your pantry, fridge, and shopping list foods that contain the following ingredients:
- high-fructose corn syrup
- hydrogenated or partially hydrogenated oils, trans fats
- number symbols (e.g., red #40)
- flavor enhancers, especially MSG and its aliases (see page 122)
- artificial sweeteners: aspartame, sucralose
- chemical preservatives

❑ 2. **Eat the sixteen superfoods for prime-time health.** Make the sixteen superfoods the mainstay of your real-food diet (see chapter 13).

❑ 3. **Go fish.** Eat a 6-ounce serving of wild salmon twice a week or take an omega-3

OUR FAVORITE RECIPES

Over the years Martha and I have accumulated many recipes that are delicious and nutritious. And we continue to add to our collection. You will find our best recipes at AskDrSears.com.

---

supplement containing at least 600 milligrams total of DHA and EPA daily. Remember, *go fish* are two of the most important words in preparing for prime time. (Review the health benefits of seafood, page 308.)

❏ 4. **Give yourself an oil change.** Eat more fish, flax, and olive oils and less processed oils. See list of healthy and unhealthy oils on page 80. Eat more omega-3s and less omega-6s.

❏ 5. **Graze**. Follow the rule of twos: eat twice as often, eat half as much, and chew twice as long. (See why and how, page 86.)

❏ 6. **Snack smart.** Aim for 3 grams of protein and fiber for most snacks. (See why, page 585.)

❑ 7. **Enjoy smoothies.** Try the sipping solution as your breakfast, midmorning snack, lunch, and midafternoon snack. (See why smoothies are smart, page 148.) Begin with one day a week. As your gut gets used to this new way of eating, increase to four or five days a week. In addition, enjoy a normal evening meal chosen from the sixteen superfoods. The sipping solution is the number one change you can make with the quickest health benefits. In my medical practice, I have gotten more positive feedback about the sipping solution than any other dietary change. This is the most effective way to get your gut accustomed to being satisfied with smaller meals of real foods. While to some, sipping rather than eating many of your meals may sound somewhat extreme, it works; and it's necessary for folks who need a major change in their eating habits.

❑ 8. **Fill up with fiber.** Strive to average 25 to 35 grams daily.

❑ 9. **Enjoy your "instead of..." list.** As you are easing into your healthier way of living, make *small changes* each day:

Instead of...	Try...
Soda	1 part juice in 4 parts sparkling water
Sweetened yogurt	Plain yogurt sweetened with blueberries, honey
White bread	100 percent whole-grain bread
Orange juice	Eating a real orange
Mayonnaise	Mustard
Sugar, artificial sweeteners, added salt	Fruit toppings, cinnamon, honey, spices (turmeric, rosemary)

Eliminating an extra 100 calories per day of junk food can translate into a loss of 10 pounds of excess body fat within a year.

Prime-Time Nutrition Tip: EAT *REAL* FOODS!

SAMPLE WEEKLY MENU

Day 1

BREAKFAST: Omelet, fruit

SNACKS: Nuts, 1 palmful; banana

LUNCH: Spinach salad, olive oil, feta cheese

DINNER: Salmon (4–6 ounces), broccoli, wild rice, spinach salad

BEFORE BED: 4-ounce Greek yogurt gelato

Day 2

BREAKFAST: Yogurt, granola, fruit

SNACKS: Baby carrots dipped in hummus, apple

LUNCH: Organic peanut butter, fruit concentrate, and sprouts on whole-wheat bread

DINNER: Lentil soup (homemade), parmesan cheese, salad

BEFORE BED: Homemade oatmeal-raisin cookie, glass of milk

Day 3

BREAKFAST: Steel-cut oatmeal, yogurt, blueberries, cinnamon

SNACKS: Homemade trail mix, edamame

LUNCH: Pita pocket sandwich: falafel with hummus

DINNER: Tuna steak, asparagus, Caesar salad

BEFORE BED: Hard-boiled egg

Day 4

BREAKFAST: Scrambled eggs, guacamole, fruit

SNACKS: Celery with organic peanut butter

LUNCH:	Tuna sandwich on whole-wheat bread
DINNER:	Chicken (free-range, organic), potatoes, onions, salad
BEFORE BED:	Cottage cheese and fruit

Day 5

BREAKFAST:	Whole-wheat French toast, blueberry topping
SNACKS:	Apple slices with almond butter, bean dip/carrots
LUNCH:	Lettuce roll-up: turkey, tomato
DINNER:	Bean and cheese burrito, guacamole, Greek yogurt
BEFORE BED:	Homemade muffin and milk

Day 6

BREAKFAST:	Smoothie: fruit, yogurt, tofu, ground flaxseeds, pomegranate juice
SNACKS:	Sip on smoothie
LUNCH:	Rest of smoothie
DINNER:	Salmon, spinach salad, mashed sweet potatoes
BEFORE BED:	Greek yogurt and blueberries

Day 7

BREAKFAST:	Greek yogurt parfait: fruit, granola
SNACKS:	Cherry tomatoes, hummus, whole-grain pita chips
LUNCH:	Three-bean chili
DINNER:	Veggie omelet, guacamole, whole-grain toast
BEFORE BED:	Frozen yogurt, blueberries

WEEK 3: MOVE MORE

During Weeks 1 and 2, you started moving more, didn't you? Now put together your personal fitness program.

❑ 1. **Put together your own home gym.** You may think you don't have the space, but like so many other decisions it's a question of priorities. You make space for your bed, the kitchen, and the bathroom. Your space for exercise is no less important. As your kitchen becomes your home pharmacy, so does your playroom (gym).

❑ 2. **Design a schedule and routine.**
  • Make time each day to move. Set aside at least a 20-minute block of time for exercise six days a week.
  • If possible, hire a personal trainer for six sessions or so to get you safely started with your exercise routine.
  • Each day incorporate three components into your exercise routine:
    • strength training (weight lifting), especially the 1-2-3-4 technique (see page 640)

695

- endurance (cardio) exercises (walking, swimming, dancing)
- flexibility exercises (stretching, yoga, Pilates)

- At least three times a day, enjoy anytime, anywhere exercises. (See suggestions, page 622.) For example:
  - Flex stretch bands while watching TV.
  - Do finger flex and squeeze-ball exercises while sitting.
  - Flex up and down on toes while standing.
  - Pump knees while standing.
  - Flex muscles while just hanging out.
- Take up a new sport such as ballroom dancing, golf, or cycling. Movement is good for your muscles, but it's also good for your mind. New movements build new cerebral pathways.
- Put on a pedometer. Aim for an average of 10,000 steps per day.

Prime-Time Fitness Tip: **CREATE AND USE A HOME GYM.**

WEEK 4: STRESS LESS

In addition to working out a routine for the health of your body, it's equally important to work out a routine for the health of your mind.

- Identify the stressors in your life that you can get rid of, or at least minimize.
- Practice the stress busters listed on pages 404–12.
- Make humor an important part of your daily living.
- Practice the 1-2-3 deep-breathing technique explained on page 210.
- Meditate for at least 5 minutes a day (see page 413).

Prime-Time Stress Buster: FOCUS ON SOLUTIONS, NOT PROBLEMS.

WEEK 5: SLEEP SOUNDLY

All the changes you've made in the previous weeks should result in better sleep. Healthy eating, healthy exercise, and happy thoughts are the ingredients of a good night's sleep. Practice the fifteen sleep-tight tips on page 377 and devote this week to improving the quality and quantity of your sleep.

Prime-Time Sleep Aid: **ALLOW ONLY HAPPY THOUGHTS AND HAPPY TALK IN THE BEDROOM.**

WEEK 6: CONNECT

One of the hallmarks of prime timers who live healthier, happier, and longer lives is the depth of their social connections.

- **Love.** Giving love and feeling loved is therapeutic. Take time and effort to strengthen the love relationships in your life.
- **Meet.** Make new relationships. Join clubs. Get more involved at your place of worship. When you meet a new person you like, invite him/her over. Make an effort to deepen the relationship.
- **Heal** troubled relationships with family members. Remember, in healing others, you heal yourself.

- **Serve.** Enjoy the *helper's high* (see page 412). The best way to relieve your stress is to help others relieve theirs. In helping others, you help yourself. Our friend Sandy told us this story: "As a hospice worker, I brought a bouquet of flowers to a bedridden person with a note that said, 'You can't get outside to enjoy spring, so I'll bring spring inside to you.'" Both Sandy and her patient had happy hearts that day.

Prime-Time Relationship Tip: **ENJOY THE HELPER'S HIGH.**

WEEK 7: DO A MAINTENANCE CHECK

During this week, focus on those body parts that don't work as well as you wish they did. Consider this your preventive maintenance head-to-toe checklist for your heart, brain, gut, eyes, ears, lungs, gums, bones, joints, and skin.

- Did you give yourself an *oil change?*
- Do you eat more *seafood?*
- Do you eat more *plant-based* and fewer animal-based foods?

699

- Do you *graze* or gorge your meals?
- Do you practice *relaxation* and meditation strategies?
- Do you *exercise* vigorously for *at least* 20 minutes a day?
- Do you eat more *blueberries, nuts,* and *greens?*
- Do you avoid *artificial food additives?*
- Do you drink *alcohol* in moderation?
- Do you eat mostly *fresh,* pure foods and fewer packaged, processed foods?
- Do you *chew* your food more slowly?
- Do you eat *fiber-rich, protein-packed* foods?
- Do you strive to stay *lean?*
- Do you wear sunglasses when necessary?
- Do you rest your eyes when strained?
- Do you *avoid loud noises* as much as possible?
- Do you *"hose your nose"* and enjoy a *"steam clean"* when your nasal passages are stuffy?
- Do you try to *breathe clean air* at home, work, and at play?

- Do you limit your use of *heavily chlorinated indoor* hot tubs?
- Do you do the 1-2-3 *deep breathing* at least six times a day?
- Do you have *good dental hygiene:* swish, brush, floss, scrape, and irrigate?
- Do you eat foods rich in *calcium* and *vitamin D?*
- Do you keep your *leg muscles* strong to protect your knees?
- Do you do *knee-pumping* movements?
- Do you *cushion* your heels when walking or running on hard surfaces?
- Do you have less of a *heel-pounding* gait?
- Do you swim as often as possible?
- Do you try to maintain a healthy *posture?*
- Do you *sit smart?*
- Do you use caution when *lifting* heavy objects?
- Do you *stoop* or bend over *properly?*
- Do you *warm up cold muscles* before using them strenuously?
- Do you *moisturize* your skin?
- Do you *drink* enough water to keep yourself well hydrated?

Prime-Time Body Tip: REDUCE YOUR WAIST.

WEEK 8: REVIEW YOUR PRIME-TIME MEDICAL CARE

Now that you have put together your personal Prime-Time Health plan, you are ready to take charge of your medical care. Try these steps:

- List what health problems you have. Do a part-by-part maintenance check. What hurts? What doesn't work as well as you wish it did? Using the index as a guide, reread the sections that address your issues.
- Have you been able to take fewer medications? In partnership with your health-care provider, try to wean yourself off some of your medications, or at least lower the dosages.
- Do you practice the pills-and-skills medical mind-set? (See chapter 17.)
- Have you reviewed your medications with your doctor lately? Have you consulted your doctor on alternative self-help skills to replace or reduce

List Your Pills	What Skills Have You Done Instead?
e.g., cholesterol-lowering medicines	Eat right, move more, trim waist

the pills? Make a long appointment with your health-care provider. Open your office visit by saying, "Doctor, I'm ready to take a more active role in my own health care. I need your help in getting off [name of medicine]. I'm ready to do whatever it takes to get off [name of medication]." You'll notice a smile on your doctor's face; perhaps you'll even get a hug or a handshake.

Prime-Time Self-Care Tip: PRACTICE THE PILLS-AND-SKILLS MIND-SET.

A CLOSING WORD FROM DR. BILL

While there is no guarantee of a prime time free of disease and disability, I can assure you that the more parts of the Prime-Time Health plan you practice, the greater are your chances of feeling younger and living longer. My wishes for you are that you:

- awaken in the morning refreshed after a good night's sleep, and you don't hurt.
- begin each day with clarity of mind, clarity of vision, good gut feelings, and mobility.
- make health your hobby and take charge of your medical care.
- recognize that prime time is the time in your life when you can reap the rewards of your individual retirement plan for health.

Prime-time health is more than feeling good and looking good. It's about doing good. Many fitness programs, like cosmetic surgery, only change a person on the outside. And with most makeovers it's easy to be caught up in self-improvement. *Prime-Time Health* transcends time on the treadmill and having the right cholesterol. Once you experience inner health the way it was meant to feel, you will be excited to use your newfound wisdom to help others. An inner voice will say, "I feel so good, I *have to* share my success with others." Do it! That feeling is priceless.

Here's to your prime-time health!

ACKNOWLEDGMENTS

As I tried to satisfy my voracious appetite for credible health and nutrition information, I found that much of the so-called science was unsettling. One journal article would make a claim, only for it to be retracted in another article. Prime timers are victims of information overload and sometimes information distrust. I was even more frustrated by the difficulty that many brilliant scientists had in translating their very important findings into language that would motivate the average person to make changes in their diet and lifestyle. I vowed that "science made simple" would be one of the hallmarks of this book.

I practiced what I preached. A bit of fatherly advice I give my kids: "Surround yourselves with people who know more than you do, and have the wisdom to listen to them." That's what I did.

ACKNOWLEDGMENTS

I realized that since my health and life depended on getting the right science, I had to surround myself with the right scientists. Over the years, I had the opportunity to befriend, work on projects with, and sit on advisory boards with some of the top scientists throughout the world. Their contributions, directly or indirectly, influenced the information in this book. I wish to thank my fellow members of the PepsiCo Advisory Board: Dr. Dean Ornish, founder and president of the Preventive Medicine Research Institute and Clinical Professor of Medicine at the University of California, San Francisco; Dr. David Heber, Professor of Medicine and Nutrition, UCLA School of Medicine; and Dr. Ken Cooper, Director of the Cooper Institute in Dallas, Texas. A special thanks also to Dr. Jorn Dyerberg, past president of the International Society for the Study of Fatty Acids and Lipids (ISSFAL), for teaching me the health benefits of omega-3s; Dr. David Katz, Professor of Preventive Medicine, Yale University; Dr. Louis Ignarro, Nobel Laureate and Professor of Physiology, UCLA; Dr. Inchel Yeam, medical director of Pacific Sleep Lab, San Clemente, California; Dr. Allen Walker, Professor of Nutrition, Harvard Medical School; Robert Orr, founder of Ocean

Nutrition Canada; my trainer, Sean Foy; and finally, Dr. Vincent Fortanasce, Professor of Neurology, University of Southern California.

My heartfelt thanks goes to my favorite nurse, and wife of forty-three years, Martha Sears, RN. Martha practiced all the Prime-Time Health tips you learned in this book, and early in our marriage tried to teach them to me. Yet, it took a midlife health crisis before I learned to listen.

I also wish to thank my editors Denise Marcil, Tracy Behar, Marie Salter, Pamela Marshall, Janet Chan, Deborah Bruce, and my research assistants Tracee Zeni and Rachelle Duvall, for their patience and inspiration. Without the help of all these "health advisers," this book could not have been written as well.

Whether they realize it or not, all of these people were in some minor or major way coauthors of *Prime-Time Health,* and to them I am grateful.